# Progress in Inflammation Research

## Series Editor

Prof. Dr. Michael J. Parnham
PLIVA
Research Institute
Prilaz baruna Filipovica 25
10000 Zagreb
Croatia

**Forthcoming titles:**

*TGF-β and Related Cytokines in Inflammation*, S.N. Breit, S. Wahl (Editors), 2001
*Mechanisms and Mediators of Neuropathic Pain*, A.B. Malmberg, S.R. Chaplan (Editors), 2001
*Nitric Oxide and Inflammation*, D. Salvemini (Editor), 2001
*Migraine: A Neuroinflammatory Disease?* E.L.H. Spierings, M. Sanchez del Rio (Editors), 2001
*NMDA Antagonists as Potential Analgesic Drugs*, R.G. Hill, D.J.S. Sirinathsinghji (Editors), 2001
*Disease-modifying Therapy in Vasculitides*, C.G.M. Kallenberg, J.W. Cohen Tervaert (Editors), 2001
*Neuroinflammatory Mechanisms in Alzheimer's Disease*, J. Rogers (Editor), 2001

(Already published titles see last page.)

# Inflammatory and Infectious Basis
# of Atherosclerosis

Jay L. Mehta

Editor

Birkhäuser Verlag
Basel · Boston · Berlin

Editor

Prof. Jay L. Mehta
University of Arkansas for Medical Sciences
Division of Cardiovascular Disease
4301 West Markham
Mail Slot 532
Little Rock, AR 72205-7199
USA

A CIP catalogue record for this book is available from the Library of Congress, Washington D.C., USA

Deutsche Bibliothek Cataloging-in-Publication Data
Inflammatory and infectious basis of atherosclerosis / ed. by Jay L. Mehta. - Basel ; Boston ; Berlin :
Birkhäuser, 2001
    (Progress in inflammation research)
    ISBN 3-7643-6154-9

## ISBN 3-7643-6154-9 Birkhäuser Verlag, Basel – Boston – Berlin

© 2001 Birkhäuser Verlag, P.O. Box 133, CH-4010 Basel, Switzerland
Birkhäuser is a member of the BertelsmannSpringer Publishing Group
Printed on acid-free paper produced from chlorine-free pulp. TCF ∞
Cover design: Markus Etterich, Basel
Cover illustration: Hypothetical sequence of events in atherosclerosis, advanced lesion. Art by John K. Richardson, Medical Media Production Service, Malcom Randall V.A. Medical Center, Gainesville, Florida (chapter by Romeo et al.).
Printed in Germany
ISBN 3-7643-6154-9

9 8 7 6 5 4 3 2 1

# Contents

# List of contributors

Dominick J. Angiolillo, Institute of Cardiology, Catholic University, Largo Vito, 00168 Roma, Italy

Anupam Agarwal, Division of Nephrology, Hypertension and Transplantation, Box 100224 JHMHC, 1600 SW Archer Road, University of Florida, Gainesville, FL 32610, USA; e-mail: agarwal@nersp.nerdc.ufl.edu

Luigi M. Biasucci, Institute of Cardiology, Catholic University, Largo Vito, 00168 Roma, Italy; e-mail: biasucci@tiscalinet.it

Allen P. Burke, Department of Cardiovascular Pathology, Armed Forces Institute of Pathology, 6825 16th Street, N.W., Washington, DC 20306-600, USA

Anton E. Becker, Department of Cardiovascular Pathology, Academic Medical Center, University of Amsterdam, P.O. Box 22700, 1100 DE Amsterdam, The Netherlands

Onno J. de Boer, Department of Cardiovascular Pathology, Academic Medical Center, University of Amsterdam, P.O. Box 22700, 1100 DE Amsterdam, The Netherlands

Hongjiang Chen, Cardivascular Medicine, Central Arkansas Veteran's Healthcare System and University of Arkansas for Medical Sciences, 4301 West Markham, Slot 532, Little Rock, AR 72205-7199, USA

Mingyi Chen, National Cardiovascular Center Research Institute, Suita, Osaka 565-8565, Japan; e-mail: cmy6@yahoo.com

Fabrizio Clementi, Department of Cardiology, University of Rome "Tor Vergata", Rome, Italy

Rory Collins, Clinical Trial Service Unit and Epidemiological Studies Unit, Nuffield Department of Clinical Medicine, University of Oxford, Radcliffe Infirmary, Oxford OX2 6HE, UK

John Danesh, Clinical Trial Service Unit and Epidemiological Studies Unit, Nuffield Department of Clinical Medicine, University of Oxford, Radcliffe Infirmary, Oxford OX2 6HE, UK; e-mail: john.danesh@dphpc.ox.ac.uk

Helmut Drexler, Abteilung Kardiologie und Angiologie, Medizinische Hochschule Hannover, Carl Neuberg Strasse 1, Germany; e-mail: Drexler.Helmut@MH-Hannover.de

Mark L. Entman, Department of Medicine, Section of Cardiovascular Sciences, Baylor College of Medicine, One Baylor Plaza, M.S. F-602, Houston, TX 77030, USA; e-mail: mentman@bcm.tmc.edu

Andrew Farb, Department of Cardiovascular Pathology, Armed Forces Institute of Pathology, 6825 16th Street, N.W., Washington, DC 20306-600, USA

Nikolaos Frangogiannis, Department of Medicine, Section of Cardiovascular Sciences, Baylor College of Medicine, One Baylor Plaza, M.S. F-602, Houston, TX 77030, USA; e-mail: ngf@bcm.tmc.edu

Nathalie Hill-Kapturczak, Department of Medicine, Box 100224 JHMHC, 1600 SW Archer Road, University of Florida, Gainesville, FL 32610, USA

Shuntaro Kagiyama, Physiology College of Medicine, Box 100274, University of Florida, Gainesville, FL 32610, USA

Frank D. Kolodgie, Department of Cardiovascular Pathology, Armed Forces Institute of Pathology, 6825 16th Street, N.W., Washington, DC 20306-600, USA

Giovanna Liuzzo, Institute of Cardiology, Catholic University, Largo Vito, 00168 Roma, Italy

Antonino Mazzone, Unità di Cardiologia, Medicina Generale II, Ospedale Civile di Legnano, Via Candiani 2, 20025 Legnano (Milan), Italy

David A. Morrow, Cardiovascular Division, Brigham and Women's Hospital, 75 Francis Street, Boston, MA 02115, USA; e-mail: damorrow@bics.bwh.harvard.edu

Harry S. Nick, Department of Neuroscience, University of Florida, Gainesville FL 32610, USA

M. Ian Phillips, Physiology College of Medicine, University of Florida, Gainesville, FL 32610, USA; e-mail: MIP@Phys.med.ufl.edu

Paul M. Ridker, Cardiovascular Division, Brigham and Women's Hospital, 75 Francis Street, Boston, MA 02115, USA; e-mail: pridker@rics.bwh.harvard.edu

Francesco Romeo, Department of Cardiology, University of Rome "Tor Vergata", Rome, Italy

Tom Saldeen, Department of Surgical Sciences, University of Uppsala, Dag Hammarskjölds väg 17, 75237 Uppsala, Sweden; e-mail: tom.saldeen@rattsmed.uu.se

Tatsuya Sawamura, National Cardiovascular Center Research Institute, Suita, Osaka 565-8565, Japan; e-mail: sawamura@ri.ncvc.go.jp

Bernhard Schieffer, Abteilung Kardiologie und Angiologie, Medizinische Hochschule Hannover, Carl Neuberg Strasse 1, 30625 Hannover, Germany; e-mail: Schieffer.Bernhard@MH-HANNOVER.de

Gerd Schmitz, Institute for Clinical Chemistry and Laboratory Medicine, University of Regensburg, Franz-Josef-Strauss-Allee 11, D-93053 Regensburg, Germany; e-mail: gerd.schmitz@klinik.uni-regensburg.de

Stefano De Servi, Unità di Cardiologia, Ospedale Civile di Legnano, Via Candiani 2, 20025 Legnano (Milan), Italy; e-mail: emodinamica.legnano@calcol.it

Heraldo P. Souza, Molecular and Cellular Biophysics Laboratories, Department of Medicine, Division of Cardiology and The Electron Paramagnetic Resonance Center, The Johns Hopkins University School of Medicine, 5501 Hopkins Bayview Circle, Baltimore, Maryland 21224, USA; Disciplina de Emergências Clínicas, Faculdade de Medicina, Universidade de São Paulo, São Paulo, Brazil; e-mail: heraldop@welch-link.welch.jhu.edu

Michael Torzewski, Institute for Clinical Chemistry and Laboratory Medicine, University of Regensburg, Franz-Josef-Strauss-Allee 11, D-93053 Regensburg, Germany; e-mail: michael.torzewski@klinik.uni-regensburg.de

Allard C. van der Wal, Department of Cardiovascular Pathology, Academic Medical Center, University of Amsterdam, P.O. Box 22700, 1100 DE Amsterdam, The Netherlands; e-mail: a.c.vanderwal@amc.uva.nl

Renu Virmani, Department of Cardiovascular Pathology, Armed Forces Institute of Pathology, 6825 16th Street, N.W., Washington, DC 20306-600, USA; e-mail: virmani@afip.osd.mil

Keith A. Youker, Department of Medicine, Section of Cardiovascular Sciences, Baylor College of Medicine, One Baylor Plaza, M.S. F-602, Houston, TX 77030, USA; e-mail: kyouker@bcm.tmc.edu

Dani S. Zander, Department of Pathology, Immunology, and Laboratory Medicine, University of Florida College of Medicine, Box 100275, Gainesville, FL 32610, USA; e-mail: zander@pathology.ufl.edu

Jay L. Zweier, Molecular and Cellular Biophysics Laboratories, Department of Medicine, Division of Cardiology and The Electron Paramagnetic Resonance Center, The Johns Hopkins University School of Medicine, 5501 Hopkins Bayview Circle, Baltimore, MD 21224, USA; e-mail: jlzweier@jhmi.edu

# Preface

There has been a major decline in mortality from atherosclerotic cardiovascular disease in the last three decades. Much of this decline has come from identification of so called "risk factors", and better control of smoking, diabetes mellitus, high blood pressure, and hyperlipidemia. Major strides have been made in developing effective medical and surgical strategies for primary and secondary prevention of atherosclerosis and related diseases. However, atherosclerosis is still the major cause of mortality in the Western world, and rapidly replacing malnutrition and infectious disease in the developing world as the cause of morbidity and mortality.

Interestingly, over the last decade there has been a resurgence of interest in inflammation that accompanies atherosclerosis. Publication of several papers on this subject in several journals in the last few years would suggest a relatively recent discovery of this concept. Virchow and Rokitanksy actually made the observation of inflammation accompanying atherosclerotic vascular disease in the1850s. Cregg in 1894 and Oster in 1908 commented on the potential infectious etiology of atherosclerosis along with smoking, diabetes, obesity and aging.

The medical and lay literature is emphasizing the role of anti-infectious agents as potential ground-breaking novel therapy for atherosclerosis. The foundation of this concept lies in the fact that the decline in cardiovascular mortality over the last half-century parallels the advent and frequent use of a variety of antibiotics. However, a similar parallelism can be shown with a number of other treatment modalities.

The late Russell Ross started his last review in the *New England Journal of Medicine* (1999) with a provocative statement: "Atherosclerosis is an inflammatory disease". I believe the cause and effect relationship between inflammation and atherosclerosis is far from proven. Inflammation in atherosclerosis could well be a response, and a protective one, to arterial injury.

This book attempts to bring together worldwide experts on inflammation in atherosclerosis to present their thoughts in this area. The first four chapters deal with the theoretical and pathological aspects of inflammation. The next six chapters discuss the contribution of free radicals, oxidized low-density lipoproteins, and angiotensin II in inflammation and possibly atherosclerosis. The last four chapters are focused on the description of the clinical aspects of inflammation and infection, and the prognostic value of inflammatory mediators. I invited Drs. Danesh and Saldeen to present a review of two interesting modes of combating inflammation by antibiotics and n-3 polyunsaturated fatty acids.

All authors have done a phenomenal job in meeting the challenge. I hope this volume will be useful to investigators, basic scientists and clinicians alike in further defining the pathophysiologic role of inflammation in atherosclerosis.

Little Rock, autumn 2000                                                        J.L. Mehta

# Atherosclerosis: an inflammatory disease

*Gerd Schmitz and Michael Torzewski*

Institute of Clinical Chemistry and Laboratory Medicine, University of Regensburg, Franz-Josef-Strauß-Allee 11, 93053 Regensburg, Germany

## Introduction

Cellular processes in atherogenesis with the exception of calcification and thrombotic events are principally no different to those found in chronic inflammatory-fibroproliferative diseases such as liver cirrhosis, rheumatoid arthritis, glomerulosclerosis, pulmonary fibrosis, or chronic pancreatitis [1]. Atherosclerotic lesions are the result of a series of highly specific cellular and molecular responses to various endogenous risk factors and potential exogenous antigens. These responses are mediated by endothelial cells, monocyte-derived macrophages, smooth muscle cells and specific subtypes of T lymphocytes. Activation of these cells leads to the release of a wide spectrum of inflammatory hydrolases, cytokines, chemokines and growth factors followed by cellular lipid accumulation and proliferation of smooth muscle cells as well as formation of fibrous tissue [2]. The modified response-to-injury hypothesis of atherosclerosis that emphasizes endothelial dysfunction rather than denudation as the first step in atherosclerosis [1] was recently extended suggesting that the key initiating event in early atherosclerosis is the subendothelial retention of cholesterol-rich, atherogenic lipoproteins bound to arterial proteoglycans (response-to-retention hypothesis) [3]. Following adherence to endothelial cells, defined subpopulations of circulating monocytes that express the lipopolysaccharide (LPS) receptor CD14 and the FcγRIII/CD16 (CD14$^{bright}$ CD16$^+$) might extravasate into the subendothelial space [4–6]. Within the vessel wall phagocytic monocytes rapidly transform to foam cells characterized by the excessive uptake of atherogenic lipoproteins by receptor-mediated endocytosis. Cellular uptake of these lipids and lipoproteins is mediated by charge and motif receptors (scavenger receptors) directly recognizing non-opsonized ligands. Alternatively, modified lipids and lipoproteins may be opsonized by either innate (complement components, C-reactive protein (CRP), serum amyloid P (SAP), serum amyloid A (SAA)) and/or specific opsonins (immunoglobulins) prior to cellular uptake mediated by different opsonin receptors including complement receptors, pentraxin family receptors and/or Fcγ-receptors. Continuous exposure to modified lipoproteins is supposed to trigger a chronic

Inflammatory and Infectious Basis of Atherosclerosis, edited by Jay L. Mehta
© 2001 Birkhäuser Verlag Basel/Switzerland

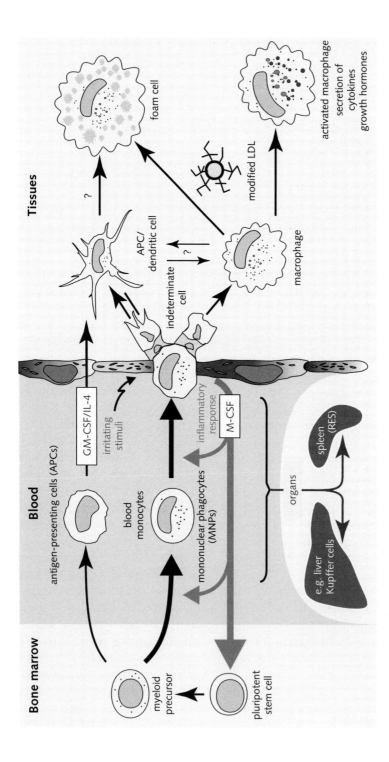

*Figure 1*

*Differentiation of monocytes and blood dendritic cells to either macrophages or antigen-presenting and dendritic cells within the vascular wall. Continuous exposure to modified lipoproteins is supposed to trigger a chronic inflammatory process within the lesion. GM-CSF, granulocyte-macrophage colony-stimulating facor; IL-4, interleukin 4; M-CSF, macrophage colony-stimulating factor; LDL, low-density lipoprotein.*

inflammatory process within the lesion. At the monocyte/macrophage level, this leads to the differentiation of either a phagocytic or an antigen-presenting pheno-type (Fig. 1) with enhanced expression of procoagulant and proinflammatory genes as well as genes associated with lipid metabolism [7]. At the smooth muscle cell (SMC) level, complement activation by CRP [8], SAA or hydrolase-modified low-density lipoprotein (LDL) [9] takes place even in the early atherosclerotic lesion. Sublytic complement attack on SMCs leads to the local release of monocyte chemo-tactic protein 1 (MCP-1), a specific monocyte chemoattractant [10].

## Monocyte subpopulations

In normal subjects, five different subpopulations of blood monocytes have been dis-criminated by cell expression densities of various antigens involved in extravasation, uptake of atherogenic lipoproteins, differentiation and inflammation. The Fcγ recep-tors, in particular CD16a/FcγRIII, together with the LPS receptor CD14, appear to be key players in defining monocyte subpopulations. Their heterogeneous expression suggested a different capacity for IgG-dependent phagocytosis [4]. The pool size of $CD14^{dim}CD16^{+}$ monocytes correlates with plasma lipids and lipoprotein metabolism as well as inflammation and the acute phase reaction (Fig. 2) stressing a link between peripheral blood monocyte heterogeneity and cardiovascular risk factors.

## Chemically-modified lipids and lipoproteins as endogenous antigens

The transformation of macrophages to foam cells *in situ* has been widely accepted as being derived from the cellular uptake of different forms of chemically-modified lipids and lipoproteins (Tab. 1). Oxidation of lipoproteins is one such modification likely occurring in lesions *in vivo* and promoting certain atherogenic processes [11]. Major questions remain, however, concerning the oxidation hypothesis, in particu-lar in terms of particle morphology, macrophage foam cell formation, and comple-ment activation. Thus, there has been increasing interest in other modifications of lipoproteins that may be important in atherogenesis. These include AGE-LDL (advanced glycosylation end-products), LDL-heparan sulfate-like and dermatan sul-fate proteoglycan complexes, LDL modified by $PLA_2$ (phospholipase $A_2$) and aggre-gated LDL [12]. In patients with diabetes, increased levels of LDL modified by AGEs have been found in the plasma as well as in atherosclerotic lesions [13]. LDL-proteoglycan complexes are internalized by cultured macrophages and smooth mus-cle cells leading to foam cell formation [14]. Uptake of LDL-proteoglycan com-plexes in human monocyte-derived macrophages is not mediated through binding to the LDL receptor, but occurs predominantly via class A scavenger receptors [15]. Recently, it was demonstrated that the secretory group II phospholipase $A_2$ expres-

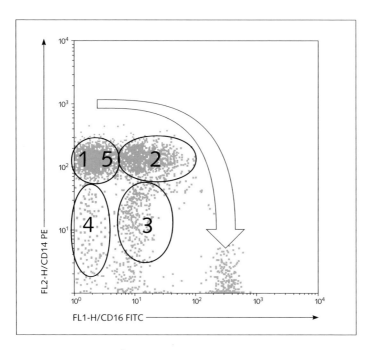

*Phenotype of CD14$^{dim}$CD16$^{+}$ peripheral blood monocytes (MNP 3) correlates*

|  | Positively to | Negatively to | Ref. |
|---|---|---|---|
| Plasma lipids and lipoproteins |  | HDL-cholesterol | [4] |
|  | plasma cholesterol and |  |  |
|  | triglycerides |  | [6] |
|  | apoE4 allele |  | [5] |
| Inflammation, acute phase reaction | M-CSF therapy |  | [81] |
|  | GM-CSF therapy |  | [82] |
|  | tuberculosis |  | [83] |
|  | solid tumors |  | [84] |
|  | sepsis |  | [85] |
|  | HIV infection |  | [86, 87] |

*Figure 2*
*Correlation of the pool size of CD14$^{dim}$CD16$^{+}$ monocytes (MNP 3) to plasma lipids and lipoprotein metabolism as well as inflammation and the acute phase reaction. Subpopulations of mononuclear phagocytes (MNP 1-5) were discriminated by flow-cytometry (top) due to their expression pattern of CD16 and CD14. M-CSF, macrophage colony-stimulating factor; GM-CSF, granulocyte-macrophage colony-stimulating facor*

Table 1 - Atherogenic lipids and lipoproteins

| Lipids/Lipoproteins | Atherogenic molecular component | Refs. |
|---|---|---|
| oxidized LDL (ox-LDL) | hydroperoxy- and hydroxy fatty acids, secondary aldehydic lipid peroxidation products, 7 β-hydroperoxycholesterol | [11, 88, 89] |
| acetylated LDL (ac-LDL) | acetylated lipids | [90] |
| enzymatically degraded LDL (E-LDL) | free cholesterol, lysophospholipids | [20] |
| LDL-proteoglycan complexes | basic amino acid residues 3359-3369 in site B of apo-B100 | [91] |
| lipoproteins aggregated by PLA$_2$, PLC | lysophosphatidylcholine, phosphatidic acid, lysophosphatidic acid | [19, 21] |
| LDL hydrolyzed by sphingomyelinase | ceramide, phosphocholine | [92] |
| LDL hydrolyzed by phospholipase C | lysophosphatidylcholine, phosphatidic acid, lysophosphatidic acid | [18] |
| LDL modified by advanced glycation end products (AGEs) | 67 amino acid domain located 1791 residues N-terminal to the LDL receptor binding site of apo-B | [93] |
| | modification of residues adjacent to the putative LDL receptor binding site | [94] |
| gangliosides (sialic acid containig glycosphingolipids) | sialic acid | [95] |

sion in human aortic tissue correlates with the degree of atherosclerosis [16]. Finally, many *in vitro* treatments of LDL, such as vortexing or extensive hydrolysis by both phospholipase A$_2$ [17] and phospholipase C [18] lead to aggregation. Aggregated lipoproteins are prominent in atherosclerotic lesions [19]. Cellular uptake of these modified lipids and lipoproteins is mediated by various members of the scavenger receptor family and the receptor for AGE (RAGE) [13]. These receptors are charge and motif receptors directly recognizing non-opsonized ligands.

Analogous to well known concepts of host defence in infectious diseases, non-oxidative, partial hydrolysis of lipids and lipoproteins by the hydrolytic host defence machinery transforms lipoproteins to an atherogenic moiety. Treatment of LDL with degrading enzymes *in vitro* converts the molecule to a complement-activating moiety (see below), which is rapidly taken up by human macrophages and thus inducing foam cell formation [20]. In correlation to these *in vitro* findings, lipoprotein particles resembling large droplet structures (10–200 nm in diameter) formed during enzymatic degradation of LDL (E-LDL) have been visualized in, and extracted from, atherosclerotic lesions [9, 21]. Moreover, E-LDL has been detected by immunohistochemistry using specific monoclonal antibodies in early atherosclerotic lesions of human coronary arteries [22].

## Potential opsonins for modified LDL and their receptors

Modified lipids and lipoproteins like E-LDL might be recognized via opsonin-mediated processes by either innate (complement components, CRP, SAP, SAA) and/or specific opsonins (immunoglobulins) prior to cellular uptake via opsonin receptors.

C-reactive protein (CRP) has recently been classified as innate recognition lectin [23]. During the last five years, the predictive association between CRP and coronary heart disease (CHD) has been extensively confirmed [24, 25]. Furthermore, CRP is emerging as a key modulator of inflammatory processes in early atherogenesis, in particular due to its known complement activating [26], lipoprotein-binding [27] and chemotactic [28] properties. Of particular importance might be calcium-dependent *in vitro* binding of CRP to E-LDL accompanied by an enhancement of complement activation [29]. Different receptors have been described for CRP. On monocytes, specific CRP binding occurs through FcγRI/CD64 [30] as well as FcγRII/CD32 [31]. However, there might be an additional "unique" CRP-receptor involved in CRP signalling [32]. At this stage additional research is needed to clarify the contribution of the different receptors to CRP binding [33].

Serum amyloid P (SAP) is the second pentraxin present in human plasma, which also has been reported to locate to atherosclerotic lesions and bind to a variety of ligands such as C4b-binding protein, CRP, complement components C1q and C3bi, and human IgG in a calcium-dependent manner. SAP specifically interacts with high-density lipoproteins as well as very low-density lipoproteins but not with low-density lipoproteins [34] and can activate the complement system [35]. The presence of glycoprotein receptors for mouse SAP on elicited, inflammatory macrophages suggests that cellular uptake of SAP might occur via specific receptors [36].

Serum amyloid A (SAA), a family of acute-phase reactants, is found on high-density lipoproteins (HDL) and displaces apolipoprotein AI from HDL particles and converts α-migrating mature HDL back to preβ$_1$-precursor HDL particles [37]. Further functions for the SAAs include participation in detoxification, depression of immune responses, and interference with platelet functions [38]. In human atherosclerotic lesions, SAA mRNA was found in most endothelial cells and some smooth muscle cells as well as macrophage-derived foam cells, adventitial macrophages, and adipocytes [39]. Formyl peptide receptor-like 1 (FPRL1), a member of the G-protein-coupled receptor family with low affinity for N-formylmethionyl-1-leucyl-1-phenylalanine (fMLP), mediates the chemotactic activity of SAA in human phagocytic cells [40].

Differential screening of a cDNA library constructed from human umbilical vein endothelial cells exposed to interleukin-1β (IL-1β) has led to the identification of

PTX3, a novel pentraxin gene. PTX3 is expressed and released from cells of the monocyte-macrophage lineage exposed to inflammatory signals and thus may represent an additional marker of inflammatory reactions, particularly those involving the vessel wall [41].

Antibodies, as specific opsonins against different epitopes of lipids and lipoproteins (charge modified phospholipids, cholesterol or cryptic protein epitopes), have been demonstrated in human plasma. Injection of silicone gel or silicone oil intraperitoneally into BALB/c mice induced the formation of antibodies that reacted with highly purified crystalline cholesterol and, to a much lesser extent, with phospholipids [42]. Human IgG1 and IgG3 autoantibodies reactive with ox-LDL have been isolated from human plasma [43]. Experimental studies demonstrated the involvement of FcγRI/CD64 in cellular uptake of LDL-immune complexes [44] and metabolism of LDL aggregates [45]. In addition, it was shown that cholesterol depletion leads to down-regulation of FcγRI/CD64 on the human monocyte-like cell line U937 [46]. The involvement of FcγRII/CD32 in cellular uptake of LDL-immune complexes is a subject being lively debated [47, 48].

Taken together, modified lipids and lipoproteins opsonized by innate and/or specific opsonins might facilitate foam cell formation (Fig. 3).

## Chronic inflammatory processes

Continuous exposure to modified lipoproteins is supposed to trigger a chronic inflammatory process within the lesion. At the monocyte/macrophage level this leads to the differentiation of either a phagocytic or an antigen-presenting phenotype with expression of procoagulant and proinflammatory genes as well as genes associated with lipid metabolism [7]. Various pathways might be responsible. The $\beta_2$ integrin CR3 (CD11b/CD18) is required for tyrosine phosphorylation initiating the focal adhesion kinase (FAK)/paxillin signal transduction pathways [49]. CRP binding to the CRP-R has been demonstrated to alter IL-8-induced signalling in neutrophils [50]. Fcγ receptors are associated with the immunoreceptor tyrosine-based activation motif (ITAM), that modulates activation of tyrosine kinases of the Src and ZAP-70 families. Subsequent events, which vary depending on the cell type and receptors involved, include activation of other enzymes such as phospholipase C, phospholipase D, phosphatidylinositol-3-kinase, and mitogen-activated protein kinase [51, 52].

## Exogenous antigens in atherogenesis

Analogous to modified lipoproteins as endogenous antigens, suggested antigenic stimuli involved in the pathogenesis and progression of atherosclerosis also include

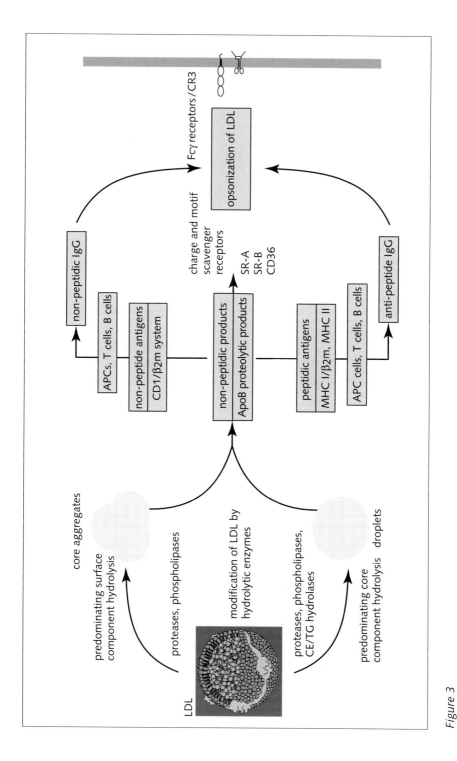

*Figure 3*

*Degradation of low-density lipoprotein (LDL) by the hydrolytic host defence machinery and cellular uptake of opsonized/non-opsonized modified lipoproteins. CE, cholesteryl ester; TG, triglyceride; β2m, β2 microglobulin.*

components of intracellular pathogens such as cytomegalovirus (CMV) and *C. pneumoniae*. Thereby, attention has focused particularly on associations with coronary heart disease (CHD) [53].

The association between anti-CMV antibodies and cardiovascular disease has been reported in several epidemiological studies. However, the majority of the studies were small and the results not necessarily adjusted for confounding factors [54]. CMV might be a cause of accelerated atherosclerosis sometimes observed in heart transplant patients [55]. Despite detection of antigens and DNA from CMV in atherosclerotic lesions [56], the evidence for a causative role in primary atherosclerosis is weak [57].

Circulating *C. pneumoniae*-specific complexes have been found in a high proportion of CHD patients [58] and the organism was demonstrated in advanced atherosclerotic lesions [59]. However, macrophages might be primed by inflammatory stimuli in the lungs and reach the atheromatous lesion via the blood stream, so that the association between the presence of *C. pneumoniae* and atherosclerosis might be purely coincidental. Furthermore, up to now, there has been no convincing and regular demonstration of *C. pneumoniae* in early atherosclerotic lesions. Nevertheless, these findings have stimulated widespread interest in the role of infection in coronary artery disease and cardiovascular events. Even if a direct involvement of this organism in early atherogenesis is doubtful, it might trigger the inflammatory changes seen during lesion progression [53].

## T, B and NK cells in atherogenesis

T lymphocytes, of both helper and suppressor phenotypes, have been identified within human atherosclerotic lesions [60, 61] displaying a shift during lesion progression. In early atherosclerotic lesions, T lymphocytes of suppressor phenotype appeared to predominate over helper cells. However, initial stages in the development of atherosclerosis also involve the infiltration of the arterial intima with Th1 cells reactive to heat shock protein (hsp) 65/60, expressed by endothelial cells in areas that are subject to increased hemodynamic stress [61] and Th1 cells responding to ox-LDL by proliferation and cytokine secretion [62]. In these early lesions, the ratio between T cells and macrophages is approximately 1:8 [60]. In advanced atherosclerotic lesions, macrophages outnumber T cells by 10 to 50:1 and CD4[+] T cells are more than twice as frequent as CD8[+] cells. CD4[+] T cells seem to be more important for acceleration of lesion formation also due to the atherogenic role of the cytokine interferon-γ (IFNγ), which is produced by the Th1 subset of CD4[+] T cells [63] (Fig. 4). Thus, the cytokine expression in advanced human atherosclerotic plaques demonstrates the presence of a predominantly pro-inflammatory, Th1-type T-cell response [64]. Animal models, however, indicate that this cell type only modulates lesion development. Transgenic mouse models allow the conclusion that

9

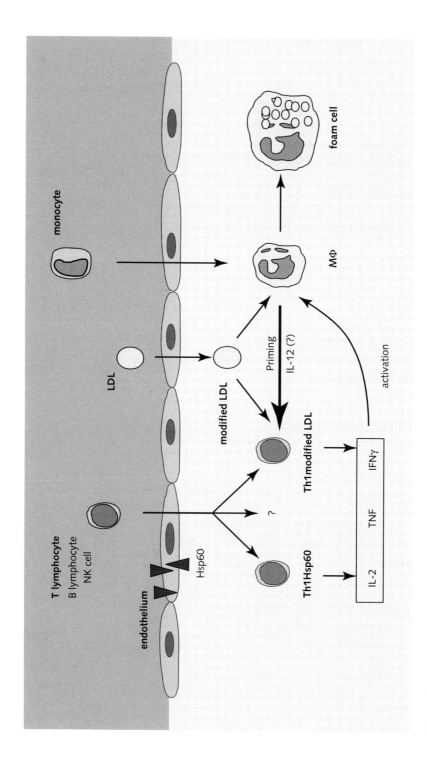

*Figure 4*

*T, B and NK cells in atherogenesis. The cytokine expression in human atherosclerotic lesions demonstrates the presence of a predominantly pro-inflammatory, Th1 T cell response. To date, Th1 cells reactive to modified LDL as well as heat shock protein (Hsp60) have been identified. IL-2, interleukin 2; TNF, tumor necrosis factor; IFNγ, interferon γ; IL-12, interleukin 12; Mφ, macrophage.*

*Table 2 - Macrophage scavenger receptors and their ligand recognition motifs*

| Class | Type | Ligands | Refs. |
|---|---|---|---|
| A | SR-AI | negatively charged macromolecules | [96, |
|  | SR-AII | like ac-LDL, ox-LDL, polyglutamic acid, | 97, |
|  | MARCO | polyinosinic acid | 98] |
| B | SR-BI/CLA-1 | anionic phospholipids, long chain fatty acids | [99, |
|  | SR-BII (CD36) |  | 100, |
|  | Macrosialin (CD68) |  | 101] |
| C | dSR-CI | negatively charged macromolecules like ac-LDL | [102, |
| endothelial | LOX-1 | ox-LDL, but not native or ac-LDL | 103] |
| receptor |  |  |  |

in the case of a lack of mature T cells the development of fatty streaks is reduced under conditions of moderate hypercholesterolemia [65]. In contrast, in the case of extreme hypercholesterolemia, no protection against the development of atherosclerosis is observed under T-cell deficiency [66]. Taken together, these results indicate that in addition to the inflammatory cascade, a specific immune response mediated by T cells may play a role in lesion progression, rather than lesion development [67].

Despite the predominance of T cells, occasional B and NK cells were observed in advanced human atherosclerotic lesions [68, 69]. Both early fatty streaks and full-blown atherosclerotic plaques of hypercholesterolemic apolipoprotein E knockout mice contained CD22[+] B cells suggesting that B cells participate in the local immune response in this experimental model [69]. In addition, the detection of antibodies as specific opsonins against different epitopes of lipids and lipoproteins in human plasma stresses the importance of a humoral immune response in atherogenesis (see above). In aortic tissue, some of the infiltrating cells consist of NK cells and it was suggested that these cells may play a critical role in vascular cell injury and rupture caused by atherosclerotic aneurysms by releasing perforin [68].

## Complement activation in atherogenesis

Complement activation significantly contributes towards atherosclerotic lesion development [29, 70]. Cholesterol-induced atherosclerotic lesion formation is reduced in complement-deficient animals [71]. The presence of the macromolecular membrane attack complex (MAC) on cell surfaces in early atherosclerotic lesions of human coronary arteries suggests that complement activation occurs even at a very early stage [72]. Due to the expression of complement regulatory

*Table 3 - Opsonins and their receptors*

| Opsonins | Receptors | Refs. |
|---|---|---|
| *inflammatory* | | |
| innate | | |
| CRP | CRP-R (putative G-protein coupled-receptor?) | [32] |
| | FcγRI/CD64 (KD $6 \times 10^{-6}$ M) | [104] |
| | FcγRII/CD32 (KD $6.6 \times 10^{-8}$ M) | [31] |
| SAP | glycoprotein receptor (mouse) | [36] |
| PTX3 | ? | |
| complement | CR1 (CD35), CR3 (CD18/CD11b), | [105] |
| components | CR4 (CD18/CD11c) | [106] |
| SAA | FPRL1 (G-protein-coupled receptor) | [40] |
| specific | | |
| IgG | FcγRI/CD64 (Ka $5.5 \times 10^8$ M$^{-1}$; IgG1=3>4>>2) | [44] |
| | FcγRII/CD32 (Ka $< 10^7$ M$^{-1}$; IgG1 = 3>>2>4) | [48] |
| IgM | IgM receptor | [107] |
| IgA | IgA receptor | [108] |
| *tissue remodelling* | | |
| proteoglycans | SR-AI, SR-AII | [15] |
| fibrinogen | glycoprotein IIb/IIIa integrin receptor | [109] |
| fibronectin | α5β1 integrin receptor | [110, 111] |
| collagen | αβ1 integrin receptor | [110] |
| | glycoprotein VI | |

molecules or other defense mechanisms, MAC does not appear to cause substantial lysis of nucleated cells. However, sublytic attack may injure vascular cells triggering various proinflammatory reactions [73]. Anaphylatoxins such as C5a are supposed to mediate cellular recruitment, especially of leukocytes. Endothelial cells, monocyte-derived macrophages and smooth muscle cells may be stimulated to release growth factors and cytokines [1]. Of these cells, smooth muscle cells are the most likely target of MAC-formation because, unlike endothelial cells, they are poorly protected by complement inhibitory proteins like CD55 or CD59. Such attack on SMC, with release of MCP-1, might explain the initial monocyte recruitment into the arterial wall [10].

In addition to potential effects of complement activation products on arterial wall cells, current research focuses on complement-activating structures in the lesion. The complement system can be activated by either the classical, the alternative or the lectin-pathway [74]. Among the potential candidates for activation by the classical pathway are the auto-immune antibodies against lipoproteins (see above). The classical pathway can also be activated in an antibody-independent manner, for example by binding some viruses [75]. The most likely candidate for complement activation via the classical pathway may be CRP [26]. It was demonstrated that the molecule is present in atherosclerotic lesions of human coronary arteries and colocalizes with the terminal complement complex C5b-9, supporting the hypothesis of its role as a complement-activating moiety in the atherosclerotic lesion [8].

Complement activation can also occur via the alternative pathway, possibly due to the exposure of free cholesterol [76], which has been shown to be an activator of the alternative C3/C5 convertase [77]. The coincidence of cholesterol accumulation and complement activation was demonstrated in the arterial wall of hypercholesterolemic rabbits [78]. As mentioned above, complement-activating lipoprotein particles resembling the characteristic micromorphology of E-LDL have been visualized in, and extracted from, human atherosclerotic lesions [9]. E-LDL has been immunohistochemically detected using specific monoclonal antibodies in all early human lesions and in colocalization with CRP. Further, CRP binds avidly to E-LDL (but not to native LDL), enhancing complement activation [79]. The alternative pathway is also activated by certain microorganisms, such as Chlamydia [80], providing a possible link between infection with *Chlamydia pneumoniae* and increased incidence of cardiovascular disease (see above).

Taken together, these data imply that complement activation could act both to initiate lesion formation and to sustain a state of chronic inflammation and lesion development.

## Conclusions and perspective

Recent work in support of the response-to-retention hypothesis [12] implicate arterial-wall molecules that promote either the subendothelial retention of lipoproteins or the response to these retained lipoproteins. Atherogenic lipoprotein modifications that convert plasma lipoproteins into particles that can induce foam cell formation are of particular interest. Extending the classical concept of cellular uptake of these lipids and lipoproteins by charge and motif scavenger receptors directly recognizing non-opsonized ligands, either innate and/or specific opsonins and their receptors are emerging as potential candidates involved in cellular uptake of modified lipids and lipoproteins. Continuous exposure to modified and opsonized lipids and lipoproteins triggers a chronic inflammatory process within the lesion. This may lead to differentiation of either a phagocytic or an antigen-presenting phenotype of monocytes/macrophages and complement attack on SMCs. The identification of atherogenic lipoprotein modifications decisive for atherogenesis *in vivo* and the identification of the opsonins and opsonin receptors relevant for cellular uptake and signalling represent important goals in cardiovascular disease research, in particular with respect to the development of therapeutic strategies to prevent or reverse lipoprotein modification or opsonization.

## References

1   Ross R (1999) Atherosclerosis – an inflammatory disease. *N Engl J Med* 340: 115–126
2   Stary HC, Chandler AB, Glagov S, Guyton JR, Insull WJ, Rosenfeld ME, Schaffer SA, Schwartz CJ, Wagner WD, Wissler RW (1994) A definition of initial, fatty streak, and intermediate lesions of atherosclerosis. A report from the Committee on Vascular Lesions of the Council on Arteriosclerosis, American Heart Association. *Circulation* 89: 2462–2478
3   Williams KJ, Tabas I (1998) The response-to-retention hypothesis of atherogenesis reinforced. *Curr Opin Lipidol* 9: 471–474
4   Rothe G, Gabriel H, Kovacs E, Klucken J, Stohr J, Kindermann W, Schmitz G (1996) Peripheral blood mononuclear phagocyte subpopulations as cellular markers in hypercholesterolemia. *Arterioscler Thromb Vasc Biol* 16: 1437–1447
5   Stohr J, Schindler G, Rothe G, Schmitz G (1998) Enhanced upregulation of the Fc gamma receptor IIIa (CD16a) during *in vitro* differentiation of ApoE4/4 monocytes. *Arterioscler Thromb Vasc Biol* 18: 1424–1432
6   Rothe G, Herr AS, Stohr J, Abletshauser C, Weidinger G, Schmitz G (1999) A more mature phenotype of blood mononuclear phagocytes is induced by fluvastatin treatment in hypercholesterolemic patients with coronary heart disease [In Process Citation]. *Atherosclerosis* 144: 251–261
7   Schmitz G, Orso E, Rothe G, Klucken J (1997) Scavenging, signalling and adhesion coupling in macrophages: implications for atherogenesis. *Curr Opin Lipidol* 8: 287–300
8   Torzewski J, Torzewski M, Bowyer DE, Frohlich M, Koenig W, Waltenberger J, Fitzsimmons C, Hombach V (1998) C-reactive protein frequently colocalizes with the terminal complement complex in the intima of early atherosclerotic lesions of human coronary arteries. *Arterioscler Thromb Vasc Biol* 18: 1386–1392
9   Seifert PS, Hugo F, Tranum-Jensen J, Zahringer U, Muhly M, Bhakdi S (1990) Isolation and characterization of a complement-activating lipid extracted from human atherosclerotic lesions. *J Exp Med* 172: 547–557
10  Torzewski J, Oldroyd R, Lachmann P, Fitzsimmons C, Proudfoot D, Bowyer D (1996) Complement-induced release of monocyte chemotactic protein-1 from human smooth muscle cells. A possible initiating event in atherosclerotic lesion formation. *Arterioscler Thromb Vasc Biol* 16: 673–677
11  Steinberg D (1997) Lewis A. Conner Memorial Lecture. Oxidative modification of LDL and atherogenesis. *Circulation* 95: 1062–1071

12  Tabas I (1999) Nonoxidative modifications of lipoproteins in atherogenesis. *Annu Rev Nutr* 19: 123–139

13  Lopes-Virella MF, Klein RL, Virella G (1996) Modification of lipoproteins in diabetes. *Diabetes Metab Rev* 12: 69–90

14  Vijayagopal P, Glancy DL (1996) Macrophages stimulate cholesteryl ester accumulation in cocultured smooth muscle cells incubated with lipoprotein-proteoglycan complex. *Arterioscler Thromb Vasc Biol* 16: 1112–1121

15  Vijayagopal P, Srinivasan SR, Radhakrishnamurthy B, Berenson GS (1993) Human monocyte-derived macrophages bind low-density-lipoprotein-proteoglycan complexes by a receptor different from the low-density- lipoprotein receptor. *Biochem J* 289 (Pt 3): 837–844

16  Schiering A, Menschikowski M, Mueller E, Jaross W (1999) Analysis of secretory group II phospholipase A2 expression in human aortic tissue in dependence on the degree of atherosclerosis. *Atherosclerosis* 144: 73–78

17  Oorni K, Hakala JK, Annila A, Ala-Korpela M, Kovanen PT (1998) Sphingomyelinase induces aggregation and fusion, but phospholipase A2 only aggregation, of low density lipoprotein (LDL) particles. Two distinct mechanisms leading to increased binding strength of LDL to human aortic proteoglycans. *J Biol Chem* 273: 29127–29134

18  Suits AG, Chait A, Aviram M, Heinecke JW (1989) Phagocytosis of aggregated lipoprotein by macrophages: low density lipoprotein receptor-dependent foam-cell formation. *Proc Natl Acad Sci USA* 86: 2713–2717

19  Aviram M, Maor I, Keidar S, Hayek T, Oiknine J, Bar-El Y, Adler Z, Kertzman V, Milo S (1995) Lesioned low density lipoprotein in atherosclerotic apolipoprotein E- deficient transgenic mice and in humans is oxidized and aggregated. *Biochem Biophys Res Commun* 216: 501–513

20  Bhakdi S, Dorweiler B, Kirchmann R, Torzewski J, Weise E, Tranum-Jensen J, Walev I, Wieland E (1995) On the pathogenesis of atherosclerosis: enzymatic transformation of human low density lipoprotein to an atherogenic moiety. *J Exp Med* 182: 1959–1971

21  Frank JS, Fogelman AS (1989) Ultrastructure of the intima in WHHL and cholesterol-fed rabbit aortas prepared by ultra-rapid freezing and freeze-etching. *J Lipid Res* 30: 967–978

22  Torzewski M, Klouche M, Hock J, Messner M, Dorweiler B, Torzewski J, Gabbert HE, Bhakdi S (1998) Immunohistochemical demonstration of enzymatically modified human LDL and its colocalization with the terminal complement complex in the early atherosclerotic lesion. *Arterioscler Thromb Vasc Biol* 18: 369–378

23  Fearon DT, Locksley RM (1996) The instructive role of innate immunity in the acquired immune response. *Science* 272: 50–53

24  Haverkate F, Thompson SG, Pyke SD, Gallimore JR, Pepys MB (1997) Production of C-reactive protein and risk of coronary events in stable and unstable angina. European Concerted Action on Thrombosis and Disabilities Angina Pectoris Study Group. *Lancet* 349: 462–466

25  Ridker PM, Cushman M, Stampfer MJ, Tracy RP, Hennekens CH (1997) Inflammation,

aspirin, and the risk of cardiovascular disease in apparently healthy men. *N Engl J Med* 336: 973–979 [published erratum appears in *N Engl J Med* 337(5): 356]

26 Wolbink GJ, Brouwer MC, Buysmann S, Ten B, Hack CE (1996) CRP-mediated activation of complement *in vivo*: assessment by measuring circulating complement-C-reactive protein complexes. *J Immunol* 157: 473–479

27 Pepys MB, Rowe IF, Baltz ML (1985) C-reactive protein: binding to lipids and lipoproteins. *Int Rev Exp Pathol* 27: 83–111

28 Whisler RL, Proctor VK, Downs EC, Mortensen RF (1986) Modulation of human monocyte chemotaxis and procoagulant activity by human C-reactive protein (CRP). *Lymphokine Res* 5: 223–228

29 Bhakdi S (1998) Complement and atherogenesis: the unknown connection [editorial]. *Ann Med* 30: 503–507

30 Marnell LL, Mold C, Volzer MA, Burlingame RW, DuClos T (1995) C-reactive protein binds to Fc gamma RI in transfected COS cells. *J Immunol* 155: 2185–2193

31 Bharadwaj D, Stein MP, Volzer M, Mold C, DuClos T (1999) The major receptor for C-reactive protein on leukocytes is fcgamma receptorII. *J Exp Med* 190: 585–590

32 Tebo JM, Mortensen RF (1990) Characterization and isolation of a C-reactive protein receptor from the human monocytic cell line U-937. *J Immunol* 144: 231–238

33 Mortensen RF, Zhong W. Regulation of phagocytic activities by C-reactive protein. *J Leukocyte Biol; in press*

34 Li XA, Hatanaka K, Ishibashi-Ueda H, Yutani C, Yamamoto A (1995) Characterization of serum amyloid P component from human atherosclerotic lesions. *Arterioscler Thromb Vasc Biol* 15: 252–257

35 Hicks PS, Saunero-Nava L, Du CT, Mold C (1992) Serum amyloid P component binds to histones and activates the classical complement pathway. *J Immunol* 149: 3689–3694

36 Siripont J, Tebo JM, Mortensen RF (1988) Receptor-mediated binding of the acute-phase reactant mouse serum amyloid P-component (SAP) to macrophages. *Cell Immunol* 117: 239–252

37 Miida T, Yamada T, Yamadera T, Ozaki K, Inano K, Okada M (1999) Serum amyloid A protein generates prebeta1 high-density lipoprotein from alpha-migrating high-density lipoprotein. *Biochemistry* 38: 16958–16962

38 Uhlar CM, Whitehead AS (1999) Serum amyloid A, the major vertebrate acute-phase reactant. *Eur J Biochem* 265: 501–523

39 Meek RL, Urieli-Shoval S, Benditt EP (1994) Expression of apolipoprotein serum amyloid A mRNA in human atherosclerotic lesions and cultured vascular cells: implications for serum amyloid A function. *Proc Natl Acad Sci USA* 91: 3186–3190

40 Su SB, Gong W, Gao JL, Shen W, Murphy PM, Oppenheim JJ, Wang JM (1999) A seven-transmembrane, G protein-coupled receptor, FPRL1, mediates the chemotactic activity of serum amyloid A for human phagocytic cells. *J Exp Med* 189: 395–402

41 Alles V, Bottazzi B, Peri G, Golay J, Introna M, Mantovani A (1994) Inducible expression of PTX3, a new member of the pentraxin family, in human mononuclear phagocytes. *Blood* 84: 3483–3493

42  Alving CR, Wassef NM, Potter M (1996) Antibodies to cholesterol: biological implications of antibodies to lipids. *Curr Top Microbiol Immunol* 210: 181–186

43  Mironova M, Virella G, Lopes-Virella MF (1996) Isolation and characterization of human antioxidized LDL autoantibodies. *Arterioscler Thromb Vasc Biol* 16: 222–229 [published erratum appears in *Arterioscler Thromb Vasc Biol* 17 (10): 2306]

44  Lopes-Virella MF, Binzafar N, Rackley S, Takei A, La Via M, Virella G (1997) The uptake of LDL-IC by human macrophages: predominant involvement of the Fc gamma RI receptor. *Atherosclerosis* 135: 161–170

45  Morganelli PM, Rogers RA, Kitzmiller TJ, Bergeron A (1995) Enhanced metabolism of LDL aggregates mediated by specific human monocyte IgG Fc receptors. *J Lipid Res* 36: 714–724

46  Bigler RD, Brown HM, Guyre PM, Lund-Katz S, Scerbo L, Esfahani M (1989) Effect of low-density lipoprotein on the expression of high affinity Fc gamma receptors. *Biochim Biophys Acta* 1011: 102–104 [published erratum appears in *Biochim Biophys Acta* 1014 (3): 333]

47  Stanton LW, White RT, Bryant CM, Protter AA, Endemann G (1992) A macrophage Fc receptor for IgG is also a receptor for oxidized low density lipoprotein. *J Biol Chem* 267: 22446–22451

48  Morganelli PM, Groveman DS, Pfeiffer JR (1997) Evidence that human Fc gamma receptor IIA (CD32) subtypes are not receptors for oxidized LDL. *Arterioscler Thromb Vasc Biol* 17: 3248–3254

49  Graham IL, Anderson DC, Holers VM, Brown EJ (1994) Complement receptor 3 (CR3, Mac-1, integrin alpha M beta 2, CD11b/CD18) is required for tyrosine phosphorylation of paxillin in adherent and nonadherent neutrophils. *J Cell Biol* 127: 1139–1147

50  Zhong W, Zen Q, Tebo J, Schlottmann K, Coggeshall M, Mortensen RF (1998) Effect of human C-reactive protein on chemokine and chemotactic factor- induced neutrophil chemotaxis and signaling. *J Immunol* 161: 2533–2540

51  Sanchez-Mejorada G, Rosales C (1998) Signal transduction by immunoglobulin Fc receptors. *J Leukoc Biol* 63: 521–533

52  Melendez A, Floto RA, Gillooly DJ, Harnett MM, Allen JM (1998) FcgammaRI coupling to phospholipase D initiates sphingosine kinase- mediated calcium mobilization and vesicular trafficking. *J Biol Chem* 273: 9393–9402

53  Gupta S (1999) Chronic infection in the aetiology of atherosclerosis – focus on *Chlamydia pneumoniae*. *Atherosclerosis* 143: 1–6

54  Melnick SL, Shahar E, Folsom AR, Grayston JT, Sorlie PD, Wang SP, Szklo M (1993) Past infection by *Chlamydia pneumoniae* strain TWAR and asymptomatic carotid atherosclerosis. Atherosclerosis Risk in Communities (ARIC) Study Investigators. *Am J Med* 95: 499–504

55  McDonald K, Rector TS, Braulin EA, Kubo SH, Olivari MT (1989) Association of coronary artery disease in cardiac transplant recipients with cytomegalovirus infection. *Am J Cardiol* 64: 359–362

56  Blasi F, Denti F, Erba M, Cosentini R, Raccanelli R, Rinaldi A, Fagetti L, Esposito G,

Ruberti U, Allegra L (1996) Detection of *Chlamydia pneumoniae* but not *Helicobacter pylori* in atherosclerotic plaques of aortic aneurysms. *J Clin Microbiol* 34: 2766–2769

57  Kol A, Sperti G, Shani J, Schulhoff N, van de Greef W, Landini MP, La Placa M, Maseri A, Crea F (1995) Cytomegalovirus replication is not a cause of instability in unstable angina. *Circulation* 91: 1910–1913

58  Linnanmaki E, Leinonen M, Mattila K, Nieminen MS, Valtonen V, Saikku P (1993) *Chlamydia pneumoniae*-specific circulating immune complexes in patients with chronic coronary heart disease. *Circulation* 87: 1130–1134

59  Kuo CC, Shor A, Campbell LA, Fukushi H, Patton DL, Grayston JT (1993) Demonstration of *Chlamydia pneumoniae* in atherosclerotic lesions of coronary arteries. *J Infect Dis* 167: 841–849

60  Munro JM, van der Walt JD, Munro CS, Chalmers JA, Cox EL (1987) An immunohistochemical analysis of human aortic fatty streaks. *Hum Pathol* 18: 375–380

61  Wick G, Kleindienst R, Schett G, Amberger A, Xu Q (1995) Role of heat shock protein 65/60 in the pathogenesis of atherosclerosis. *Int Arch Allergy Immunol* 107: 130–131

62  Stemme S, Faber B, Holm J, Wiklund O, Witztum JL, Hansson GK (1995) T lymphocytes from human atherosclerotic plaques recognize oxidized low density lipoprotein. *Proc Natl Acad Sci USA* 92: 3893–3897

63  Kishikawa H, Shimokama T, Watanabe T (1993) Localization of T lymphocytes and macrophages expressing IL-1, IL-2 receptor, IL-6 and TNF in human aortic intima. Role of cell-mediated immunity in human atherogenesis. *Virchows Arch A Pathol Anat Histopathol* 423: 433–442

64  Frostegard J, Ulfgren AK, Nyberg P, Hedin U, Swedenborg J, Andersson U, Hansson GK (1999) Cytokine expression in advanced human atherosclerotic plaques: dominance of pro-inflammatory (Th1) and macrophage-stimulating cytokines. *Atherosclerosis* 145: 33–43

65  Emeson EE, Shen ML, Bell CG, Qureshi A (1996) Inhibition of atherosclerosis in CD4 T-cell-ablated and nude (nu/nu) C57BL/6 hyperlipidemic mice. Am J Pathol 149: 675–685

66  Dansky HM, Charlton SA, Harper MM, Smith JD (1997) T and B lymphocytes play a minor role in atherosclerotic plaque formation in the apolipoprotein E-deficient mouse. *Proc Natl Acad Sci USA* 94: 4642–4646

67  Schmitz G, Herr AS, Rothe G (1998) T-lymphocytes and monocytes in atherogenesis. *Herz* 23: 168–177

68  Seko Y, Sato O, Takagi A, Tada Y, Matsuo H, Yagita H, Okumura K, Yazaki Y (1997) Perforin-secreting killer cell infiltration in the aortic tissue of patients with atherosclerotic aortic aneurysm. *Jpn Circ J* 61: 965–970

69  Zhou X, Hansson GK (1999) Detection of B cells and proinflammatory cytokines in atherosclerotic plaques of hypercholesterolaemic apolipoprotein E knockout mice. *Scand J Immunol* 50: 25–30

70  Torzewski J, Bowyer DE, Waltenberger J, Fitzsimmons C (1997) Processes in atherogenesis: complement activation. *Atherosclerosis* 132: 131–138

71   Schmiedt W, Kinscherf R, Deigner HP, Kamencic H, Nauen O, Kilo J, Oelert H, Metz J, Bhakdi S (1998) Complement C6 deficiency protects against diet-induced atherosclerosis in rabbits. *Arterioscler Thromb Vasc Biol* 18: 1790–1795

72   Torzewski M, Torzewski J, Bowyer DE, Waltenberger J, Fitzsimmons C, Hombach V, Gabbert HE (1997) Immunohistochemical colocalization of the terminal complex of human complement and smooth muscle cell alpha-actin in early atherosclerotic lesions. *Arterioscler Thromb Vasc Biol* 17: 2448–2452

73   Morgan BP (1992) Effects of the membrane attack complex of complement on nucleated cells. *Curr Top Microbiol Immunol* 178: 115–140

74   Morgan BP (1999) Regulation of the complement membrane attack pathway. *Crit Rev Immunol* 19: 173

75   Marschang P, Ebenbichler CF, Dierich MP (1994) HIV and complement: role of the complement system in HIV infection. *Int Arch Allergy Immunol* 103: 113–117

76   Alving CR, Richards RL, Guirguis AA (1977) Cholesterol-dependent human complement activation resulting in damage to liposomal model membranes. *J Immunol* 118: 342–347

77   Vogt W, von Z, Damerau IB, Hesse D, Luhmann B, Nolte R (1985) Mechanisms of complement activation by crystalline cholesterol. *Mol Immunol* 22: 101–106

78   Seifert PS, Hugo F, Hansson GK, Bhakdi S (1989) Prelesional complement activation in experimental atherosclerosis. Terminal C5b-9 complement deposition coincides with cholesterol accumulation in the aortic intima of hypercholesterolemic rabbits. *Lab Invest* 60: 747–754

79.  Bhakdi S, Torzewski M, Klouche M, Hemmes M (1999) Complement and atherogenesis: Binding of CRP to degraded, nonoxidized LDL enhances complement activation. *Arterioscler Thromb Vasc Biol* 19: 2348–2354

80   Hall RT, Strugnell T, Wu X, Devine DV, Stiver HG (1993) Characterization of kinetics and target proteins for binding of human complement component C3 to the surface-exposed outer membrane of *Chlamydia* trachomatis serovar L2. *Infect Immun* 61: 1829–1834

81   Weiner LM, Li W, Holmes M, Catalano RB, Dovnarsky M, Padavic K, Alpaugh RK (1994) Phase I trial of recombinant macrophage colony-stimulating factor and recombinant gamma-interferon: toxicity, monocytosis, and clinical effects. *Cancer Res* 54: 4084–4090

82   Schmid I, Baldwin GC, Jacobs EL, Isacescu V, Neagos N, Giorgi JV, Glaspy JA (1995) Alterations in phenotype and cell-surface antigen expression levels of human monocytes: differential response to *in vivo* administration of rhM-CSF or rhGM-CSF. *Cytometry* 22: 103–110

83   Vanham G, Edmonds K, Qing L, Hom D, Toossi Z, Jones B, Daley CL, Huebner B, Kestens L, Gigase P, Ellner JJ (1996) Generalized immune activation in pulmonary tuberculosis: co-activation with HIV infection. *Clin Exp Immunol* 103: 30–34

84   Saleh MN, Goldman SJ, LoBuglio AF, Beall AC, Sabio H, McCord MC, Minasian L, Alpaugh RK, Weiner LM, Munn DH (1995) CD16+ monocytes in patients with cancer:

spontaneous elevation and pharmacologic induction by recombinant human macrophage colony-stimulating factor. *Blood* 85: 2910–2917

85  Fingerle G, Pforte A, Passlick B, Blumenstein M, Strobel M, Ziegler-Heitbrock HW (1993) The novel subset of CD14+/CD16+ blood monocytes is expanded in sepsis patients. *Blood* 82: 3170–3176

86  Nockher WA, Bergmann L, Scherberich JE (1994) Increased soluble CD14 serum levels and altered CD14 expression of peripheral blood monocytes in HIV-infected patients. *Clin Exp Immunol* 98: 369–374

87  Allen JB, Wong HL, Guyre PM, Simon GL, Wahl SM (1991) Association of circulating receptor Fc gamma RIII-positive monocytes in AIDS patients with elevated levels of transforming growth factor-beta. *J Clin Invest* 87: 1773–1779

88  Steinberg D, Parthasarathy S, Carew TE, Khoo JC, Witztum JL (1989) Beyond cholesterol. Modifications of low-density lipoprotein that increase its atherogenicity. *N Engl J Med* 8320: 915–924

89  Colles SM, Irwin KC, Chisolm GM (1996) Roles of multiple oxidized LDL lipids in cellular injury: dominance of 7 beta-hydroperoxycholesterol. *J Lipid Res* 37: 2018–2028

90  Goldstein JL, Ho YK, Basu SK, Brown MS (1979) Binding site on macrophages that mediates uptake and degradation of acetylated low density lipoprotein, producing massive cholesterol deposition. *Proc Natl Acad Sci USA* 76: 333–337

91  Boren J, Olin K, Lee I, Chait A, Wight TN, Innerarity TL (1998) Identification of the principal proteoglycan-binding site in LDL. A single-point mutation in apo-B100 severely affects proteoglycan interaction without affecting LDL receptor binding. *J Clin Invest* 101: 2658–2664

92  Schissel SL, Jiang X, Tweedie-Hardman J, Jeong T, Camejo EH, Najib J, Rapp JH, Williams KJ, Tabas I (1998) Secretory sphingomyelinase, a product of the acid sphingomyelinase gene, can hydrolyze atherogenic lipoproteins at neutral pH. Implications for atherosclerotic lesion development. *J Biol Chem* 273: 2738–2746

93  Bucala R, Makita Z, Koschinsky T, Cerami A, Vlassara H (1993) Lipid advanced glycosylation: pathway for lipid oxidation *in vivo*. *Proc Natl Acad Sci USA* 90: 6434–6438

94  Wang X, Bucala R, Milne R (1998) Epitopes close to the apolipoprotein B low density lipoprotein receptor-binding site are modified by advanced glycation end products. *Proc Natl Acad Sci USA* 95: 7643–7647

95  Wen FQ, Jabbar AA, Patel DA, Kazarian T, Valentino LA (1999) Atherosclerotic aortic gangliosides enhance integrin-mediated platelet adhesion to collagen. *Arterioscler Thromb Vasc Biol* 19: 519–524

96  Kodama T, Freeman M, Rohrer L, Zabrecky J, Matsudaira P, Krieger M (1990) Type I macrophage scavenger receptor contains alpha-helical and collagen-like coiled coils. *Nature* 343: 531–535

97  Rohrer L, Freeman M, Kodama T, Penman M, Krieger M (1990) Coiled-coil fibrous domains mediate ligand binding by macrophage scavenger receptor type II. *Nature* 343: 570–572

98  Elomaa O, Sankala M, Pikkarainen T, Bergmann U, Tuuttila A, Raatikainen-Ahokas A,

Sariola H, Tryggvason K (1998) Structure of the human macrophage MARCO receptor and characterization of its bacteria-binding region. *J Biol Chem* 273: 4530–4538

99   Acton SL, Scherer PE, Lodish HF, Krieger M (1994) Expression cloning of SR-BI, a CD36-related class B scavenger receptor. *J Biol Chem* 269: 21003–21009

100  Abumrad NA, el-Maghrabi MR, Amri EZ, Lopez E, Grimaldi PA (1993) Cloning of a rat adipocyte membrane protein implicated in binding or transport of long-chain fatty acids that is induced during preadipocyte differentiation. Homology with human CD36. *J Biol Chem* 268: 17665–17668

101  Ramprasad MP, Terpstra V, Kondratenko N, Quehenberger O, Steinberg D (1996) Cell surface expression of mouse macrosialin and human CD68 and their role as macrophage receptors for oxidized low density lipoprotein. *Proc Natl Acad Sci USA* 93: 14833–14838

102  Pearson A, Lux A, Krieger M (1995) Expression cloning of dSR-CI, a class C macrophage-specific scavenger receptor from *Drosophila melanogaster*. *Proc Natl Acad Sci USA* 92: 4056–4060

103  Sawamura T, Kume N, Aoyama T, Moriwaki H, Hoshikawa H, Aiba Y, Tanaka T, Miwa S, Katsura Y, Kita T, Masaki T (1997) An endothelial receptor for oxidized low-density lipoprotein. *Nature* 386: 73–77

104  Crowell RE, Du CT, Montoya G, Heaphy E, Mold C (1991) C-reactive protein receptors on the human monocytic cell line U-937. Evidence for additional binding to Fc gamma RI. *J Immunol* 147: 3445–3451

105  Seifert PS, Hansson GK (1989) Complement receptors and regulatory proteins in human atherosclerotic lesions. *Arteriosclerosis* 9: 802–811

106  Netea MG, Demacker PN, Kullberg BJ, Boerman OC, Verschueren I, Stalenhoef AF, Van Der Meer JW (1998) Increased interleukin-1alpha and interleukin-1beta production by macrophages of low-density lipoprotein receptor knock-out mice stimulated with lipopolysaccharide is CD11c/CD18-receptor mediated. *Immunology* 95: 466–472

107  Wu R, Lefvert AK (1995) Autoantibodies against oxidized low density lipoproteins (oxLDL): characterization of antibody isotype, subclass, affinity and effect on the macrophage uptake of oxLDL. *Clin Exp Immunol* 102: 174–180

108  Mironova M, Virella G, Virella-Lowell I, Lopes-Virella MF (1997) Anti-modified LDL antibodies and LDL-containing immune complexes in IDDM patients and healthy controls. *Clin Immunol Immunopathol* 85: 73–82

109  Szuwart T, Zhao B, Fritsch A, Mertens K, Dierichs R (1999) Oxidized low-density lipoprotein inhibits the binding of monoclonal antibody to platelet glycoprotein IIB-IIIA. *Thromb Res* 96: 85–90

110  Falcone DJ, Salisbury BG (1988) Fibronectin stimulates macrophage uptake of low density lipoprotein- heparin-collagen complexes. *Arteriosclerosis* 8: 263–273

111  Hillis GS, Mlynski RA, Simpson JG, MacLeod AM (1998) The expression of beta 1 integrins in human coronary artery. *Basic Res Cardiol* 93: 295–302

# Inflammation in coronary atherosclerosis – pathological aspects

*Renu Virmani, Frank D. Kolodgie, Allen P. Burke and Andrew Farb*

Department of Cardiovascular Pathology, Armed Forces Institute of Pathology, 6825 16th Street N.W., Washington, DC 20306-600, USA

## Introduction

Inflammation is an important mechanism in the initiation and progression of a developing atherosclerotic plaque [1–3]. The first cell to adhere to the intact endothelium is the circulating monocyte, which eventually migrates between endothelial cells, locates itself in the subendothelial space, and transforms into the foamy macrophage through the ingestion of lipids. The recruitment of macrophages within the intima is governed by a myriad of adhesion molecules, chemotactic agents, growth factors, and cytokines, all critical to the induction of atherosclerosis. The processes by which lipids accumulate and recruit inflammatory cells to sites of predilection for coronary atherosclerosis are under intense investigation. In addition, the possibility of infectious agents as initiators of coronary inflammation is also currently being explored [1]. The purpose of this review is to focus on the pathological aspects of inflammation in the coronary atherosclerotic plaque. Because the role of inflammation varies as a function of the stage and type of atherosclerotic plaque, the inflammatory milieu will be considered in context of plaque progression; early intimal thickening to complex symptomatic lesions that may be fatal. Plaques will be classified according the terminology of our recent review [4]; conventional definitions provided by the American Heart Association (AHA) classification [5, 6] will also be stated.

## Intimal thickening (intimal mass lesions)

While some atherosclerotic lesions may begin as intimal xanthomata, there is substantial evidence that most adult human lesions originate from pre-existing intimal masses [5, 6]. Because these lesions in children occur in similar locations as obstructive lesions in adults, intimal masses are thought to be a precursor of the majority of obstructive lesions. Unlike intimal xanthomas, there is little evidence that the inti-

Inflammatory and Infectious Basis of Atherosclerosis, edited by Jay L. Mehta
© 2001 Birkhäuser Verlag Basel/Switzerland

mal mass lesion may regress, and atherosclerotic lesions in the hyperlipidemic swine model almost exclusively arise from these lesions [7].

Ikari et al. reported that the intimal layer in the proximal left anterior descending coronary artery is rarely formed before 30 weeks of gestation8. In this study, 35% of coronary arteries show intimal cells between 36 weeks gestation and birth, and all coronary arteries show intimal masses by three months after birth. The ratio of intima to media is 0.1 after birth and it continues to increase ($0.247 \pm 0.667$) in the second post-natal year [8]. The replication index of smooth muscle cells in the media is high during fetal development. Although proliferation rates decrease between birth and two years-of-age, they remain relatively high (2–5%) despite the absence of inflammatory cells. Therefore, the coronary artery intima forms rapidly after birth and may be a major determinant of the atherosclerotic process that will smolder for decades, and may eventually cause symptomatic disease. Thus, it appears that intimal cell masses maintain unique properties that promote the focal accumulation of lipids and/or macrophages (Fig. 1). These pathological changes in early atherosclerosis may be related to wound healing, or occur at sites of inflammation as proposed by Libby and Hansson [9].

There is very little known about the initiation of the intimal mass lesion, other than that the process is clonal [7, 10]. The stimulus for the monoclonal proliferation of smooth muscle cells is likely related to endothelial injury and accumulation of lipid within the intima [11]. The nature of endothelial injury is most likely multifactorial, although contradictory to early studies it does not involve desquamation but for the most part, the endothelium becomes dysfunctional. Significant numbers of inflammatory cells associated with pre-existing intimal cell masses are uncommon and the relationship between the development and progression of this lesion and inflammation is unclear.

## Intimal xanthomas (fatty streaks)

The intimal xanthoma is another potential non-progressive lesion of coronary atherosclerosis [4]. Pathologically, this lesion is composed of foamy macrophages within the intima containing smooth muscle cells within a proteoglycan-collagenous matrix (Fig. 2). There is no significant smooth muscle cell proliferation, calcification, accumulation of lipid pools, or necrotic core formation. Although T lymphocytes have been identified in fatty streak lesions, they are not as prominent as macrophages. Mast cells have also been identified in intimal xanthomas both in the intima and adventitia.

Intimal xanthomas are known to develop focally at lesion prone sites where more advances lesions appear later with aging. However, there are areas where fatty streak lesions will disappear with advancing age referred to as lesion-resistant. In human atherosclerosis, sites of regression are common in the thoracic aorta [12, 13].

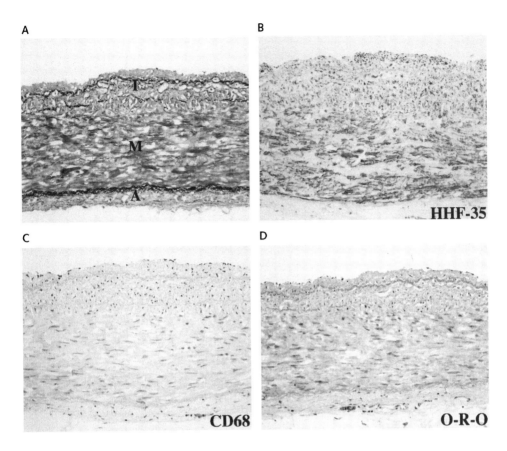

Figure 1
*Intimal thickening. Coronary artery showing high power view of the arterial wall; media (m),
intima (i), and adventitia (a). There is intimal thickening with splitting of the internal elastic
lamina with smooth muscle cells interspersed in a proteoglycan rich matrix (A, Movat Stain).
B shows HHF-35 staining of intimal and medial smooth muscle cells. No macrophages (CD-
68) or oil-red-O positive areas identified (C and D, respectively).*

In the right coronary artery, it is within the first 2 cm where fibroatheroma form.
This is the lesion-prone area whereas fatty streaks extend into the proximal one-half
to two-thirds of the vessel [5, 14].

## Expression of adhesion molecules: relevance to human disease

Atherosclerosis is considered by many as a chronic inflammatory process since inflammatory cells are recognized at all stages of lesion development. The entity of

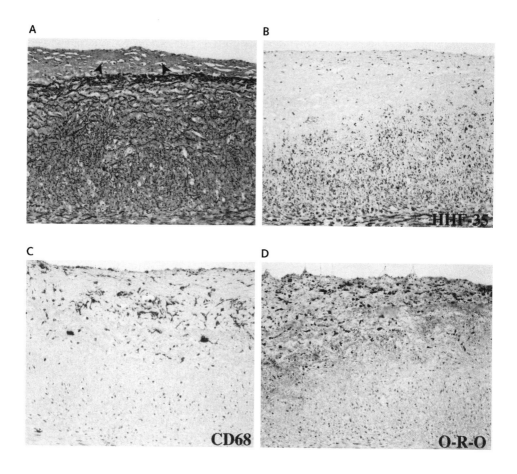

Figure 2

(A) Early xanthomatous lesion with hard to discern macrophages (arrowheads) infiltrating the area of intimal thickening (Movat stain); there is splitting of the internal elastic lamina. (B) shows HHF-35 staining of the intima. Note the most superficial layers do not stain positive for smooth muscle cells. (C) Positive macrophage staining (CD68) in the superficial layers of the plaque. (D) Similar layers to C staining positive for oil-red-O; both intracellular and extracellular lipid is present.

plaque erosion, however, places doubt on this hypothesis since this lesion appears to have little inflammatory component. Nonetheless, the binding and recruitment of circulating leukocytes to the vascular endothelium is considered a fundamental step in the developing atherosclerotic lesion, in particular those that go on to develop plaque rupture.

It must be emphasized that the process of inflammation during atherogenesis is under the surveillance of a complex immunological network presenting an abundance of positive and negative feedback mechanisms. Although the role of inflammation in the development of early lesions is well established, its function in advanced disease becomes less clear, especially in plaques associated with symptomatic disease

The fundamental process of recruitment and transendothelial migration of circulating leukocytes at sites of atherosclerosis is mediated through a family of adhesion molecules. The expression patterns of endothelial leukocyte-adhesion molecules, in particular vascular cell adhesion molecule-1 (VCAM-1), was initially established in hypercholesterolemic rabbits [15, 16]. In this experimental model, VCAM-1 is expressed locally in the aortic endothelium overlying early foam cell lesions and at sites of lesion formation. Other cell types, such as neointimal smooth muscle cells, deep within the plaque also express VCAM-1. Another adhesion molecule, intercellular adhesion molecule-1 (ICAM-1) is also found in foam cell lesions in endothelium expressing VCAM-1, and unlike VCAM-1, ICAM-1 expression extends into noninvolved regions. The expression of ICAM-1 is also not restricted to the endothelium, since it can be found on macrophages and smooth muscle cells within the intimal foam cell lesions. In contrast, the expression of E-selectin in foam cell lesions is very low [16].

Studies on the expression of vascular adhesion-molecules in human atherosclerotic tissue are mostly restricted to the autopsy material. Furthermore, the majority of reports of adhesion molecules in human atherosclerosis focus on advanced chronic disease

Unlike the rabbit atherosclerosis model, expression of adhesion molecules in human lesions is highly variable and is consistent with the morphological heterogeneity associated with symptomatic coronary plaques. Early studies by O'Brien et al. [17] demonstrated VCAM-1 expression in all atherosclerotic plaques (fibroatheromas) and 45% of control segments with nonatherosclerotic diffuse intimal thickening. In contrast to that in the rabbit, VCAM-1 was infrequently found on luminal endothelial cells, and was most prevalent in the areas of neovascularization, localized to endothelial and smooth muscle cells and inflammatory infiltrate in the base of plaques. Similar findings were reported by Davies et al. in human coronary arteries from explanted hearts [18]. Lesion types in this study were referred to, as fibrous plaques and plaques containing extracellular lipid. Although nonatherosclerotic control arteries showed no VCAM-1 staining, ICAM-1 and E-selectin were focally expressed on luminal endothelium. ICAM-1 was strongly present in the endothelium overlying all types of plaques and in macrophages; VCAM-1 and E- selectin expression on luminal surface of endothelium was variable. Adventitial vessel endothelium adjacent to plaques showed expression of ICAM-1 and E-selectin and VCAM-1 staining in similar areas was associated with lymphoid aggregates.

A follow-up study by O'Brien et al. suggested that recruitment of circulating leukocytes is mediated through adhesion molecules expressed on the intimal neovasculature rather than the main arterial lumen [19]. Macrophage accumulations were associated with expression of VCAM-1, whereas T-lymphocyte deposition was associated with expression of both ICAM-1 and VCAM-1. These data are consistent with the hypothesis that plaque neovascularization represents a significant route for infiltration of leukocytes and inflammatory activation in the atherosclerotic plaque.

A number of factors seem to regulate the expression of adhesion molecules. Some of these factors include, cholesterol [20, 21], cytokines [22], oxidative stress [23], sheer stress [24], Lp(a) [25] and advanced glycosylation end-products [26]. The latter may provide part of the explanation for the enhanced atherosclerosis associated with diabetes mellitus. Many of these stimuli act synergistically. Further, the expression of the adhesion molecules may be differentially regulated [20]. There is some evidence that adhesion molecules are developmentally regulated proteins that are expressed in fetal tissue, lost in the adult, and re-expressed in pathological processes, such as atherosclerosis [27]. This may explain why intimal cells of advanced lesions show expression of adhesion molecules. At least experimentally, the level of VCAM-1 expression correlates directly with circulating cholesterol levels and macrophage infiltrates [28].

Although the cellular expression of adhesion molecules is difficult to assess clinically, soluble forms measured in the circulation may serve as molecular markers of subclinical coronary disease. Circulating forms of VCAM-1, E-selectin, and ICAM-1, possibly arising from the shedding or proteolytic cleavage from endothelial cells, have been detected in plasma and are elevated in atherosclerosis. Although a recent clinical study suggested that shed VCAM-1 levels correlated with the overall extent of atherosclerotic disease [29], ICAM-1 and E-selectin levels may be more predictive markers of coronary atherosclerosis [30]. In addition to their clinical value, soluble adhesion molecules, at least *in vitro*, have been shown to reduce the adhesion of monocytes to activated endothelial cells presenting a negative feedback role in atherosclerosis progression.

Once the moncytes infiltrate the vascular wall, they transform into lipid-laden foam cells which is the characteristic lesion of early atherosclerosis. Two growth factors that enhance monocyte migration and lesion progression include monocyte chemotactic protein-1 (MCP-1) and macrophage colony-stimulating factor (MCSF). These factors further induce the proliferation and differentiation of monocytes. Both interleukin-1$\alpha$ (IL-1$\alpha$) and tumor necrosis factor $\alpha$ (TNF$\alpha$) induce MCP-1 and MCSF mRNA expression in both endothelial and smooth muscle cells in a concentration-dependent manner [31]. As evidence for the role of growth factors, formation of fatty streaks is diminished by blockade of MCSF function by antibodies as well as in mice that are apo-E or low-density lipoprotein (LDL) and MCSF-receptor deficient [32]. However, this effect does not appear to be mediated by circulating lipoproteins.

## Fibroatheromas (fibrous cap atheroma)

The transition between early lesions of atherosclerosis and the well-developed fibroatheroma is marked by an intermediate or preatheroma (Type III) as defined by the AHA classification [5, 6]. The preatheroma is characterized by the presence of extracellular lipid pools, which form between layers of smooth muscle cells. These pools tend to occur at sites of adaptive intimal thickening (Fig. 2). The lipid pools lie below the macrophage foam-cell layers and are located in the proteoglycan matrix and among collagen fibers. However, no necrotic core is identified in these regions. These lesions show large numbers of lipid droplets with or without peripheral laminated membranes and remnants of extracellular matrix components. The smooth muscle cells show lipid droplets in the cytoplasm. The preatheromas are rich in free cholesterol, fatty acids, sphingomyelin, lysolecithin, and triglycerides. The glycosaminogylcan with the highest affinity for plasma LDL is dermatan sulfate, which consists of biglycan and decorin [33]. In addition to macrophages, the deposition of intimal T lymphocytes is common in these lesions.

The fibrous cap atheroma also referred to as Type IV lesion as per the AHA classification is the first of the advanced lesions of coronary atherosclerosis (Fig. 3). Virchow likened this lesion to a dermal cyst (e.g. a sebaceous cyst, "Grutzbalg"), a fatty mass encapsulated by fibrous tissue [34]. Thus, since the 1850s, the defining feature of the "atheroma" has been the presence of a necrotic, fatty mass encapsulated by a fibrous tissue. This feature is analogous to the capsule containing an abscess and, like an abscess, the plaque can rupture. The relationship between inflammation and the development of the fibroatheroma is complex. The definition of fibroatheroma includes the presence of a lipid- rich core and the origin and development of this core is the key towards the understanding of the disease progression. As the atherosclerotic plaque enlarges, the lipid core becomes consolidated into one or more masses of extracellular lipid, cholesterol crystals, and necrotic debris. Only a few studies exist on the mechanisms of progression of a cellular xanthoma into a fibrous cap atheroma with a necrotic core [35].

Cholesterol in the fibrous cap atheroma occurs in intra- or extracellular droplets, liposomes, and crystals. Extracellular sources (e.g., plasma lipid) are especially important for accumulation of cholesteryl esters (predominantly cholesteryl linoleate) which predominate in later lesions and are similar to plasma LDL. The origin of the extracellular lipid, especially free cholesterol, has been long debated. Two theories have been suggested; one maintains that lipase-mediated hydrolysis of phospholipids and cholesterol esters in the extracellular space leads to the production of free cholesterol, which, when concentrated, will crystallize [36]; the second suggests that cholesterol ester lipid droplets within macrophages form cholesterol crystals from hydrolysis within lysosomes [37]. Alternatively, we have proposed that excessive free cholesterol also comes from the breakdown of erythrocyte cell membranes, contributing to the free cholesterol pool within the advanced plaque [38].

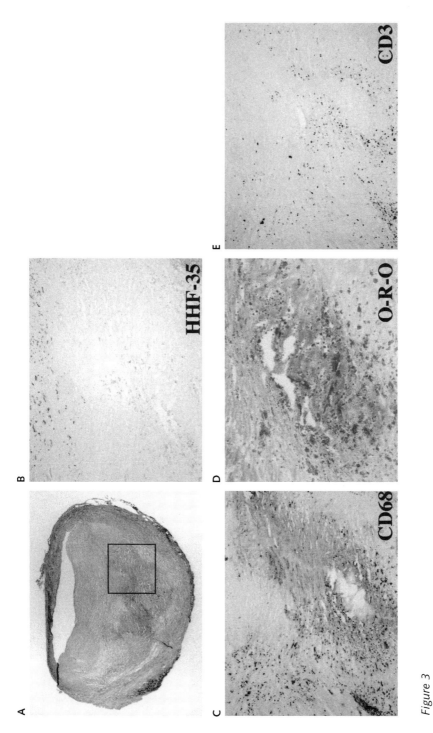

*Figure 3*
*Fibrous cap atheroma. (A) Hematoxylin and eosin stained section of a coronary artery showing early necrotic core formation (area within the box) with an overlying thick fibrous cap. The fibrous cap contains α-actin positive smooth muscle cells, (B), while the early necrotic core stains positive for macrophages (CD68 and oil-red-O (C and D, respectively). The necrotic core shows both intra and extracellular oil-red-O positive areas (D). (E) Few CD-3 positive T lymphocytes are found in the same area.*

## Thin cap fibroatheroma (a vulnerable plaque)

A common mechanism of disruption of the fibrous cap atheroma involves the thinning, or weakening, of the fibrous cap, resulting in fissures and ruptures. These breaks in the fibrous cap expose tissue factor to the lumen. The subsequent luminal thrombosis is the basis of luminal narrowing, vasospasm, and clot embolization.

We have previously defined thin-capped fibroatheroma as a lesion with a fibrous cap of 65 μm or less that is infiltrated by foam cells and T lymphocytes [39]. The thin-capped fibroatheroma typically contains a large necrotic core with cholesterol clefts and may also contain intraplaque hemorrhage and calcification. Prior areas of rupture may be evident, often resulting in multiple compartments of lipid-rich core and mild to moderate calcification. Coronary lesions also show variants of a thin-capped fibroatheroma with large collections of superficial macrophages overlying an intimal mass lesion without significant lipid rich core. Saphenous vein grafts commonly show these types of lesions and may represent processes important to the progression of atherosclerotic plaques [40].

Although the macrophage is often considered the most important inflammatory cell in the progression of atherosclerosis, there has been increased attention to the role of T ymphocytes. Because both macrophages and T cells are present in the fibrous cap, antigen presentation with immune activation is likely to occur. Many T cells in the developing atheroma express IL-2 receptors and human leukocyte antigen-DR (HLA-DR). The presence of the latter in plaques provides indirect evidence for local interferon-γ (INFγ) secretion. In early lesions, macrophages outnumber lymphocytes by a factor of 10 to 50, and CD8 cells predominate over CD4 cells with a ratio of 2:1 [41]. However, there is a switch to a greater number of CD4 lymphocytes, with activation of HLA class II antigens, in advanced plaques.

The progression of a stable fibroatheroma into a rupture-prone thin cap fibroatheroma is under intense investigation. There are a number of proteases which, have been implicated in thinning of the fibrous cap. Serpin proteinase inhibitors or "serpins" may participate in remodeling, regulation of blood pressure, inflammation, cell migration and differentiation, fibrinolysis, and blood coagulation. Those involved in atherogenesis include α1-proteinase inhibitor, which acts on leukocyte elastase and cathapsin G, α1-antitripsin and α2-macroglobulin regulators of lipoprotein catabolism; α2-antiplasmin and plasminogen activator inhibitor (PAI-1) regulators of fibrinolysis, and antithrombin III, an inhibitor of blood coagulation. The serpins may also affect the atherosclerotic pathway via matrix metalloproteinase stromelysin-3.

Although a number of matrix metalloproteinases (MMPs) have been implicated in thinning of the fibrous cap, it is unclear when they become critical to lesion instability since they are present in abundance in early plaque [42]. However, one such MMP, Stromelysin-3, a member of the serpin family has been shown to colocalize with CD40 expression on endothelial cells, smooth muscle cells, and monocytes in advanced human atheroma. Activated T lymphocytes express the CD40 ligand surface molecule, which, when activated, promotes the expression of adhesion molecules, cytokines, MMPs, and tissue factor [43]. The regulation of stromelysin-3 by CD40 ligand (CD40L) may be crucial to the progression of a stable plaque to one prone to rupture and thrombosis [44].

Interruption of CD40-CD40L signaling by an anti-CD40L antibody has been demonstrated to limit experimental autoimmune diseases, such as collagen-induced arthritis, lupus nephritis, acute or chronic graft-versus-host disease, multiple sclerosis and thyroiditis. Mach et al. [43] showed reduction of atherosclerosis by inhibition of CD 40 signaling (antibody directed against CD154 pathway) in mice. Furthermore, atheroma of mice treated with anti-CD40L antibody contained significantly fewer macrophages and T lymphocytes, and exhibited decreased expression of VCAM-1 [43]. Lutgens et al. showed that genetic disruption of CD154 in apo E-deficient mice resulted in a marked reduction in plaque area, along with less lipid and collagen and a reduction in T cells and macrophages in advanced plaques [45].

## Plaque rupture

Fibrous cap disruption (Fig. 4) resulting in continuity between the overlying thrombus and the necrotic core defines plaque rupture. Ruptured lesions typically have a large necrotic core and a disrupted fibrous cap infiltrated by macrophages. The trigger for plaque rupture is the object of intense study, and is likely related to those conditions that result in thinning of the fibroatheromatous cap (see above).

## Inflammation and plaque rupture

The density of macrophages at the site of rupture is typically very high, although in some cases macrophages may be relatively sparse. In our experience, occasional neutrophils are seen in regions of plaque rupture. Studies of carotid plaque ruptures

---

*Figure 4*
*Plaque rupture. This lesion is the most frequent cause of coronary thrombosis and is characterized by a thin fibrous cap (A, within arrows, and D, Movat stain). (B) The fibrous cap at the rupture site heavily infiltrated by CD68 positive macrophages. (C) shows a paucity of UCHL positive T lymphocytes interspersed within the fibrous cap. Only few smooth muscle cells are seen (E) and most cells in the fibrous cap are HLA-DR positive (F). (Abbreviations: NC, necrotic core; Th, thrombus)*

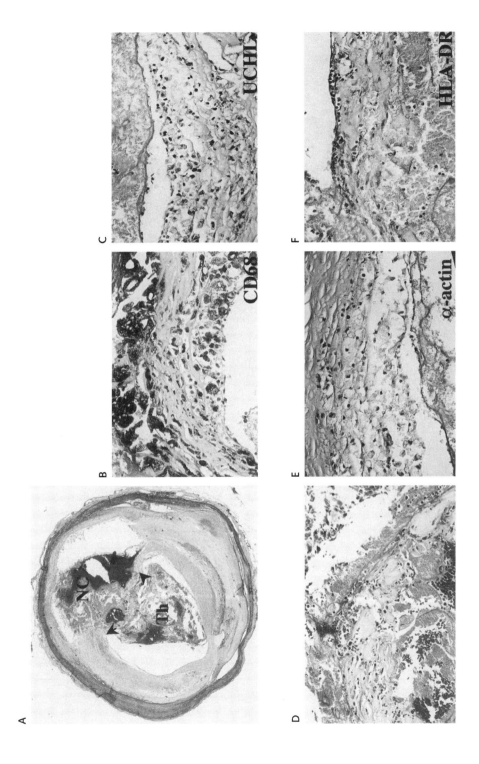

show that the fibrous cap at the site of interruption contains approximately 2/3rds of cells that are macrophages, 1/3rd T lymphocytes, and a few B lymphocytes [46]. In our own laboratory, we have shown that macrophages are present in virtually all cases of plaque ruptures near the rupture site, and T lymphocytes were demonstrated in 75% of ruptures [47]. Although macrophage density is maximal in plaque rupture, the number of T lymphocytes does not vary among culprit lesions. The smooth muscle cell content within the fibrous cap at the rupture site is typically low. Risk factors most predictive for this type of lesion are hypercholesterolemia, low serum HDL, and a high TC/HDL-C ratio. In women older that 50 years, ruptured plaques comprise the majority of atherosclerotic lesions associated with acute thrombi [39].

## The role of interferon

What converts a collagen-rich fibrous cap to one that ruptures is under extensive investigation in many laboratories. The majority of investigators have emphasized the importance of cytokine-mediated degradation of the fibrous cap. For example, Libby and colleagues have shown the importance of IFNγ, which markedly decreases the ability of human smooth muscle cells to express interstitial collagen genes [48]. INFγ is secreted by T lymphocytes [41]. Other studies have shown the presence of HLA-DRα expression suggesting activation of T cells and macrophages in the fibrous cap of plaque ruptures [47, 49]. We have shown that the fibrous cap in plaque rupture is infiltrated by macrophages and T cells with a ratio of 7.6 ± 6.1 [50]. Besides the inhibition of collagen synthesis, IFNγ may also inhibit proliferation and promote apoptosis of smooth muscle cells (SMCs) [48]. Moreover, IFNγ activates macrophages, which are rich in MMPs, which may promote the breakdown of collagen, proteoglycans and elastins [51].

## Matrix metalloproteinases

The MMPs consist of at least 16 zinc-dependent endopeptidases that possess catalytic activity against extracellular matrix. *In vitro* studies have shown that several inflammatory mediators modulate the expression of MMPs [52]. TNFα and IL-1 increase MMP-1, MMP-3 and MMP-9 expression in SMCs and macrophages [51, 53], while IL-4, IFNγ and IL-10 inhibit their synthesis [54]. MMPs are also inhibited by endogenous tissue inhibitors of metalloproteinases (TIMPs) [52, 55]. Breakdown of fibrous cap collagen by MMPs released from monocyte-derived macrophages have been shown *in vitro* and lipid-laden macrophages from atherosclerotic plaques elaborate MMP-1 and MMP-3 [56]. Although MMPs are a common finding in animal models of atherosclerosis, to our knowledge no one has been able to demonstrate plaque rupture in lesions where a necrotic core and fibrous cap are known to be present.

There is, however, direct evidence for collagenolysis within the fibrous cap from a study by Libby and colleagues, demonstrating collagenase-cleaved type I collagen by a novel cleavage-specific antibody [57]. It is well known that the triple helix of the intersitial collagen fibrils is resistant to degradation by most proteinases. The breakdown of collagen by collagenases yields characteristic fragments of 75% and 25% of the span of the intact collagenases. Antibodies have been developed that recognize the larger collagen fragment of the collagenase-cleaved type-1 collagen within the atheroma. Interestingly, type I collagen fragments are colocalized with MMP-1 and MMP-13-positive macrophages. Moreover, increased collagenolysis has been found in atheromatous versus fibrous plaques associated with higher levels of proinflammatory cytokines, activators of MMPs.

## Myeloperoxidase (MPO)

There is experimental evidence that macrophage MPO may be responsible for disruption of the fibrous cap in plaque rupture [58]. Subsets of macrophages rich in myeloperoxidase are present in the fibrous cap and constitute approximately 13% of the total population. Myeloperoxidase (MPO), an enzyme responsible for hypochlorous acid/hypochlorite (HOCl) production *in vivo*, is actively present in human atherosclerotic lesions, and HOCl aggregates and transforms LDL into a high-uptake form for macrophages *in vitro* [59]. Many MPO positive cells have been shown to contain cathepsin G, leucocyte elastase, and MMP-9 enzymes, which can potentially destroy the fibrous cap. HOCl can inhibit TIMP-1 in a concentration dependent manner and can degrade collagen and elastin *in vitro*. Finally, HOCl also induces death of SMCs where as taurine prevents the cytotoxic effect of HOCl. Thus, there appears to be a redundancy of pathways by which the fibrous cap may rupture provided all the cellular elements at the site of rupture are present.

## Apoptosis in plaque rupture

Apoptosis may also play a role in plaque rupture. There is extensive apoptosis of macrophages at rupture sites relative to remote non-ruptured areas of the fibrous cap [60]. Areas of macrophage apoptosis at plaque rupture sites showed intense immunoreactivity to caspase-1/IL-1β converting enzyme (ICE), a mediator of apoptosis. In addition, ICE activation is more pronounced in ruptured plaques compared to stable lesions without thrombi. Other investigators have demonstrated apoptosis in smooth muscle cells and macrophages of unstable atheromas, with the predominant apoptotic cell being the macrophage [61].

## Plaque erosion

Erosion is a mechanism of plaque disruption that does not involve thinning of the fibrous cap (Fig. 5). The morphological characteristics of plaque erosion include the abundance of smooth muscle cells and proteoglycans, and disruption of the surface endothelium without a prominent lipid core [47, 49]. Compared to rupture sites in the thin capped fibroatheroma, plaque erosion contains relatively few or no macrophages, and the numbers of T lymphocytes are decreased compared to those found in ruptures [47]. Erosions account for approximately 40% of cases of thrombotic sudden coronary death, and are especially common in young women and men. These lesions are usually eccentric, rarely show calcification, and normally result in less severe narrowing than plaque rupture [47]. Currently, we have limited understanding of the mechanism(s) of erosion. Besides the thrombus, the most striking aspects of this lesion are the absence of endothelium and the "activated" appearance of the underlying smooth muscle cells. Smooth muscle cells at the site of erosion are bizarre in shape and contain hyperchromatic nuclei with prominent nucleoli. It has been postulated that erosions result from vasospasm, and are often found in cigarette smokers [39]. The role of inflammation in the pathogenesis of erosion, especially that of lymphocytic infiltrates has yet to be elucidated.

## Healed plaque rupture

There is little information about plaques that rupture and heal without resulting in death of the individual (Fig. 6). Mann and Davies suggest that healed plaque ruptures may be important in plaque progression [62]. In a recent autopsy series, healed ruptures were found in 61% of cases of sudden coronary death with an increased incidence in patients with hypercholesterolemia and diabetes mellitus [62, 63]. Healed ruptures are characterized by a disrupted fibrous cap filled in by smooth muscle cells, proteoglycans, and collagen. The matrix within the healed fibrous cap defect may consist of a proteoglycan-rich mass or a collagen-rich scar, depending on the phase of healing. The typical wound-healing response characterized by the degradation of the thrombus, transient infiltration of the vessel wall and thrombus itself by inflammatory cells and capillaries with the progressive removal of the necrotic debris is thought to be a paradigm for the healing of arterial thrombi. Although there are few studies of the healing of thrombi in human coronary disease an angioplasty study in non-human primates fed a high cholesterol diet demonstrate an elaborate time-dependent array of proteoglycans and procollagen with persistent healing [64]. This healing response was associated with the expression of integrins $\alpha_V\beta_3$ and $\alpha_2\beta_1$ in the developing neointima. In a rabbit model of double balloon injury, Courtman et al. have shown that negative remodeling of the aorta can be blocked with an active site-inhibited recombinant human factor VIIa, an inhibitor

A

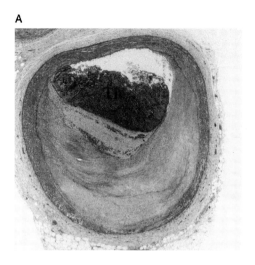

B

C

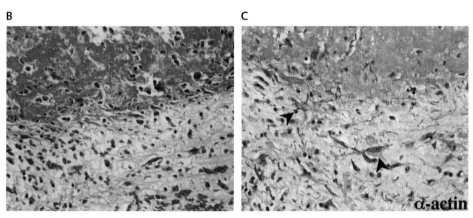

*Figure 5*
*Plaque erosion. This lesion accounts for 40% of cases of coronary thrombosis in patients with sudden coronary death. Note the luminal thrombus (Th), absence of necrotic core and underlying proteoglycan-rich plaque (green stain on Movat stain). (B) High power view of the area of thrombus and the underlying plaque shows large spindle-shaped cells with interspersed rare inflammatory cells (H&E stain). (C) The spindle-shaped cells in B containing vesicular nuclei with prominent nucleoli are α-actin positive smooth muscle cells.*

of tissue factor [65]. We have shown that healed human coronary plaques are smaller in size (negative remodeling) compared with acute ruptures. This response may result from activation of the extrinsic pathway of coagulation resulting in thrombus formation and subsequent healing. In human disease, lesions with healed ruptures may exhibit multi-layering of lipid and necrotic core suggestive of repetitive episodes

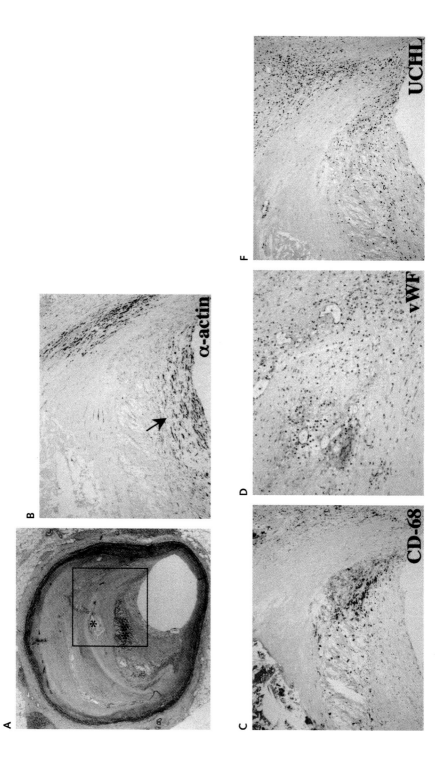

of thrombosis [66]. Obviously, the role of healed rupture, ongoing inflammation, and angiogenesis in the enlargement of the coronary atherosclerotic plaque warrants further study.

## Inflammation and plaque remodeling

### Medial atrophy

The pioneering work of Glagov demonstrated that the human coronary artery expands with increasing volume of atherosclerotic plaque [67]. The complex inter-action, however, between healing of plaque rupture, inflammation, and arterial remodeling has yet to be fully elucidated. Luminal narrowing that results in clinical syndromes may result not only in the progression of atherosclerosis but also in a failure of arterial remodeling. We have demonstrated that a failure of remodeling may play a role in increasing atherosclerotic disease in men with low levels of high-density lipoprotein cholesterol [68]. It appears likely that arterial remodeling is mediated by an inflammatory mechanism. Studies performed on aortic atheroscle-rosis in the human demonstrate that T lymphocytes elaborate perforin and Fas, pos-sibly resulting in death of smooth muscle cells, a source of elastin and collagen [69]. Elastolytic enzymes, such as cathepsin S and K, are expressed by smooth muscle cells exposed to cytokines, and may contribute to elastin digestion and arterial remodeling [70]. As mentioned above, activation of the extrinsic coagulation cas-cade may also result in negative remodeling [65].

### Adventitial inflammation

Although the role of adventitial fibrosis and inflammation in the progression of plaque is poorly characterized, there is some evidence in the literature implicating adventitial inflammation as a mechanism of luminal narrowing. This seems coun-

---

*Figure 6*
*Healed plaque rupture. (A) Movat-stained section of a coronary plaque showing hemorrhage into a necrotic core (\*\*) with an overlying layer of smooth muscle cells and proteoglycans representing the healed site after the rupture. The underlying plaque shows another area of necrotic core (\*) with overlying fibrous tissue, which likely represents an area of prior rup-ture. (B) High power view of the area close to the lumen showing newly formed smooth muscles (α-actin stain, arrow). (C) shows the necrotic core surrounded by CD-68 positive macrophages. Note the neovascularization (von Willebrand factor (vWF) positive capillaries in D) and UCHL positive T lymphocytes (E) in the shoulder region of the plaque.*

terintuitive however, since adventitial inflammation is usually associated with aneurysm formation [71]. Intriguingly, one recent study showed that adventitial inflammation correlated well with luminal narrowing in peripheral lesions in apo E knockout mice [72]. Similarly, arterial balloon injury models in rabbit and pig demonstrate that adventitial fibrosis is a more important determinant of lumen loss than intimal mass [73, 74]. In another report, Katsumata and colleagues demonstrated that chronic application of IL-1β to the adventitia alone caused lumen narrowing in pig coronary arteries [75].

Along with animal data, the role of inflammation in coronary narrowing is supported by a few autopsy studies. Kohchi et al. reported findings from a quantitative analysis of adventitial inflammation of the coronary artery with intimal lesions in 12 patients who suffered coronary death with a history of unstable angina [76]. In patients with unstable angina, the incidence of adventitial inflammation correlated with the degree of luminal narrowing and was significantly greater than that in angina patients who died of noncardiac causes and also in patients without angina.

## Plaque calcification and inflammation

Calcification of the extracellular matrix of atherosclerotic plaques is considered an active process [77]. Mineralization of vesicles released from apoptotic smooth muscle cells may be one of the initiating events in plaque calcification [78]. A number of proteins, including bone morphogenic protein [79], osteocalcin, and matrix gla protein are involved in the regulation of calcium within the atherosclerotic plaque [80]. Expression of osteopontin and matrix gla protein has been demonstrated in foam cells of the fibroatheromatous plaque [81]. Osteonectin, osteopontin, and osteocalcin have been shown to co-localize with calcium deposits, apoB, fibrin, and MMP-3 in advanced, symptomatic carotid lesions, suggesting that plaque calcification in the carotid arteries may be related to hemorrhage and thrombosis [82]. The role of inflammation in plaque calcification, however, remains to be elucidated.

*Note*
The opinions or assertions contained herein are the private views of the authors and are not to be construed as official or reflecting the views of the Department of the Army, the Department of the Air Force, or the Department of Defense.

## References

1    Mehta JL, Saldeen TG, Rand K (1998) Interactive role of infection, inflammation and traditional risk factors in atherosclerosis and coronary artery disease. *J Am Coll Cardiol* 31: 1217–1225

2    Whicher J, Biasucci L, Rifai N (1999) Inflammation, the acute phase response and atherosclerosis. *Clin Chem Lab Med* 37: 495–503

3    Zhou J, Chew M, Ravn HB, Falk E (1999) Plaque pathology and coronary thrombosis in the pathogenesis of acute coronary syndromes. *Scand J Clin Lab Invest* (Suppl) 230: 3–11

4    Virmani R, Kolodgie FD, Burke AP, Farb A, Schwartz SM (2000) Lessons from sudden coronary death: A comprehensive morphologic classification scheme for atherosclerotic lesions. *Atheroscler Thromb Vasc Biol* 20: 1262–1275

5    Stary HC, Chandler AB, Glagov S, Guyton JR, Insull W Jr, Rosenfeld ME, Schaffer SA, Schwartz CJ, Wagner WD, Wissler RW et al (1994) A definition of initial, fatty streak, and intermediate lesions of atherosclerosis. A report from the Committee on Vascular Lesions of the Council on Arteriosclerosis, American Heart Association. *Arterioscler Thromb* 14: 840–856

6    Stary HC, Chandler AB, Dinsmore RE, Guyton JR, Insull W Jr, Rosenfeld ME, Schaffer SA, Schwartz CJ, Wagner WD, Wissler RW et al (1995) A definition of advanced types of atherosclerotic lesions and a histological classification of atherosclerosis. A report from the Committee on Vascular Lesions of the Council on Arteriosclerosis, American Heart Association. *Arterioscler Thromb Vasc Biol* 15: 1512–1531

7    Schwartz SM, deBlois D, O'Brien ER (1995) The intima. Soil for atherosclerosis and restenosis. *Circ Res* 77: 445–465

8    Ikari Y, McManus BM, Kenyon J, Schwartz SM (1999) Neonatal intima formation in the human coronary artery. *Arterioscler Thromb Vasc Biol* 19: 2036–2040

9    Libby P, Hansson GK (1991) Involvement of the immune system in human atherogenesis: current knowledge and unanswered questions. *Lab Invest* 64: 5–15

10   McCaffrey TA, Du B, Consigli S, Szabo P, Bray PJ, Hartner L, Weksler BB, Sanborn TA, Bergman G, Bush HL Jr et al (1997) Genomic instability in the type II TGF-beta1 receptor gene in atherosclerotic and restenotic vascular cells. *J Clin Invest* 100: 2182–2188

11   Chatterjee SB, Dey S, Shi WY, Thomas K, Hutchins GM (1997) Accumulation of glycosphingolipids in human atherosclerotic plaque and unaffected aorta tissues. *Glycobiology* 7: 57–65

12   Velican D, Velican C (1980) Atherosclerotic involvement of the coronary arteries of adolescents and young adults. *Atherosclerosis* 36: 449–460

13   Strong JP, Malcom GT, McMahan CA, Tracy RE, Newman WP 3rd, Herderick EE, Cornhill JF (1999) Prevalence and extent of atherosclerosis in adolescents and young adults: implications for prevention from the Pathobiological Determinants of Atherosclerosis in Youth Study. *Jama* 281: 727–735

14   Stary HC (1987) Macrophages, macrophage foam cells, and eccentric intimal thickening in the coronary arteries of young children. *Atherosclerosis* 64: 91–108

15   Li H, Cybulsky MI, Gimbrone MA Jr, Libby P (1993) An atherogenic diet rapidly induces VCAM-1, a cytokine-regulatable mononuclear leukocyte adhesion molecule, in rabbit aortic endothelium. *Arterioscler Thromb* 13: 197–204

16   Richardson M, Kurowska EM, Carroll KK (1994) Early lesion development in the aor-

tas of rabbits fed low-fat, cholesterol-free, semipurified casein diet. *Atherosclerosis* 107: 165–178

17   O'Brien KD, Allen MD, McDonald TO, Chait A, Harlan JM, Fishbein D, McCarty J, Ferguson M, Hudkins K, Benjamin CD et al (1993) Vascular cell adhesion molecule-1 is expressed in human coronary atherosclerotic plaques. Implications for the mode of progression of advanced coronary atherosclerosis . *J Clin Invest* 92: 945–951

18   Davies MJ, Gordon JL, Gearing AJ, Piyott R, Woolf N, Katz D, Kyriakopoulos A (1993) The expression of the adhesion molecules ICAM-1, VCAM-1, PECAM, and E- selectin in human atherosclerosis. *J Pathol* 171: 223–229

19   O'Brien KD, McDonald TO, Chait A, Allen MD, Alpers CE (1996) Neovascular expression of E-selectin, intercellular adhesion molecule-1, and vascular cell adhesion molecule-1 in human atherosclerosis and their relation to intimal leukocyte content. *Circulation* 93: 672–682

20   Nakashima Y, Raines EW, Plump AS, Breslow JL, Ross R (1998) Upregulation of VCAM-1 and ICAM-1 at atherosclerosis-prone sites on the endothelium in the ApoE-deficient mouse. *Arterioscler Thromb Vasc Biol* 18: 842–851

21   Allen S, Khan S, Al-Mohanna F, Batten P, Yacoub M (1998) Native low density lipoprotein-induced calcium transients trigger VCAM- 1 and E-selectin expression in cultured human vascular endothelial cells. *J Clin Invest* 101: 1064–1075

22   Couffinhal T, Duplaa C, Moreau C, Lamaziere JM, Bonnet J (1994) Regulation of vascular cell adhesion molecule-1 and intercellular adhesion molecule-1 in human vascular smooth muscle cells. *Circ Res* 74: 225–234

23   Khan BV, Parthasarathy SS, Alexander RW, Medford RM (1995) Modified low density lipoprotein and its constituents augment cytokine-activated vascular cell adhesion molecule-1 gene expression in human vascular endothelial cells. *J Clin Invest* 95: 1262–1270

24   Nagel T, Resnick N, Atkinson WJ, Dewey CF Jr, Gimbrone MA Jr (1994) Shear stress selectively upregulates intercellular adhesion molecule-1 expression in cultured human vascular endothelial cells. *J Clin Invest* 94: 885–891

25   Allen S, Khan S, Tam S, Koschinsky M, Taylor P, Yacoub M (1998) Expression of adhesion molecules by lp(a): a potential novel mechanism for its atherogenicity. *Faseb J* 12: 1765–1776

26   Schmidt AM, Hori O, Chen JX, Li JF, Crandall J, Zhang J, Cao R, Yan SD, Brett J, Stern D et al (1995) Advanced glycation endproducts interacting with their endothelial receptor induce expression of vascular cell adhesion molecule-1 (VCAM-1) in cultured human endothelial cells and in mice. A potential mechanism for the accelerated vasculopathy of diabetes. *J Clin Invest* 96: 1395–1403

27   Printseva O, Peclo MM, Gown AM (1992) Various cell types in human atherosclerotic lesions express ICAM-1. Further immunocytochemical and immunochemical studies employing monoclonal antibody 10F3. *Am J Pathol* 140: 889–896

28   Truskey GA, Herrmann RA, Kait J, Barber KM (1999) Focal increases in vascular cell adhesion molecule-1 and intimal macrophages at atherosclerosis-susceptible sites in the

rabbit aorta after short-term cholesterol feeding. *Arterioscler Thromb Vasc Biol* 19: 393–401

29    Peter K, Nawroth P, Conradt C, Nordt T, Weiss T, Boehme M, Wunsch A, Allenberg J, Kubler W, Bode C et al (1997) Circulating vascular cell adhesion molecule-1 correlates with the extent of human atherosclerosis in contrast to circulating intercellular adhesion molecule-1, E-selectin, P-selectin, and thrombomodulin. *Arterioscler Thromb Vasc Biol* 17: 505–512

30    Hwang SJ, Ballantyne CM, Sharrett AR, Smith LC, Davis CE, Gotto AM, Boerwinkle E (1997) Circulating adhesion molecules VCAM-1, ICAM-1, and E-selectin in carotid atherosclerosis and incident coronary heart disease cases: the Atherosclerosis Risk In Communities (ARIC) study. *Circulation* 96: 4219–4225

31    Wang J, Wang S, Lu Y, Weng Y, Gown AM (1994) GM-CSF and M-CSF expression is associated with macrophage proliferation in progressing and regressing rabbit atheromatous lesions. *Exp Mol Pathol* 61: 109–118

32    Qiao JH, Tripathi J, Mishra NK, Cai Y, Tripathi S, Wang XP, Imes S., Fishbein MC, Clinton SK, Libby P et al (1997) Role of macrophage colony-stimulating factor in atherosclerosis: studies of osteopetrotic mice. *Am J Pathol* 150: 1687–1699

33    Evanko SP, Raines EW, Ross R, Gold LI, Wight TN (1998) Proteoglycan distribution in lesions of atherosclerosis depends on lesion severity, structural characteristics, and the proximity of platelet-derived growth factor and transforming growth factor-beta. *Am J Pathol* 152: 533–546

34    Virchow R (ed) (1858) *Cellular pathology based on physiological and pathological histology*. Alabama: Classics of Medicine Library, Birmingham

35    Guyton JR, Klemp KF (1996) Development of the lipid-rich core in human atherosclerosis. *Arterioscler Thromb Vasc Biol* 16: 4–11

36    Kruth HS (1997) Cholesterol deposition in atherosclerotic lesions. *Subcell Biochem* 28: 319–362

37    Tangirala RK, Jerome WG, Jones NL, Small DM, Johnson WJ, Glick JM, Mahlberg FH, Rothblat GH (1994) Formation of cholesterol monohydrate crystals in macrophage-derived foam cells. *J Lipid Res* 35: 93–104

38    Kruth HS (1984) Localization of unesterified cholesterol in human atherosclerotic lesions. *Am J Pathol* 114: 201–208

39    Burke AP, Farb A, Malcom GT, Liang Y-H, Smialek J, Virmani R (1997) Coronary risk factors and plaque morphology in patients with coronary disease dying suddenly. *N Engl J Med* 336: 1276–1282

40    Farb A, Weber DK, Burke AP, Kolodgie F, Virmani R (1999) Morphology of stenosis progression and rupture in saphenous vein bypass grafts (abstract). *Circulation* 100: I-599

41    Hansson GK, Holm J, Jonasson L (1989) Detection of activated T lymphocytes in the human atherosclerotic plaque. *Am J Pathol* 135: 169–175

42    Schonbeck U, Mach F, Bonnefoy JY, Loppnow H, Flad HD, Libby P (1997) Ligation of CD40 activates interleukin 1beta-converting enzyme (caspase-1) activity in vascular

smooth muscle and endothelial cells and promotes elaboration of active interleukin 1beta. *J Biol Chem* 272: 19569–19574

43    Mach F, Schonbeck U, Sukhova GK, Atkinson E, Libby P (1998) Reduction of atherosclerosis in mice by inhibition of CD40 signalling. *Nature* 394: 200–203

44    Mach F, Schonbeck U, Bonnefoy JY, Pober JS, Libby P (1997) Activation of monocyte/macrophage functions related to acute atheroma complication by ligation of CD40: induction of collagenase, stromelysin, and tissue factor. Circulation 96: 396–399

45    Lutgens E, Gorelik L, Daemen MJ, de Muinck ED, Grewal IS, Koteliansky VE, Flavell RA (1999) Requirement for CD154 in the progression of atherosclerosis. *Nat Med* 5: 1313–1316

46    Milei J, Parodi JC, Fernandez Alonso G, Barone A, Beigelman R, Ferreira LM, Arrigoni G, Mattussi L (1996) Carotid atherosclerosis. Immunocytochemical analysis of the vascular and cellular composition in endarterectomies. *Cardiologia* 41: 535–542

47    Farb A, Burke AP, Tang AL, Liang TY, Mannan P, Smialek J, Virmani R (1996) Coronary plaque erosion without rupture into a lipid core. A frequent cause of coronary thrombosis in sudden coronary death. *Circulation* 93: 1354–1363

48    Hansson GK, Jonasson L, Holm J, Clowes MM, Clowes AW (1988) Gamma-interferon regulates vascular smooth muscle proliferation and Ia antigen expression *in vivo* and *in vitro*. *Circ Res* 63: 712–719

49    van der Wal AC, Becker AE, van der Loos CM, Das PK (1994) Site of intimal rupture or erosion of thrombosed coronary atherosclerotic plaques is characterized by an inflammatory process irrespective of the dominant plaque morphology. *Circulation* 89: 36–44

50    Burke AP, Kolodgie F, Farb A, Liang Y-H, Malcom G, Virmani R (1999) Macrophage density within the fibrous cap correlates with the etiology of thrombus, diabetes, and serum cholesterol. *J Am Coll Cardiol* 33: 323A

51    Galis ZS, Muszynski M, Sukhova GK, Simon-Morrissey E, Unemori EN, Lark MW, Ameto E, Libby P (1994) Cytokine-stimulated human vascular smooth muscle cells synthesize a complement of enzymes required for extracellular matrix digestion. *Circ Res* 75: 181–189

52    Galis ZS, Sukhova GK, Lark MW, Libby P (1994) Increased expression of matrix metalloproteinases and matrix degrading activity in vulnerable regions of human atherosclerotic plaques. *J Clin Invest* 94: 2493–2503

53    Fabunmi RP, Baker AH, Murray EJ, Booth RF, Newby AC (1996) Divergent regulation by growth factors and cytokines of 95 kDa and 72 kDa gelatinases and tissue inhibitors or metalloproteinases-1, -2, and - 3 in rabbit aortic smooth muscle cells. *Biochem J* 315: 335–342

54    Sasaguri T, Arima N, Tanimoto A, Shimajiri S, Hamada T, Sasaguri Y (1998) A role for interleukin 4 in production of matrix metalloproteinase 1 by human aortic smooth muscle cells. *Atherosclerosis* 138: 247–253

55    Lee E, Grodzinsky AJ, Libby P, Clinton SK, Lark MW, Lee RT (1995) Human vascular

smooth muscle cell-monocyte interactions and metalloproteinase secretion in culture. *Arterioscler Thromb Vasc Biol* 15: 2284–2289

56  Shah PK, Falk E, Badimon JJ, Fernandez-Ortiz A, Mailhac A, Villareal-Levy G, Fallon JT, Regnstrom J, Fuster V (1995) Human monocyte-derived macrophages induce collagen breakdown in fibrous caps of atherosclerotic plaques. Potential role of matrix-degrading metalloproteinases and implications for plaque rupture. *Circulation* 92: 1565–1569

57  Sukhova GK, Schonbeck U, Rabkin E, Schoen FJ, Poole AR, Billinghurst RC, Libby P (1999) Evidence for increased collagenolysis by interstitial collagenases-1 and 13 in vulnerable human atheromatous plaques. *Circulation* 99: 2503–2509

58  Sugiyama S, Okada Y, Sukhova GK, Heinecke JW, Virmani R, Libby P (1998) A distinct proinflammatory subpopulation of macrophages in human atherosclerosis (abstract). *Circulation* 98: I–315

59  Hazell LJ, Arnold L, Flowers D, Waeg G, Malle E, Stocker R (1996) Presence of hypochlorite-modified proteins in human atherosclerotic lesions. *J Clin Invest* 97: 1535–1544

60  Kolodgie FD, Narula J, Burke AP, Haider N, Farb A, Hui-Liang Y, Smialek J, Virmani R (2000) Localization of apoptotic macrophages at the site of plaque rupture in sudden coronary death. *Am J Pathol* 157: 1259–1268

61  Bjorkerud S, Bjorkerud B (1996) Apopotosis is abundant in human atherosclerotic lesions, especially in inflammatory cells (macrophages and T cells) and may contribute to the accumulation of gruel and plaque instability. *Am J Pathol* 149: 367–380

62  Mann J, Davies MJ (1999) Mechanisms of progression in native coronary artery disease: role of healed plaque disruption. *Heart* 82: 265–268

63  Burke A, Farb A, Kolodgie FD, Malcom GT, Virmani R (1997) Healed plaque ruptures are frequent in men with severe coronary disease and are associated with elevated total/high density lipoprotein (HDL) cholesterol. *Circulation* 96: SI–235

64  Geary RL, Nikkari ST, Wagner WD, Williams JK, Adams MR, Dean RH (1998) Wound healing: a paradigm for lumen narrowing after arterial reconstruction. *J Vasc Surg* 27: 96–106; discussion –108

65  Courtman DW, Schwartz SM, Hart CE (1998) Sequential injury of the rabbit abdominal aorta induces intramural coagulation and luminal narrowing independent of intimal mass: extrinsic pathway inhibition eliminates luminal narrowing. *Circ Res* 82: 996–1006

66  Davies MJ (1996) Stability and instability: two faces of coronary atherosclerosis. The Paul Dudley White Lecture 1995. *Circulation* 94: 2013–2020

67  Glagov S, Weisenberg E, Zarins CK, Stankunavicius R, Kolettis GJ (1987) Compensatory enlargement of human atherosclerotic coronary arteries. *N Engl J Med* 16: 1371–1375

68  Taylor AJ, Yousefi P, Malcom GT, Smialek J, Virmani J (1999) Arterial remodeling in the left coronary system: the role of high-density lipoprotein cholesterol. *J Am Coll Cardiol.* 34: 760–767

69   Henderson EL, Geng YJ, Sukhova GK, Whittemore AD, Knox J, Libby P (1999) Death of smooth muscle cells and expression of mediators of apoptosis by T lymphocytes in human abdominal aortic aneurysms. *Circulation* 99: 96–104

70   Sukhova GK, Shi GP, Simon DI, Chapman HA, Libby P (1998) Expression of the elastolytic cathepsins S and K in human atheroma and regulation of their production in smooth muscle cells. *J Clin Invest* 102: 576–583

71   Freestone T, Turner RJ, Higman DJ, Lever MJ, Powell JT (1997) Influence of hypercholesterolemia and adventitial inflammation on the development of aortic aneurysm in rabbits. *Arterioscler Thromb Vasc Biol* 17: 10–17

72   Seo HS, Lombardi DM, Polinsky P, Powell-Braxton L, Bunting S, Schwartz SM, Rosenfeld ME (1997) Peripheral vascular stenosis in apolipoprotein E-deficient mice. Potential roles of lipid deposition, medial atrophy, and adventitial inflammation. *Arterioscler Thromb Vasc Biol* 17: 3593–3601

73   Andersen HR, Maeng M, Thorwest M, Falk E (1996) Remodeling rather than neointimal formation explains luminal narrowing after deep vessel wall injury: insights from a porcine coronary (re)stenosis model. *Circulation* 93: 1716–1724

74   Kakuta T, Usui M, Coats WD Jr, Currier JW, Numano F, Faxon DP (1998) Arterial remodeling at the reference site after angioplasty in the atherosclerotic rabbit model. *Arterioscler Thromb Vasc Biol* 18: 47–51

75   Katsumata N, Shimokawa H, Seto M, Kozai T, Yamawaki T, Kuwata K, Egashira K, Ikegaki I, Asano T, Sasaki Y et al (1997) Enhanced myosin light chain phosphorylations as a central mechanism for coronary artery spasm in a swine model with interleukin-1beta. *Circulation* 96: 4357–4363

76   Kohchi K, Takebayashi S, Hiroki T, Nobuyoshi M (1985) Significance of adventitial inflammation of the coronary artery in patients with unstable angina: results at autopsy. *Circulation* 71: 709–716

77   Schinke T, McKee MD, Kiviranta R, Karsenty G (1998) Molecular determinants of arterial calcification. *Ann Med* 30: 538–541

78   Kockx MM, Herman AG (1998) Apoptosis in atherogenesis: implications for plaque destabilization. *Eur Heart J* 19 (Suppl) G: G23–G28

79   Parhami F, Bostrom K, Watson K, Demer LL (1996) Role of molecular regulation in vascular calcification. *J Atheroscler Thromb* 3: 90–94

80   Shanahan CM, Proudfoot D, Farzaneh-Far A, Weissberg PL (1998) The role of Gla proteins in vascular calcification. *Crit Rev Eukaryot Gene Expr* 8: 357–375

81   Shanahan CM, Cary NR, Metcalfe JC, Weissberg PL (1994) High expression of genes for calcification-regulating proteins in human atherosclerotic plaques. *J Clin Invest* 93: 2393–2402

82   Bini A, Mann KG, Kudryk BJ, Schoen FJ (1999) Noncollagenous bone matrix proteins, calcification, and thrombosis in carotid artery atherosclerosis. *Arterioscler Thromb Vasc Biol* 19: 1852–1861

# Pathology of acute coronary syndromes

*Allard C. van der Wal, Onno J. de Boer and Anton E. Becker*

Department of Cardiovascular Pathology, Academic Medical Center, University of Amsterdam, P.O. Box 22700, 1100 DE Amsterdam, The Netherlands

## Introduction

Acute coronary syndromes include several distinct clinical entities such as various forms of unstable angina, acute myocardial infarction and sudden (coronary) cardiac death. Despite the variation in clinical presentation, most of these syndromes have the same pathological substrate: an unstable atherosclerotic plaque. The unstable plaque is a lesion complicated by spontaneous disruption of the plaque, always followed by at least some degree of thrombus formation [1]. Over the past ten years or so, numerous clinical, angiographical and pathological studies have led to novel insights into the sequence of plaque disruption, thrombus formation and myocardial ischemia [2–4]. Intrinsic plaque features determine the vulnerability of a lesion to rupture development. So called "rupture triggers" (vasospasms or elevated blood pressure) may affect the time of onset of disruption in such a vulnerable plaque. The extent of plaque disruption, degree of luminal narrowing and the systemic thrombotic state (systemic activation of the coagulation system, increased platelet reactivity) determine if there will be: (1) a complete thrombotic occlusion of the vessel lumen; (2) a mural thrombus with critical flow reduction; or (3) a minute thrombus in the vessel lumen, in many instances clinically silent.

In this chapter, the distinctive morphological features of unstable plaques and the cellular mechanisms that underlie plaque vulnerability will be outlined from a pathologist's point of view.

## Pathology of plaque disruption and thrombus formation

Arterial thrombus formation over atherosclerotic plaques is primarily a platelet and thrombin-dependent process. Platelets adhere to areas devoid of endothelium and become activated through various mediators that are locally present at the rupture site. These mediators include von Willebrand factor, thrombin and collagen. Conformational activation of surface glycoprotein (GP) IIb/IIIa enables platelets to bind

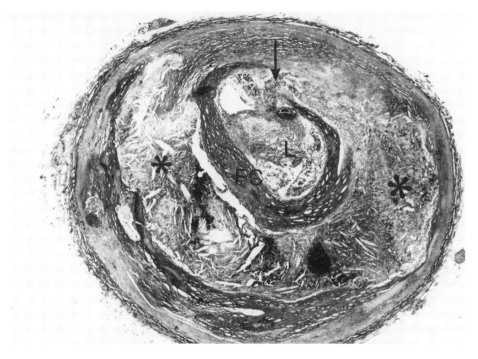

Figure 1
*Cross section of an atherosclerotic coronary artery with a thrombotic occlusion of the lumen. Thrombosis is due to complete disruption of the fibrous cap of the plaque (arrow), and blood has entered the lipid core. L indicates lumen. FC indicates fibrous cap. Asterisks are in the lipid core.*

fibrinogen, which cross links them to one another. At the same time, generation of thrombin is initiated by locally exposed tissue factor (TF), resulting in additional platelet activation and conversion of fibrinogen to fibrin [5]. The ensuing thrombotic response to plaque rupture develops in several stages with a varied make up of the thrombus. Later stages of the mural thrombus show, in addition to the platelet component, large amounts of densely packed fibrin (white clots), whereas large occluding arterial thrombi, secondary to locally reduced flow, have a component of loose fibrin networks filled with erythrocytes (red clots).

Several pathological studies have identified two distinct types of plaque disruption in thrombosed segments of coronary arteries [2–4]. The first consists of deep ruptures that extend through the fibrous cap of the lesion and reach into the lipid-rich core; this is called thrombogenic debris (Fig. 1). These rupture sites vary in size from a single disruption to complex lacerations of the lesion. In its major form, deep

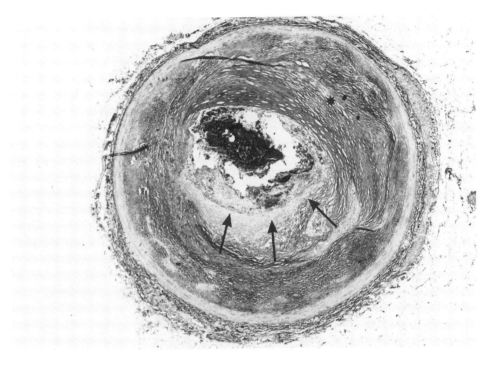

*Figure 2*
*Cross section of a coronary artery with a high grade stenosing plaque and thrombotic occlu-*
*sion of the lumen. Thrombus is due to endothelial erosions of the plaque surface (arrows),*
*the plaque is otherwise intact.*

rupture enables blood to enter the lipid core causing a rapid expansion of the lesion. Highly thrombogenic materials are also projected into the lumen of the coronary artery, which generally leads to massive thrombus formation. In many instances, the result is a complete thrombotic obstruction of the vessel.

A second type of plaque complication that came to attention more recently is the superficial erosion. Erosions are involved in about 40% of plaque complications [4, 6] and represent areas of endothelial denudation of a plaque which remains otherwise intact (Fig. 2). These lessions underlie many examples of mural, non-occlusiv,e platelet-rich thrombi, characteristic for patients with less severe acute coronary syndromes, such as unstable angina. These mural thrombi are also a potential source for embolization of the distal coronary artery bed, resulting in small foci of myocardial necrosis that form a pathological substrate for dangerous ventricular arrhytmias, as has been noticed in cases of sudden cardiac death [7]. Moreover, in high grade stenosing lesions with more than 75% lumen reduction, such erosions may also lead to complete obstruction, a complication more frequently seen in young victims of sudden cardiac death [8] and in diabetic patients [4] for reasons thus far unknown.

However, not all episodes of endothelial discontinuity will necessarily lead to clinical disease. Minor plaque disruptions with microscopic evidence of thrombosis have been observed in patients who died of non-cardiac diseases [9], indicating clinically silent events. Further, fragments of thrombi in up to 20% of atherectomy specimens obtained from patients with chronic stable angina must have resulted from plaque disruptions which went clinically unnoticed [10].

## Plaques at risk: stenosis rate and plaque composition

Over a lifetime, many atherosclerotic plaques may develop in a given patient, and of those the great majority will remain clinically unnoticed, whereas only one or a few give rise to dangerous thrombotic obstructions. Initially most attention was focused on the degree of lumen stenosis at sites of plaque formation in order to estimate the risk of coronary occlusion in a patient. Although thrombus formation superimposed on severely stenotic lesions will readily lead to complete obstruction, it is now well appreciated that many, if not most, acute thrombotic complications occur in mildly to moderately stenotic lesions. This phenomenon is partly explained by a local compensatory dilation of the vessel segment, which places the bulk of the plaque volume outside the vascular lumen, invisible to angiograms [11]. Still, the fact remains that about 50% of all thrombosed plaques that cause myocardial infarction are not critically stenotic lesions [12], which implies that intrinsic morphological features of the plaque are of greater importance than the degree of stenosis. Towards this end, a detailed insight into the morphology of plaques is required.

Atherosclerotic plaques show a tissue composition which allows us to distinguish them from any other arterial disease. The fully developed atherosclerotic plaque is a focal lesion with a central lipid core, the "atheroma", encaged by a fibrous cap covered by the arterial endothelium. Fibrous tissues in the cap, mainly collagens produced by smooth muscle cells (SMC), provide the structural integrity of the plaque. Inflammatory cells, which are macrophages, T lymphocytes and mast cells, reside in the fibrous cap and are recruited from the arterial circulation or, in advanced plaques only, from newly formed microvessels present at the base and in the shoulder region of the lesion. The atheroma, rich in extracellular lipids and cellular debris, is soft and highly thrombogenic and often bordered by a rim of foam cells. The foam cells result from unlimited scavenger receptor-dependent uptake of modified lipoproteins by macrophages, one of the most distinctive pathological processes in atherogenesis (Fig. 3). Dystrophic calcification of the plaque tissue can

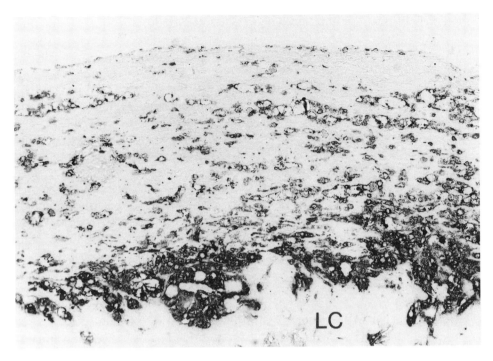

*Figure 3*
*Detail of an atherosclerotic plaque showing the fibrous cap and part of the lipid core (LC).*
*Macrophages are immunostained with anti-CD68. There is a rim of large, swollen immuno-*
*positive cells visible around the atheroma, representing lipid-laden foam cells.*

be quite extensive in the advanced stages of plaque formation, and may serve as a marker for atherosclerosis on angiograms.

These structural components are basically present to some extent in all plaques. However, it is an important feature of the advanced stages of atherosclerosis that plaques show huge variations in the relative amounts of these components, even when different plaques within one and the same coronary artery of a patient are compared. Any combination of fibrous cap thickness, atheroma size and degree of calcification may occur. Moreover, major differences in the ratios of smooth muscle cells and inflammatory cells (including foam cells) between plaques and even between different areas within one plaque have been observed in immunocyto-chemical studies of large series of plaques [13, 14]. These variations in relative amounts of tissue components have important implications for the stability of plaques.

## Vulnerable atherosclerotic plaques: lipids and inflammation

Important denominators in the vulnerability of a plaque to develop ruptures are the size of the atheroma and the thickness of the fibrous cap. Fibrous plaques are lesions largely composed of fibrocellular or fibrosclerotic tissue. They may cause high grade stenosis in coronary arteries, but most of them remain clinically unnoticed or may only cause stable angina pectoris. In contrast, lipid rich plaques with only a thin fibrous cap are the lesions frequently found in thrombosed coronary arteries of symptomatic patients. Intrinsic mechanical forces contribute to plaque rupture in such vulnerable "rupture prone" plaques. Circumferential wall stress, the most important stress factor involved in ruptures, is increased in such lesions with a large atheroma and a thin cap [15]. However, not only physical but also structural properties of the cap appear to be crucial. Richardson et al demonstrated that apart from high stress regions, the actual sites of rupture are also influenced by variations in the mechanical strength of the fibrous cap due to accumulations of foam cells [16].

A role for inflammation in plaque rupture emerged from studies on thrombosed coronary arteries of patients who died instantly or within two days after the onset of the infarct. We noticed abundant infiltration of activated T cells and macrophages at places where the plaques had ruptured, often with a marked decrease in collagen content at the immediate site of rupture (Fig. 4). Acute plaque complications in a series of patients were either deep ruptures (60%) or erosions of the plaque surface (40%). Also, in the case of plaque erosions we frequently noticed the presence of large accumulations of lipid-loaded macrophages and T cells in continuity with the thrombus, indicating a role for inflammation (Fig. 5) [6]. It seems likely that large amounts of tissue factor produced by foam cells act as thrombogenic substrate in these instances [17]. However, in an autopsy study by Farb et al, erosions were also found in proteoglycan and smooth muscle cell-rich types of plaques. These lesions, which occurred more often in younger individuals and in women, showed inflammation less often [7].

The use of coronary atherectomy has further enabled the study of the relationships between plaque inflammation, plaque disruption and thrombosis, in patients with less life threatening forms of myocardial ischemia. These studies have correlated several histopathological parameters of inflammation in the excised tissues of lesions with the clinical status of the patients. These studies have documented not only a clear relationship between the amount of inflammatory cells in plaque tissues of patients and the severity of the ischemic coronary syndrome (increasing from chronic stable angina through unstable angina to acute myocardial infarction), but also between the abundant production of several inflammatory proteins including gelatinases and cytokines, vasoreactive substances and tissue factor by the macrophages present in culprit lesions of patients with acute coronary syndromes. All these observations indicate active inflammation as an important determinant in plaque instability [10, 17–19].

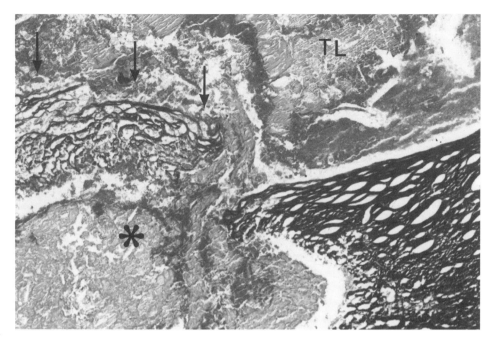

*Figure 4*
*Detail of the ruptured fibrous cap of a coronary atherosclerotic plaque. Blood has entered the lipid core of the lesion (asterisk). TL indicates thrombosed lumen. There is an abrupt change in collagen content (arrows) at the site where plaque had ruptured.*

Recently, an interesting relationship has been elucidated between the morphology of plaques and the geometry of the arterial wall. Geometric remodeling, defined as a change in the arterial circumference, ranges from compensatory enlargement to shrinkage of the vessel wall at sites of plaque formation. Obviously, enlargement compensates for the stenosis at sites of plaque formation, whereas shrinkage aggravates the effect of plaque growth on blood flow. Detailed histomorphometric and immunohistochemical characterization of atherosclerotic femoral arteries has revealed a relationship between the type of remodeling of the vessel wall and the tissue composition of the local plaque. Lipid-rich plaques with many inflammatory cells ("rupture prone") are often associated with local arterial dilation, whereas fibrous plaques ("stable") often colocalize with segments of arterial shrinkage [20]. Recently, *in vivo* angioscopic studies in patients with symptomatic coronary artery disease have revealed complex irregular lesions, with or without thrombus, predominantly in compensatory enlarged segments (unstable angina patients), whereas smooth lesions are more frequently seen in shrunken segments (stable angina

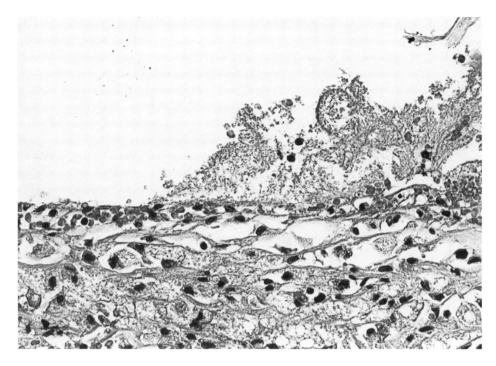

*Figure 5*
*Detail of a superficial erosion with superimposed mural thrombosis. Lipid-laden foam cells are in continuity with the platelet rich thrombus.*

patients), which suggests a relationship between arterial remodeling and plaque vulnerability also in coronary arteries [21]. The association of vulnerable inflamed lipid lesions with local vessel dilation further explains why many ruptured plaques are only mildly stenotic on angiograms.

## Inflammatory and repair mechanisms in the plaque

The risk of plaque disruption critically depends on the presence of inflammation, and secretory products of inflammatory cells in the fibrous cap. The inflammatory cells may affect the stability of plaques in various ways.

Inhibition of collagen synthesis in the plaque is initiated by the T cell cytokine interferon-γ (IFNγ). This cytokine, produced by activated memory T lymphocytes, particularly those of the $T_{H1}$ subtype, inhibits the proliferation of smooth muscle cell, and decreases their capability of producing collagen, leading to destabilization of a plaque [22].

Other cytokines, such as interleukin-1 (IL-1) and tumor necrosis factor $\alpha$ (TNF$\alpha$), induce apoptosis [23], an intrinsically programmed mode of cell death, which has now been recognized as a mechanism of smooth muscle cell death in plaques, thus introducing a second mechanism for impaired collagen synthesis.

Plaque macrophages, especially when loaded with lipids (foam cells), produce several matrix degrading metalloproteinases (MMPs), including interstitial collagenase (MMP-1), stromelysin (MMP-3) and the gelatinases MMP-2 and MMP-9, a process which is under the control of inflammatory cytokines (TNF and IL-1). Once activated by plasmin or mast cell products in the extracellular space, the MMPs are capable of lysing all the connective tissue components of a fibrous cap. Several tissue inhibitors of MMPs (TIMP 1–3) are also produced in plaques. Generally, there appears to be a net effect in favor of tissue breakdown due to the presence of MMPs, as has been demonstrated with the use of *in situ* zymography of human plaque materials. Examination of frozen sections of atherosclerotic plaques on a gelatin gel revealed proteolysis of the gelatin at sites corresponding to macrophage accumulations in vulnerable sites of the plaque [24]. This proteolytic degradation of plaque tissue is presently considered the most powerful mechanism of plaque destabilization. Finally, pro-inflammatory cytokines with angiogenic properties, also secreted by macrophages and T cells, may stimulate the formation of microvessels, which has been noted to occur preferentially in lipid-rich lesions. The capillary sprouts, located in the shoulder regions of advanced lesions, often amidst inflammatory infiltrates, provide an alternative pathway for leukocyte recruitment in rupture prone sites of plaques, which is perhaps more easily accessible than the arterial endothelium [25].

The overall effect of these processes is to favour tissue degradation, basically similar to many other inflammatory diseases with a chronic longstanding course, such as pulmonary fibrosis or rheumatoid arthritis. Thus a process of tissue repair is introduced in the coronary arteries.

Stimulation of the proliferative and synthetic capacity of SMC initiates this repair reaction, which results in the deposition of various matrix components, such as proteoglycans, elastin and collagens. Growth factors, including transforming growth factor-$\beta$ (TGF$\beta$), platelet-derived growth factor (PDGF) and basic fibroblast growth factor (bFGF), which are produced by "injured" endothelial cells and macrophages, or released from thrombus attached to the plaque surface are also involved [26]. Smooth muscle cell proliferation and extracellular matrix synthesis is a slowly progressive mechanism of plaque growth and may significantly contribute to the plaque volume in a time span of many years. Nevertheless, repair has a beneficial effect on the plaque integrity. Collagens produced by SMC serve to encapsulate the soft and thrombogenic lipid core and thus may stabilize the plaque. Arterial thrombus due to plaque rupture, if not spontaneously lysed, will soon be organized and incorporated into the plaque mass through ingrowth of SMC and deposition of matrix. In all instances the final result is a reparative and stabilizing effect on the plaque structure [2].

## Inflammation: a smouldering or an acute process?

A slowly progressive increase in the number of inflammatory cells may gradually induce a smouldering destabilizing effect on the plaque, which eventually leads to development of vulnerable regions in the plaque. Alternatively, acute activation of the inflammatory process, with a concomitant burst of secretion of cytokines, vasoactive molecules and proteases by inflammatory cells, could lead to rapid progression of the destabilizing process. Such processes are characterized by expression of IL-2 receptors (IL-2R) on lymphocytes, which serve as a marker for acute activation of T cells in the plaque tissues. IL-2R appear on the cell surface of T cells shortly (within 2–24 h) after antigenic stimulation and persist for only a few days after the stimulus is gone. During this period a wide variety of inflammatory mediators are produced, particularly by cytokine-activated macrophages and the T cells themselves [27]. It has been shown in randomly selected plaques of non-symptomatic patients that the average numbers of these IL-2R positive cells are very low (2–5%). However, in atherectomy specimens obtained from patients with acute syndromes (refractory unstable angina and acute myocardial infarction), we have found that IL-2R positive cells may account for up to 18% of the total number of T cells in lesions. In specimens obtained from patients with mild cardiac symptoms (stable angina or "stabilized" unstable angina), these numbers were again significantly lower [28]. These observations indeed suggest a local burst of inflammatory activity around the time of onset of acute syndromes. Raised levels of systemic markers for T cell-mediated inflammation, particularly increased numbers of HLA-DR positive T cells and increased levels of soluble IL-2R in the circulating blood, have been reported in patients with unstable angina by Neri Serneri et al. [29]. The activation markers decrease gradually over a period of eight weeks after the onset of the event, indicating that acute T-cell activation can also be detected in the serum of patients around the time of onset of the acute event [29]. However, it is not presently clear whether the systemic inflammatory parameters really reflect the inflammatory state of atherosclerotic plaques, or whether other inflammatory stimuli (such as infections) as discussed elsewhere in the text, may be involved.

## Initiation of plaque inflammation and acute syndromes

The identity of the initiators of plaque inflammation is presently not entirely clear. The presence of large concentrations of inflammatory cells, particularly in lipid rich lesions, suggests that lipids may act as a principal driving force for the inflammatory process. Scavenger receptor-dependent phagocytosis of oxidized-LDL (ox-LDL) by foam cell macrophages, with a consequent release of several potent inflammatory mediators (including MMPs and tissue factor), indeed represents an important lipid-related inflammatory reaction in the plaque. In addition, specific T cell-mediated immune responses may be involved since a sub-population of the human plaque T cells can be stimulated with ox-LDL [30]. Outcomes of several lipid-lowering trials also suggest an effect on the biological activity of lipids in plaques. Most of these studies showed a modest reduction in diameter stenosis between baseline and follow up angiograms in the long term, yet a marked decrease in clinical cardiac events even shortly after the initiation of therapy. These observations suggest that plaque biology is altered by improvement of the lipid profiles [31]. Plaque stabilization can also be explained by a reduction in lipid-promoted oxidative stress and inflammatory responses [22].

Several additional offending agents have also been suggested to play a role in the initiation of plaque inflammation. Among these, infection with *Chlamydia pneumoniae* has received the most attention. Several seroepidemiological studies have revealed a relationship between *C. pneumoniae* and the onset of acute coronary artery disease. Moreover, *C. pneumoniae* elementary bodies and DNA have been detected *in situ* in atherosclerotic plaques by several investigators [32,33]. However, there is presently still no conclusive evidence for a causal relationship between microorganisms and the inflammatory response in the plaque.

## Conclusions

Plaque composition and biological activity of the plaque rather than plaque volume or degree of stenosis determine the vulnerability to rupture. Lipid-related inflammation in the plaque leads to degradation and weakening of the plaque tissue. In contrast, SMC proliferations and collagen synthesis exert reparative and stabilizing effects. It thus appears that the biological state of lesions, with particular reference to inflammation, must be considered of prime importance in the clinical outcome of coronary atherosclerosis. Inflammation may, therefore, serve as a desirable target for prevention of ischemic coronary syndromes. Controlling the tissue damaging effects of inflammation, either by specific inhibition of components of the inflammatory response or alternatively by elimination of inflammatory stimuli such as ox-LDL or possibly C pneumoniae, may result in a biologically stable plaque, and hence, prevention of acute atherosclerotic syndromes.

## References

1   Davies MJ, Thomas AC (1985) Plaque fissuring – the cause of acute myocardial infarction, sudden ischemic death and crescendo angina. *Br Heart J* 53: 363–373

2   van der Wal AC, Becker AE (1999) Atherosclerotic plaque rupture – the pathologic basis of plaque stability and instability. *Cardiovasc Res* 41: 334–344

3   Falk E, Shah PK, Fuster V (1995) Coronary plaque disruption. *Circulation* 92: 657–671

4    Davies MJ (1996) Stability and instability: two faces of coronary atherosclerosis. *Circulation* 94: 2013–2020

5    Davie EW (1995) Biochemical and molecular aspects of the coagulation cascade. *Thrombosis Haemost* 74: 1–6

6    van der Wal AC, Becker AE, van der Loos CM, Das PK (1994) Site of intimal rupture or erosion of thrombosed coronary atherosclerotic plaques is characterized by an inflammatory process irrespective of the dominant plaque morphology. *Circulation* 89: 36–44

7    Farb A, Burke AP, Tang AL, Liang Y, Mannan P, Smialek J, Virmani R (1996) Coronary plaque erosion without rupture into a lipid core: a frequent cause of coronary thrombosis in sudden coronary death. *Circulation* 93: 1354–1363

8    Davies MJ (1999) The investigation of sudden cardiac death. *Histopathology* 34: 93–98

9    Davies MJ, Bland J, Hangartner, Angelini A, Thomas A (1989) Factors influencing the presence or absence of acute coronary artery thrombi in sudden ischemic death. *Eur Heart J* 10: 203–208

10   van der Wal AC, Becker AE, Koch KT, Piek JJ, Teeling P, van der Loos CM, David GK (1996) Clinically stable angina is not necessarily associated with histologically stable atherosclerotic plaques. *Heart* 76: 112–117

11   Glagov S, Weisenberg E, Zarins CK, Stanunavicius R, Kolettis G (1987) Compensatory enlargment of human atherosclerotic coronary arteries. *N Engl J Med* 316: 1371–1375

12   Fishbein, MJ, Siegel RJ (1996) How big are coronary atheosclerotic plaques that rupture? *Circulation* 94: 2662–2666

13   Gown AM, Tsukada T, Ross R (1986) Human atherosclerosis. II. Immunocytochemical analysis of the cellular composition of human atherosclerotic lesions. *Am J Pathol* 125: 191–207

14   van der Wal AC, Becker AE, Tigges AJ, Loos CM van der, Das PK (1994) Fibrous and lipid-rich atherosclerotic plaques are part of interchangeable morphologies related to inflammation – a concept. *Cor Art Dis* 5: 463–469

15   Cheng GC, Loree HM, Kamm RD, Fishbein MC, Lee RT (1993) Distribution of circumferential stress in ruptured and stable atherosclerotic lesions: a structural analysis with histopathologic correlation. *Circulation* 87: 1179–1187

16   Richardson PD, Davies MJ, Born GVR (1989) Influence of plaque configuration and stress distribution on fissuring of coronary atherosclerotic plaques. *Lancet* 2: 941–944

17   Moreno PR, Bernardi CH, Lopez-Cuellar J, Muria AM, Palacios IF, Gold HK, Mehran R, Sharma SK, Nemerson Y, Fuster V, Fallon JT (1996) Macrophages, smooth muscle cells, and tissue factors in unstable angina. Implications for cell mediated thrombogenecity in acute coronary syndromes. *Circulation* 94: 3090–3097

18   Moreno PR, Falk E, Palacios IF, Newell JB, Fuster V, Fallon J (1994) Macrophage infiltration in acute coronary syndromes: implications for plaque rupture. *Circulation* 90: 775–778

19   Kaartinen M, van der Wal AC, Piek JJ, van der Loos CM, Becker AE, Kovanen PT

(1998) Mast cell infiltration in acute coronary syndromes-implications for plaque rupture. *J Am Coll Cardiol* 32: 606–612

20 Pasterkamp G, Schoneveld AH, van der Wal AC, Haudenschild CC, Clarijs RJG, Becker AE, Hillen B, Borst C (1998) The relation of arterial geometry with luminal narrowing and histological markers for plaque vulnerability: the remodeling paradox. *J Am Coll Cardiol* 32: 655–662

21 Smits PC, Pasterkamp G, De Jaegere PT, de Feyter PJ, Borst C (1999) Angioscopic complex lesions are compensator enlarged: an angioscopy and intracoronary ultrasound study. *Cardiovasc Res* 41: 458–464

22 Libby P (1995) Molecular bases of acute coronary syndromes. *Circulation* 91: 2844–2850

23 Geng Y, Libby P (1995) Evidence for apoptosis in advanced human atheroma: co-localization with interleukin-beta converting enzyme. *Am J Pathol* 147: 251–266

24 Galis ZS, Sukhova GK, Lark MW, Libby P (1994) Increased expression of matrix metalloproteinases and matrix degrading activities in vulnerable regions of human atherosclerotic plaques. *J Clin Invest* 94: 2493–2503

25 de Boer OJ, van der Wal AC, Teeling P, Becker AE (1999) Leukocyte recruitment in rupture prone regions of lipid plaques: a prominent role for neovascularization? *Cardiovasc Res* 41: 443–449

26 Ross R (1993) The pathogenesis of atherosclerosis – a perspective for 1990's. *Nature* 362: 801–809

27 Waldman TA (1986) The structure, functionand expression of interleukin-2 receptors on normal and malignant lymphocytes. *Science* 232: 727–732

28 van der Wal AC, Piek JJ, de Boer OJ, Teeling P, van der Loos CM, Becker AE (1998) Recent onset activation of the plaque immune response in coronary lesions underlying acute coronary syndromes. *Heart* 80: 14–18

29 Neri Serneri GG, Prisco D, Martini, Gori AM, Brunelli T, Pogessi L, Rostagno C, Gensini GF, Abbate R (1997) Acute Tcell activation is detectable in unstable angina. *Circulation* 95: 1806–1812

30 Stemme S, Faber S, Holm J, Wiklund O, Witztum JL, Hansson GK (1995) T lymphocytes from human atherosclerotic plaques recognize oxidized low-density lipoprotein. *Proc Natl Acad Sci USA* 92: 3893–3897

31 Rabbani R, Topol EJ (1999) Strategies to achieve coronary arterial plaque stabilization. *Cardiovasc Res* 41: 4022–417

32 De Boer OJ, van der Wal AC, Becker AE (2000) Atherosclerosis, inflammation and infection. *J Pathol* 190: 237–243

33 Muhlestein JB, Hammond EH, Carlquist JF, Radicke E, Thomson MJ, Karagounis LA, Woods ML, Anderson JL (1996) Increased incidence of *Chlamydia* species within the coronary arteries of patients with symptomatic versus other forms of cardiovascular disease. *J Am Coll Cardiol* 27: 1551–1561

# Transplantation-associated arteriosclerosis and inflammation

*Dani S. Zander*

Department of Pathology, Immunology, and Laboratory Medicine, University of Florida College of Medicine, and the Veterans Affairs Medical Center, Box 100275, Gainesville, FL 32610, USA

## Introduction

Transplantation-associated arteriosclerosis (TAA), a complication of allotransplantation, remains the major limitation to the long-term survival of many solid organ transplant recipients. Over the last decade, particularly, our understanding of the pathogenesis of TAA grew significantly. Morphological, immunohistochemical, and molecular studies performed on human tissues combined with an expanding clinical, radiological and epidemiological database have improved our knowledge of the cellular and biochemical events that culminate in TAA. Studies using innovative animal models have added to what has been gleaned from the human studies, and allowed for trials of unique therapeutic strategies. Nonetheless, for cardiac transplant recipients, TAA continues to be the largest single cause of death after the first year post-transplantation [1]. Arteriosclerosis is also a feature of chronic renal transplant rejection [2] and chronic pulmonary allograft rejection [3], though in lung allografts it appears to be unassociated with any physiological consequences [4]. Since much of the literature regarding TAA focuses upon its manifestations in the transplanted heart, the following discussion will concentrate primarily upon TAA developing in cardiac allografts, also known as cardiac allograft vasculopathy (CAV).

Graft arteriosclerosis has been referred to as "accelerated" because of its rapid progression compared to arteriosclerosis in non-transplanted individuals. Graft vascular disease can become evident as early as three months after cardiac transplantation, and can cause death at any time thereafter, sometimes decades after transplantation [5]. Estimates of its prevalence among heart transplant recipients are influenced by the technique used for diagnosis, but one, two, and three year rates lie in the ranges of 11–18%, 17–27%, and 26–44%, respectively [6–9]. Of the numerous immunological and non-immunological risk factors for CAV that have been evaluated, higher frequencies and severities of acute rejection bear the strongest relationship to subsequent development of CAV [6, 7, 10–13]. Histocompatibility influences the frequency of rejection and the probability of graft survival, with higher rejection

Inflammatory and Infectious Basis of Atherosclerosis, edited by Jay L. Mehta
© 2001 Birkhäuser Verlag Basel/Switzerland

rates and severity associated with complete mismatch at the HLA-B and -DR loci [14] and improved graft survival with HLA matching [15, 16]. However, other studies have failed to identify relationships between HLA incompatibility, CAV, rejection, and survival after heart transplantation. This subject is addressed in two comprehensive reviews by Costanzo [14, 17]. Repeatedly positive panel reactive antibody studies have been linked to increased prevalence of TAA and lower 1-, 3-, and 5-year actuarial survival rates [18]. Scattered reports cite lipid abnormalities as risk factors for development of CAV, including high serum cholesterol [19–21], lipoprotein(a) [22] and triglyceride levels [19, 23], and low HDL-c [23]. Cytomegalovirus infection has been linked to an increased risk of TAA in some series [24–26], but not others [27, 28]. Finally, donor and recipient demographic characteristics including recipient age > 50, donor age > 40, and male recipients of female donor hearts, have been associated with development of, and graft loss from, CAV [29].

## Pathology

In the heart, the morphological features of TAA have been addressed in a large number of articles [13, 30–35]. TAA affects the major epicardial vessels and their branches, including the intramyocardial branches. The intima is thickened by a proliferation of modified smooth muscle cells with interspersed lipid-containing macrophages and variable numbers of lymphocytes (Figs. 1, 2). Intimal fibrosis and fibrofatty plaques are also seen. The process tends to be concentric and diffuse, involving arteries and veins [36], with less frequent calcification and grumous atheroma formation than coronary artery disease in individuals without transplants [30]. Also, in contrast to naturally occurring atherosclerosis, the internal elastic lamina is often intact. Perivascular lymphocytes commonly accompany the intimal abnormalities. Secondary ischemic myocardial pathology (subendocardial myocyte vacuolization and coagulative myocyte necrosis) can be seen in endomyocardial biopsies from patients with TAA [37].

## Pathogenesis

### Immunological factors

TAA is believed to represent the outcome of a chronic immunological reaction directed against donor cells. In the evolution of TAA, T lymphocytes and macrophages accumulate in the intimal regions of coronary arteries adjacent to endothelial cells. The coronary endothelium suffers lymphocyte-mediated injury and there is local synthesis of proinflammatory cytokines, chemokines, and growth factors by endothelial and inflammatory cells, and other intimal cells. The result of these com-

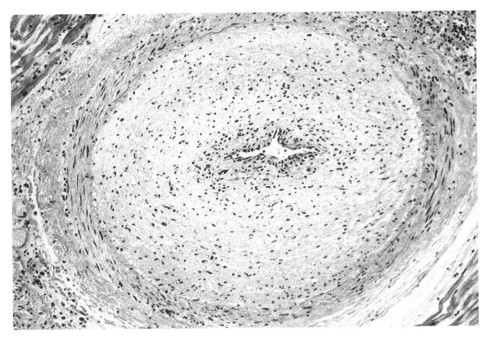

*Figure 1*
*TAA in a coronary artery branch causing severe stenosis. There is prominent concentric inti-*
*mal thickening caused by proliferation of modified smooth muscle cells with deposition of*
*collagen and mild mononuclear cell infiltrates (hematoxylin-eosin; original magnification*
*× 200).*

plex interactions is a stenotic vessel with a thickened intima rich in modified smooth muscle cells.

Cellular immunity is central to the pathogenesis of TAA. Data derived from human and animal studies testifies to the essential role T lymphocytes play in the sequence of events leading to TAA. In human cardiac allografts, CD4+ and CD8+ T cells infiltrate the intimal regions of coronary arteries, targeting endothelial cells expressing HLA and other potentially stimulatory antigens [38, 39]. Arteries often demonstrate a lymphocytic endothelialitis in which most of the lymphocytes are CD8+ T cells [40]. Using a murine heart transplant model, sustained anti-CD4/CD8 therapy markedly reduces intimal thickening and inflammatory cell activation [41]. Allograft arteries in mice deficient in both T-cell receptors and humoral immunity show minimal neointimal formation, while arteries grafted into mice deficient in only CD4+ T cells, humoral immunity, or macrophages develop small neointimas with reduced numbers of smooth muscle cells and less collagen than control animals

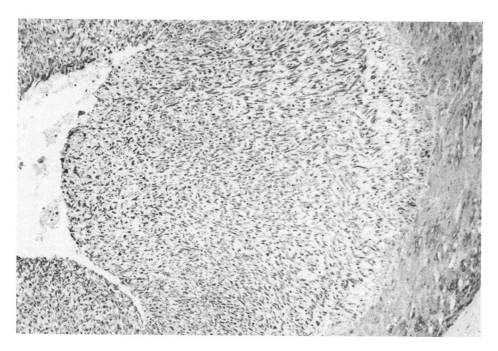

*Figure 2*

*Immunohistochemical stain for actin highlights numerous modified smooth muscle cells in the intima of this coronary artery branch with TAA (streptavidin-biotin-complex; original magnification × 200).*

[42]. In rat and mouse models of chronic cardiac and renal allograft rejection, treatment of graft recipients with CTLA4Ig, a fusion protein that blocks CD28-B7-mediated T-cell costimulation, inhibits the development of TAA [43–45]. The reduction in TAA is accompanied by decreased lymphocyte and macrophage infiltration [45] and decreased expression of T-cell interferon-γ (IFNγ), and the macrophage activation factors monocyte chemoattractant protein-1 (MCP-1) and inducible nitric oxide synthase (iNOS), as well as transforming growth factor-β (TGFβ) [43].

Endothelial cell activation, accomplished primarily via T lymphocytes in allograft rejection, initiates alterations in cellular and soluble factors that are believed to represent steps towards TAA. In clinically significant human acute cardiac allograft rejection, there is upregulation of endothelial HLA antigens, increased expression of the adhesion molecules P-selectin and intercellular adhesion molecule-1 (ICAM-1), expression of the pro-inflammatory cytokines interleukin-1β (IL-1β) and tumor necrosis factor-α (TNFα), and increased expression of platelet-derived growth factor-AA and -BB (PDGF-AA and -BB) [46]. Endothelial cell damage has been reported to proceed through a Fas-mediated apoptotic pathway involving CD4-positive cytolytic T cells [47], though perforin-expressing lymphocytes have also been observed in subendothelial locations in coronary arteries with TAA [48]. Alloantibody-stimulated endothelial cell activation is suppressed *in vitro* by induction of heme oxygenase-1 (HO-1) or Bcl-xL, and induction of HO-1 *in vivo* protects mouse cardiac allografts against chronic vascular injury [49].

Leukocyte adhesion molecules facilitate rejection by promoting leukocyte accumulation in the graft vasculature. In transplantation, the most important adhesion molecules are the immunoglobulins ICAM-1 and vascular cell adhesion molecule (VCAM-1), the β-2 and β-1 integrins including lymphocyte function-associated antigen-1 (LFA-1) and very late antigen-4 (VLA-4), and the selectins. In transplanted mouse hearts, there is high expression of ICAM-1 (CD54) by endothelial cells and its ligand LFA-1 (CD11a) on infiltrating mononuclear cells, and treatment with monoclonal antibodies to ICAM-1 and LFA-1 effectively reduces TAA [50, 51]. Similarly, hyperbaric transfection of antisense oligodeoxynucleotides blocks ICAM-1 expression and reduces cardiac allograft TAA [52]. In rat cardiac allografts, early P-selectin expression on microvascular endothelial cells is characteristic of acute rejection, while the intensity of arterial intimal thickening in chronic vascular rejection correlates with the intensity of endothelial P-selectin and VCAM-1 expression [53]. Binding of VLA-4 on circulating lymphocytes and monocytes to fibronectin also appears to be important in the pathogenesis of TAA. Administration of peptides to block this interaction prevents development of TAA, decreases T-cell and macrophage infiltration, and decreases intragraft expression of IFNγ, IL-12, MCP-1, and TGFβ in rat cardiac allografts [54].

With progression to TAA, T cells and macrophages accumulate in the intima and there is upregulation of chemokines and cytokines. These substances participate in the recruitment and activation of leukocytes to potentiate the response to the allograft. Though the roles of chemokines and cytokines in allograft rejection have not been thoroughly explored, more studies will likely follow to define their activities more clearly. Regulated upon activation, normal T cell expressed and secreted (RANTES), a chemokine that attracts T lymphocytes, NK cells, monocytes, and eosinophils, is produced in lymphocytes, macrophages, myofibroblasts, and endothelial cells in human coronary arteries with TAA, but not in normal coronary arteries [55]. Local increases in production of MCP-1, a chemotactic factor for monocytes, correlate with increased interstitial and vascular macrophage localization [56]. Cardiac allografts in mice demonstrate early intra-allograft expression of IL-1β and IFNγ-inducible protein followed by macrophage inflammatory protein (MIP)-1α, MIP-1β, and RANTES by day 8 after transplantation, with persistence of high levels of IFNγ-inducible protein and RANTES at sixty days after transplantation [57]. In rat cardiac allografts, IFNγ, IL-6, and MCP-1 expression remain elevated in mononuclear cells [58]. Increased mRNA expression of IL-1β, IL-2, IL-6, and IFNγ in rat aortic allografts parallels the severity of graft arteriosclerosis [59].

Genetic or acquired IFNγ deficiency inhibits development of TAA in mice [60–63]. Compared with wild-type recipients, IFNγ-deficient animals show reduced MHC antigen, ICAM-1, and VCAM-1 expression [63].

Evolution of the vascular changes from an inflammatory cell-rich phenotype to one dominated by a smooth muscle cell-rich intimal proliferation requires the local elaboration of growth factors. Multiple studies have shown increased expression of the mesenchymal cell mitogen and chemotactic substance PDGF [64, 65] and its receptors in organ allografts with acute rejection or TAA, and cell culture experiments creating conditions of alloreactive lymphocyte-mediated endothelial cell injury yield increased production of PDGF. Additional evidence suggests that fibroblast growth factor (FGF), transforming growth factor (TGF), and other growth factors are related to TAA, but the roles of these substances are not as clearly defined. Insulin-like growth factor (IGF) has been studied using animal models, and these investigations suggest an association between IGF production and TAA, which can be inhibited by estradiol [66–68].

In human cardiac allografts, expression of PDGF-A and acidic FGF in vascular walls and cardiac myocytes is elevated relative to normal hearts [69]. Macrophage PDGF is increased in transplanted hearts with evidence of vascular rejection, CAV, or global ischemia [70], and increased cardiac levels of aFGF are strongly associated with CAV [71]. In human renal chronic vascular rejection, PDGF-A chain is expressed by a population of intimal smooth muscle cells, while in acute rejection, endothelial cell expression of PDGF-A chain is up-regulated and PDGF-B chain is produced in monocytes infiltrating the rejecting arteries [72]. In rat cardiac allografts, PDGF-AA, PDGF-receptor α and PDGF-receptor β expression in intimal cells and PDGF-BB expression in interstitial mononuclear inflammatory cells correlate with intimal thickening. As in humans, smooth muscle cells and macrophages in the intima express PDGF-AA, and PDGF-receptor α and β expression is found in arterial endothelial cells and interstitial mononuclear inflammatory cells. High-dose cyclosporine A treatment diminishes the increased levels of PDGF-AA and PDGF-receptor α expression observed in intimal cells [73]. Inhibition of PDGF receptor tyrosine kinase reduces smooth muscle cell migration and proliferation *in vitro* and after rat carotid artery ballooning injury *in vivo* [74], and reduces the incidence and intensity of arteriosclerotic lesions in rat cardiac allograft recipients [75]. Mice that are genetically deficient in TGFβ develop increased luminal occlusion in cardiac allograft arteries compared with wild-type recipients, and this effect is associated with attenuation of the Th1 response [76].

Cell culture studies also shed light on the effects of endothelial cell injury on synthesis of growth factors. Allogeneic lymphocytes induce human aortic endothelial cells to release products that cause smooth muscle cell proliferation and produce increased mRNA for PDGF-A and -B, TGFα and -β, and basic FGF [77]. When peripheral blood mononuclear cells from cardiac transplant recipients are co-cultured with donor-specific human aortic endothelial cells, mononuclear cells from only those transplant recipients with TAA cause endothelial cell upregulation of PDGF-A and TGFα [78].

In contrast to the role of cellular immunity in the pathogenesis of TAA, the role of humoral immunity is less established. Panel reactive antibodies (anti-HLA antibodies) develop in up to 82% [18, 79, 80] of heart transplant recipients, and are associated with significantly lower 1-, 3-, and 5-year actuarial survival rates and an increased prevalence of CAV [18, 79]. However, antibodies discovered by screening against a panel of reference cells are of unknown specificity relative to the recipient's donor, and have been suggested to be a marker of generally increased recipient alloreactivity against the donor graft rather than a primary agent of rejection [81]. In one study, donor-specific anti-endothelial cell antibodies assessed by flow cytometry developed in only 15% of the heart transplant recipients evaluated, and were not associated with angiographically detectable CAV [81]. In another study, however, cardiac transplant recipients who had specific donor-reactive antibodies in the first six months posttransplantation required significantly more antirejection therapy than crossmatch negative recipients [80]. Likewise, animal and cell culture studies offer conflicting results. In a mouse aortic allograft model, recipient mice lacking humoral immunity (targeted deletion of the joining region gene segments for the immunoglobulin heavy chain) develop TAA, while mice lacking donor-specific immune responses (severe combined immunodeficient mice and recombination activating gene-1-deficient mice) show a virtual absence of graft neointimal formation [82]. Conversely, TAA can be produced by injecting murine recipients of heart allografts with an antiserum directed to antigens of the donor [83]. Using cultured cells, antibody ligation of class I HLA molecules on endothelial cells causes increased high-affinity FGF receptor mRNA expression, enhanced basic FGF ligand binding, increased cell proliferation, and augmented smooth muscle cell proliferation is produced by antibody binding to class I molecules on smooth muscle cells [84]. Though further studies are needed to define the role of humoral immunity in TAA, antibodies may represent one pathway to endothelial activation that leads to secondary changes in expression of growth factors, adhesion molecules, histocompatibility antigens, and proinflammatory cytokines predisposing to TAA.

## Inducible nitric oxide synthase

Inducible nitric oxide synthase (iNOS) is an enzyme that produces large amounts of NO and is induced in macrophages, smooth muscle cells, endothelial cells, and other cells by cytokine stimulation. Human coronary arteries with TAA express large amounts of iNOS and the oxidant peroxynitrite (formed from NO and superoxide), particularly in neointimal macrophages and smooth muscle cells, in contrast to normal coronary arteries and native coronary arteries with naturally occurring atherosclerosis [85, 86]. Animal studies suggest that early immune-mediated upregulation in iNOS expression after transplantation confers some protection against development of TAA [87]. Transduction with iNOS using an adenoviral vector prevents development of TAA in rat aortic allografts [87]. Modulation of the inflammatory response using a diet deficient in essential fatty acids lessens the degree of intimal thickening and the percentage of vessels exhibiting TAA in rat cardiac allografts, and is accompanied by a parallel reduction in iNOS-expressing mononuclear cells [88]. Experiments with iNOS-deficient (knockout) mice confirm the protective role of iNOS in the development of TAA. INOS-deficient mice demonstrate significantly increased luminal occlusion and intima/media ratios in allografts, and a significant increase in neointimal smooth muscle cells compared to wild-type controls [89]. NO, via a cyclic guanosine monophosphate-mediated mechanism, inhibits proliferation of cultured rat vascular smooth muscle cells [90].

## Lipids

Arteriosclerosis in allograft vasculature differs morphologically from naturally occurring arteriosclerosis in individuals without allografts. Not surprisingly, comparisons of lipid, apolipoprotein, and proteoglycan components of arteriosclerotic lesions reveal some differences between transplant-associated and naturally-occurring arteriosclerosis. In human heart allografts, apolipoprotein (a) and apolipoprotein E deposits are more prominent in the intimas of diseased vessels than in naturally-occuring atherosclerosis, while the reverse is true for apolipoprotein B. Proteoglycan deposits, especially versican, are located very close to areas of apolipoprotein (a) and apolipoprotein E staining, suggesting that interactions between proteoglycans and apolipoproteins influence lipid retention in TAA [91]. In a study using apolipoprotein E- knockout mice, carotid artery loops allografted into hypercholesterolemic recipients had greater degrees of luminal occlusion and cross-sectional neointimal areas than carotid allografts in normocholesterolemic recipients, with most of the difference due to smooth muscle cell accumulation in the hypercholesterolemic mice [92]. In a rat aortic allograft model, elevations in very low-density lipoprotein (VLDL) and intermediate-density lipoprotein (IDL) levels and cholesterol were associated with increased severity of TAA. Grafts demonstrated significant lipid deposits and increased expression of epidermal growth factor (EGF) and IGF-1, possibly promoting smooth muscle cell proliferation [93].

## Coagulation/Fibrinolysis

In human cardiac allograft biopsies during the first three months post-transplantation, persistent depletion of vascular tissue plasminogen activator in arteriolar smooth muscle cells is associated with development of TAA [94]. Deposition of microvascular fibrin has been linked to development of TAA [95]. Homozygous plasminogen-deficient mice show reduced TAA compared to wild-type mice; carotid artery allografts have thinner intimas containing fewer smooth muscle cells and less medial necrosis, fragmentation of elastic laminae, and adventitial remodeling, suggesting a role for plasmin proteolysis in each of these changes [96]. Tissue factor is found in endothelial cells in rat cardiac allografts, but not in non-transplanted control hearts, and may contribute to TAA via alterations in coagulation [97].

## Infections

Infections have long been considered as potential etiological agents for arteriosclerosis, and the recent upsurge of interest in this area will undoubtedly yield some illuminating results over the next few years. In the area of TAA, the most extensively studied infectious agent is cytomegalovirus (CMV). Although epidemiological studies provide variable support for CMV as an etiological factor for TAA, experimental results offer suggestions about mechanisms whereby CMV can exert its effects on the graft vasculature. Many of the effects of CMV on cells and soluble mediators of inflammation replicate changes observed during rejection, and CMV may be one trigger that prompts activation of a non-specific inflammatory cascade leading to TAA. However, some of the experimental data suggests distinct mechanisms of action for CMV in the genesis of TAA. Other than CMV, however, infections do not appear to be important in the initiation or progression of TAA. Although *Chlamydia pneumoniae* infection is frequent in cardiac transplant recipients, *Chlamydia pneumoniae* does not independently predispose to TAA or have a synergistic effect with CMV in the development of TAA [98].

CMV infection causes alterations in expression of adhesion molecules, HLA antigens, and cytokines similar to those described in rejection, and has a unique role in smooth muscle cell migration. In peripheral blood mononuclear cells, CMV infection increased production of the proinflammatory cytokine IL-6 [99], and in a monocytic cell line, CMV immediate early gene products enhance the expression of IL-6 in lipopolysaccharide-stimulated cells [100]. Compared with controls, bronchoalveolar lavage cells from human lung transplant recipients with CMV pneumonia demonstrate increased IL-1$\beta$ and IL-6, and a marker of activated cytotoxic cells, serine esterase B [101]. Experiments using cell cultures reveal IFN$\gamma$ and TNF$\alpha$-mediated induction of endothelial ICAM-1 and HLA class I and DR molecules by CMV-activated donor-derived T cells [102], while another study using human umbilical vein endothelial cells favors a direct interaction of immediate early proteins with the ICAM-1 promoter elements to increase gene expression [103]. A recent report describes chemokine receptor US28-mediated migration of primary arterial smooth muscle cells in response to human CMV infection [104].

Expression of US28 in the presence of CC chemokines (RANTES, MCP-1) promoted smooth muscle cell migration by chemokinesis and chemotaxis. As discussed earlier in this chapter, RANTES and MCP-1 are increased in coronary arteries with TAA.

Intramyocardial arterioles in biopsies from CMV-infected heart allograft recipients demonstrate subendothelial infiltration of inflammatory cells ("endothelialitis"), predominantly T cells, which peaks at the onset of CMV infection and subsides slowly [105]. In rat aortic allografts, CMV infection induces similar subendothelial infiltration by T cells and macrophages followed by proliferation of intimal smooth muscle cells, which can be inhibited by triple drug immunosuppression [106]. Analysis of mRNA for growth factors in aortic allografts reveals increased mRNA for PDGF-BB, TGFβ1, acidic and basic FGF, and EGF in the CMV-infected grafts compared to noninfected grafts [107]. In aggregate, these results favor a combination of immune-mediated and direct effects of CMV on the promulgation of TAA.

## Conclusions

TAA remains a significant source of diminished life expectancy and quality of life for organ transplant recipients, particularly recipients of heart transplants. An immunologically-mediated process, TAA has a distinctive morphology and often progresses at a pace that is accelerated compared to naturally occurring arteriosclerosis. While many risk factors have been investigated, there is no single factor that has been consistently identified as essential for development of TAA. More frequent and severe episodes of acute rejection, however, bear the strongest relationship to development of TAA in heart transplant recipients.

TAA evolves through a progression of cellular and biochemical interactions between host inflammatory cells, donor endothelial and mesenchymal cells, and soluble mediators of inflammation and repair. Endothelial cell activation and injury, primarily caused by T lymphocytes, prompts increased expression of HLA antigens, adhesion molecules, proinflammatory cytokines, and chemokines, causing further accumulation of T cells and macrophages in the intima. With local synthesis of growth factors, the intima thickens primarily due to proliferation of modified smooth muscle cells. Deposition of mucopolysaccharides, collagen and lipids often accompanies the smooth muscle cells. Humoral immunity and CMV probably contribute to this cascade by causing endothelial cell injury and subsequent changes, but may also have more direct effects.

At maturity, TAA is usually diffuse. In cardiac transplant recipients, it can lead to secondary ischemic complications and is an important indication for retransplantation. While current pharmacological therapies have little effect on the progression of TAA, new therapeutic strategies geared to interrupting the immunological events culminating in TAA are under investigation. Over the next decade, our growing understanding of the pathogenesis of TAA may allow us a greater ability to prevent or ameliorate TAA.

## References

1    Hosenpud JD, Bennett LE, Keck BM, Fiol B, Boucek MM, Novick RJ (1998) The Registry of the International Society for Heart and Lung Transplantation: fifteenth official report 1998. *J Heart Lung Transplant* 17: 656–668

2    Racusen LC, Solez K, Colvin RB, Bonsib SM, Castro MC, Cavallo T, Croker BP, Demetris AJ, Drachenberg CB, Fogo AB et al (1999) The Banff 97 working classification of renal allograft pathology. *Kidney Int* 55: 713–723

3    Yousem SA, Berry GJ, Cagle PT, Chamberlain D, Husain AN, Hruban RH, Marchevsky A, Ohori NP, Ritter J, Stewart S et al (1996) Revision of the 1990 working formulation for the classification of pulmonary allograft rejection: Lung Rejection Study Group. *J Heart Lung Transplant* 15: 1–15

4    Yousem SA, Paradis IL, Dauber JH, Zeevi A, Duquesnoy RJ, Dal CR, Armitage J, Hardesty RL, Griffith BP (1989) Pulmonary arteriosclerosis in long-term human heart-lung transplant recipients. *Transplantation* 47: 564–569

5    Billingham ME (1994) Pathology and etiology of chronic rejection of the heart. *Clin Transplant* 8: 289–292

6    Wahlers T, Fieguth HG, Jurmann M, Albes J, Hausen B, Demertzis S, Schafers HJ, Oppelt P, Mugge A, Borst HG (1996) Graft coronary vasculopathy in cardiac transplantation – evaluation of risk factors by multivariate analysis. *Eur J Cardiothorac Surg* 10: 1–5

7    Uretsky BF, Murali S, Reddy PS, Rabin B, Lee A, Griffith BP, Hardesty RL, Trento A, Bahnson HT (1987) Development of coronary artery disease in cardiac transplant patients receiving immunosuppressive therapy with cyclosporine and prednisone. *Circulation* 76: 827–834

8    Gao SZ, Schroeder JS, Alderman EL, Hunt SA, Valantine HA, Wiederhold V, Stinson EB (1989) Prevalence of accelerated coronary artery disease in heart transplant survivors. Comparison of cyclosporine and azathioprine regimens. *Circulation* 80: III100–III105

9    Haverich A, Costard-Jackle A, Cremer J, Herrmann G, Simon R (1994) Cyclosporin A and transplant coronary disease after heart transplantation: Facts and fiction. *Transplant Proc* 26: 2713–2715

10   Bailey LL, Zuppan CW, Chinnock RE, Johnston JK, Razzouk AJ, Gundry SR (1995) Graft vasculopathy among recipients of heart transplantation during the first 12 years of life. The Pediatric Heart Transplant Group. *Transplant Proc* 27: 1921–1925

11   Pahl E, Fricker FJ, Armitage J, Griffith BP, Taylor S, Uretsky BF, Beerman LB, Zuberbuhler JR (1990) Coronary arteriosclerosis in pediatric heart transplant survivors: limitation of long-term survival. *J Pediatr* 116: 177–183

12  Hornick P, Smith J, Pomerance A, Mitchell A, Banner N, Rose M, Yacoub M (1997) Influence of acute rejection episodes, HLA matching, and donor/recipient phenotype on the development of 'early' transplant-associated coronary artery disease. *Circulation* 96 (9 Suppl): II-148–153

13  Liu G, Butany J (1992) Morphology of graft arteriosclerosis in cardiac transplant recipients. *Hum Pathol* 23: 768–773

14  Costanzo NM (1992) Cardiac allograft vasculopathy: relationship with acute cellular rejection and histocompatibility. *J Heart Lung Transplant* 11: S90–103

15  Opelz G, Wujciak T (1994) The influence of HLA compatibility on graft survival after heart transplantation. The Collaborative Transplant Study. *N Engl J Med* 330: 816–819

16  Smith JD, Rose ML, Pomerance A, Burke M, Yacoub MH (1995) Reduction of cellular rejection and increase in longer-term survival after heart transplantation after HLA-DR matching [see comments]. *Lancet* 346: 1318–1322

17  Costanzo MR (1995) The role of histoincompatibility in cardiac allograft vasculopathy. *J Heart Lung Transplant* 14: S180–S184

18  Rose EA, Smith CR, Petrossian GA, Barr ML, Reemtsma K (1989) Humoral immune responses after cardiac transplantation: correlation with fatal rejection and graft atherosclerosis. *Surgery* 106: 203–207

19  Escobar A, Ventura HO, Stapleton DD, Mehra MR, Ramee SR, Collins TJ, Jain SP, Smart FW, White CJ (1994) Cardiac allograft vasculopathy assessed by intravascular ultrasonography and nonimmunologic risk factors. *Am J Cardiol* 74: 1042–1046

20  Eich D, Thompson JA, Ko DJ, Hastillo A, Lower R, Katz S, Katz M, Hess ML (1991) Hypercholesterolemia in long-term survivors of heart transplantation: an early marker of accelerated coronary artery disease. *J Heart Lung Transplant* 10: 45–49

21  Hess ML, Hastillo A, Mohanakumar T, Cowley MJ, Vetrovac G, Szentpetery S, Wolfgang TC, Lower RR (1983) Accelerated atherosclerosis in cardiac transplantation: role of cytotoxic B-cell antibodies and hyperlipidemia. *Circulation* 68: II94–101

22  Barbir M, Kushwaha S, Hunt B, Macken A, Thompson GR, Mitchell A, Robinson D, Yacoub M (1992) Lipoprotein(a) and accelerated coronary artery disease in cardiac transplant recipients. *Lancet* 340: 1500–1502

23  Valantine HA (1995) Role of lipids in allograft vascular disease: a multicenter study of intimal thickening detected by intravascular ultrasound. *J Heart Lung Transplant* 14: S234–S237

24  Koskinen P, Lemstrom K, Mattila S, Hayry P, Nieminen MS (1996) Cytomegalovirus infection associated accelerated heart allograft arteriosclerosis may impair the late function of the graft. *Clin Transplant* 10: 487–493

25  Everett JP, Hershberger RE, Norman DJ, Chou S, Ratkovec RM, Cobanoglu A, Ott GY, Hosenpud JD (1992) Prolonged cytomegalovirus infection with viremia is associated with development of cardiac allograft vasculopathy. *J Heart Lung Transplant* 11: S133–S137

26  Grattan MT, Moreno CC, Starnes VA, Oyer PE, Stinson EB, Shumway NE (1989) Cytomegalovirus infection is associated with cardiac allograft rejection and atherosclerosis. *JAMA* 261: 3561–3566

27   Costanzo NM, Swinnen LJ, Fisher SG, O'Sullivan EJ, Pifarre R, Heroux AL, Mullen GM, Johnson MR (1992) Cytomegalovirus infections in heart transplant recipients: relationship to immunosuppression [see comments]. *J Heart Lung Transplant* 11: 837–846

28   Nadasdy T, Smith J, Laszik Z, Waner JL, Johnson LD, Silva FG (1994) Absence of association between cytomegalovirus infection and obliterative transplant arteriopathy in renal allograft rejection. *Mod Pathol* 7: 289–294

29   Sharples LD, Caine N, Mullins P, Scott JP, Solis E, English TA, Large SR, Schofield PM, Wallwork J (1991) Risk factor analysis for the major hazards following heart transplantation – rejection, infection, and coronary occlusive disease. *Transplantation* 52: 244–252

30   Billingham ME (1992) Histopathology of graft coronary disease. *J Heart Lung Transplant* 11: S38–S44

31   Johnson DE, Gao SZ, Schroeder JS, DeCampli WM, Billingham ME (1989) The spectrum of coronary artery pathologic findings in human cardiac allografts. *J Heart Transplant* 8: 349–359

32   Kosek JC, Bieber C, Lower RR (1971) Heart graft arteriosclerosis. *Transplant Proc* 3: 512–514

33   Uys CJ, Rose AG (1984) Pathologic findings in long-term cardiac transplants. *Arch Pathol Lab Med* 108: 112–116

34   Bieber CP, Stinson EB, Shumway NE, Payne R, Kosek J (1970) Cardiac transplantation in man. VII. Cardiac allograft pathology. *Circulation* 41: 753–772

35   Rose AG, Viviers L, Odell JA (1993) Pathology of chronic cardiac rejection: An analysis of epicardial and intramyocardial coronary arteries and myocardial alterations in 43 human allografts. *Cardiovasc Pathol* 2: 7–19

36   Oni AA, Ray J, Hosenpud JD (1992) Coronary venous intimal thickening in explanted cardiac allografts. Evidence demonstrating that transplant coronary artery disease is a manifestation of a diffuse allograft vasculopathy. *Transplantation* 53: 1247–1251

37   Winters GL, Schoen FJ (1997) Graft arteriosclerosis-induced myocardial pathology in heart transplant recipients: predictive value of endomyocardial biopsy. *J Heart Lung Transplant* 16: 985–993

38   Salomon RN, Hughes CC, Schoen FJ, Payne DD, Pober JS, Libby P (1991) Human coronary transplantation-associated arteriosclerosis. Evidence for a chronic immune reaction to activated graft endothelial cells. *Am J Pathol* 138: 791–798

39   Rose ML (1998) Endothelial cells as antigen-presenting cells: role in human transplant rejection. *Cell Mol Life Sci* 54: 965–978

40   Hruban RH, Beschorner WE, Baumgartner WA, Augustine SM, Ren H, Reitz BA, Hutchins GM (1990) Accelerated arteriosclerosis in heart transplant recipients is associated with a T-lymphocyte-mediated endothelialitis. *Am J Pathol* 137: 871–882

41   Raisanen SA, Glysing JT, Mottram PL, Russell ME (1997) Sustained anti-CD4/CD8 treatment blocks inflammatory activation and intimal thickening in mouse heart allografts. *Arterioscler Thromb Vasc Biol* 17: 2115–2122

42    Shi C, Lee WS, He Q, Zhang D, Fletcher DL Jr, Newell JB, Haber E (1996) Immuno-logic basis of transplant-associated arteriosclerosis. *Proc Natl Acad Sci USA* 93: 4051–4056

43    Russell ME, Hancock WW, Akalin E, Wallace AF, Glysing JT, Willett TA, Sayegh MH (1996) Chronic cardiac rejection in the LEW to F344 rat model. Blockade of CD28-B7 costimulation by CTLA4Ig modulates T cell and macrophage activation and attenuates arteriosclerosis. *J Clin Invest* 97: 833–838

44    Glysing JT, Raisanen SA, Sayegh MH, Russell ME (1997) Chronic blockade of CD28-B7-mediated T-cell costimulation by CTLA4Ig reduces intimal thickening in MHC class I and II incompatible mouse heart allografts. *Transplantation* 64: 1641–1645

45    Azuma H, Chandraker A, Nadeau K, Hancock WW, Carpenter CB, Tilney NL, Sayegh MH (1996) Blockade of T-cell costimulation prevents development of experimental chronic renal allograft rejection [see comments]. *Proc Natl Acad Sci USA* 93: 12439–12444

46    Salom RN, Maguire JA, Hancock WW (1998) Endothelial activation and cytokine expression in human acute cardiac allograft rejection. *Pathology* 30: 24–29

47    Dong C, Wilson JE, Winters GL, McManus BM (1996) Human transplant coronary artery disease: pathological evidence for Fas-mediated apoptotic cytotoxicity in allograft arteriopathy. *Lab Invest* 74: 921–931

48    Fox WM, Hameed A, Hutchins GM, Reitz BA, Baumgartner WA, Beschorner WE, Hruban RH (1993) Perforin expression localizing cytotoxic lymphocytes in the intimas of coronary arteries with transplant-related accelerated arteriosclerosis. *Hum Pathol* 24: 477–482

49    Hancock WW, Buelow R, Sayegh MH, Turka LA (1998) Antibody-induced transplant arteriosclerosis is prevented by graft expression of anti-oxidant and anti-apoptotic genes. *Nat Med* 4: 1392–1396

50    Russell PS, Chase CM, Colvin RB (1995) Coronary atherosclerosis in transplanted mouse hearts. IV Effects of treatment with monoclonal antibodies to intercellular adhesion molecule-1 and leukocyte function-associated antigen-1. *Transplantation* 60: 724–729

51    Suzuki J, Isobe M, Yamazaki S, Horie S, Okubo Y, Sekiguchi M (1997) Inhibition of accelerated coronary atherosclerosis with short-term blockade of intercellular adhesion molecule-1 and lymphocyte function-associated antigen-1 in a heterotopic murine model of heart transplantation. *J Heart Lung Transplant* 16: 1141–1148

52    Poston RS, Ennen M, Pollard J, Hoyt EG, Billingham ME, Robbins RC (1998) Ex vivo gene therapy prevents chronic graft vascular disease in cardiac allografts. *J Thorac Cardiovasc Surg* 116: 386–396

53    Koskinen PK, Lemstrom KB (1997) Adhesion molecule P-selectin and vascular cell adhesion molecule-1 in enhanced heart allograft arteriosclerosis in the rat. *Circulation* 95: 191–196

54    Korom S, Hancock WW, Coito AJ, Kupiec WJ (1998) Blockade of very late antigen-4 integrin binding to fibronectin in allograft recipients. II. Treatment with connecting seg-

ment-1 peptides prevents chronic rejection by attenuating arteriosclerotic development and suppressing intragraft T cell and macrophage activation. *Transplantation* 65: 854–859

55  Pattison JM, Nelson PJ, Huie P, Sibley RK, Krensky AM (1996) RANTES chemokine expression in transplant-associated accelerated atherosclerosis. *J Heart Lung Transplant* 15: 1194–1199

56  Russell ME, Adams DH, Wyner LR, Yamashita Y, Halnon NJ, Karnovsky MJ (1993) Early and persistent induction of monocyte chemoattractant protein 1 in rat cardiac allografts. *Proc Natl Acad Sci USA* 90: 6086–6090

57  Fairchild RL, VanBuskirk AM, Kondo T, Wakely ME, Orosz CG (1997) Expression of chemokine genes during rejection and long-term acceptance of cardiac allografts. *Transplantation* 63: 1807–1812

58  Russell ME, Wallace AF, Hancock WW, Sayegh MH, Adams DH, Sibinga NE, Wyner LR, Karnovsky MJ (1995) Upregulation of cytokines associated with macrophage activation in the Lewis-to-F344 rat transplantation model of chronic cardiac rejection. *Transplantation* 59: 572–578

59  Geerling RA, Ansari AA, LaFond WA, Baumgartner WA, Wesselingh S, Herskowitz A (1998) Accelerated arteriosclerosis in aortic grafts: a role for cytokines in progressive intimal lesion development. *Transplant Proc* 30: 946–947

60  Russell PS, Chase CM, Winn HJ, Colvin RB (1994) Coronary atherosclerosis in transplanted mouse hearts. III. Effects of recipient treatment with a monoclonal antibody to interferon-gamma. *Transplantation* 57: 1367–1371

61  Nagano H, Libby P, Taylor MK, Hasegawa S, Stinn JL, Becker G, Tilney NL, Mitchell RN (1998) Coronary arteriosclerosis after T-cell-mediated injury in transplanted mouse hearts: role of interferon-gamma. *Am J Pathol* 152: 1187–1197

62  Raisanen SA, Glysing JT, Koglin J, Russell ME (1998) Reduced transplant arteriosclerosis in murine cardiac allografts placed in interferon-gamma knockout recipients. *Am J Pathol* 152: 359–365

63  Nagano H, Mitchell RN, Taylor MK, Hasegawa S, Tilney NL, Libby P (1997) Interferon-gamma deficiency prevents coronary arteriosclerosis but not myocardial rejection in transplanted mouse hearts. *J Clin Invest* 100: 550–557

64  Shimokado K, Raines EW, Madtes DK, Barrett TB, Benditt EP, Ross R (1985) A significant part of macrophage-derived growth factor consists of at least two forms of PDGF. *Cell* 43: 277–286

65  Ross R, Raines EW, Bowen-Pope DF (1986) The biology of platelet-derived growth factor. *Cell* 46: 155–169

66  Saito S, Motomura N, Lou H, Ramwell PW, Foegh ML (1997) Specific effects of estrogen on growth factor and major histocompatibility complex class II antigen expression in rat aortic allograft. *J Thorac Cardiovasc Surg* 114: 803–809

67  Lou H, Zhao Y, Delafontaine P, Kodama T, Katz N, Ramwell PW, Foegh ML (1997) Estrogen effects on insulin-like growth factor-I (IGF-I)-induced cell proliferation and IGF-I expression in native and allograft vessels. *Circulation* 96: 927–933

68  Lou H, Ramwell PW, Foegh ML (1998) Estradiol 17-beta represses insulin-like growth factor I receptor expression in smooth muscle cells from rabbit cardiac recipients. *Transplantation* 66: 419–426

69  Zhao XM, Yeoh TK, Frist WH, Porterfield DL, Miller GG (1994) Induction of acidic fibroblast growth factor and full-length platelet-derived growth factor expression in human cardiac allografts. Analysis by PCR, *in situ* hybridization, and immunohistochemistry. *Circulation* 90: 677–685

70  Shaddy RE, Hammond EH, Yowell RL (1996) Immunohistochemical analysis of platelet-derived growth factor and basic fibroblast growth factor in cardiac biopsy and autopsy specimens of heart transplant patients. *Am J Cardiol* 77: 1210–1215

71  Zhao XM, Citrin BS, Miller GG, Frist WH, Merrill WH, Fischell TA, Atkinson JB, Yeoh TK (1995) Association of acidic fibroblast growth factor and untreated low grade rejection with cardiac allograft vasculopathy. *Transplantation* 59: 1005–1010

72  Alpers CE, Davis CL, Barr D, Marsh CL, Hudkins KL (1996) Identification of platelet-derived growth factor A and B chains in human renal vascular rejection. *Am J Pathol* 148: 439–451

73  Lemstrom KB, Koskinen PK (1997) Expression and localization of platelet-derived growth factor ligand and receptor protein during acute and chronic rejection of rat cardiac allografts. *Circulation* 96: 1240–1249

74  Myllarniemi M, Calderon L, Lemstrom K, Buchdunger E, Hayry P (1997) Inhibition of platelet-derived growth factor receptor tyrosine kinase inhibits vascular smooth muscle cell migration and proliferation. *FASEB J* 11: 1119–1126

75  Sihvola R, Koskinen P, Myllarniemi M, Loubtchenkov M, Hayry P, Buchdunger E, Lemstrom K (1999) Prevention of cardiac allograft arteriosclerosis by protein tyrosine kinase inhibitor selective for platelet-derived growth factor receptor. *Circulation* 99: 2295–2301

76  Koglin J, Glysing JT, Raisanen SA, Russell ME (1998) Immune sources of transforming growth factor-beta1 reduce transplant arteriosclerosis: insight derived from a knockout mouse model. *Circ Res* 83: 652–660

77  Wagner CR, Morris TE, Shipley GD, Hosenpud JD (1993) Regulation of human aortic endothelial cell-derived mesenchymal growth factors by allogeneic lymphocytes *in vitro*. A potential mechanism for cardiac allograft vasculopathy. *J Clin Invest* 92: 1269–1277

78  Hosenpud JD, Morris TE, Shipley GD, Mauck KA, Wagner CR (1996) Cardiac allograft vasculopathy. Preferential regulation of endothelial cell-derived mesenchymal growth factors in response to a donor-specific cell-mediated allogeneic response. *Transplantation* 61: 939–948

79  Rose EA, Pepino P, Barr ML, Smith CR, Ratner AJ, Ho E, Berger C (1992) Relation of HLA antibodies and graft atherosclerosis in human cardiac allograft recipients. *J Heart Lung Transplant* 11: S120–S123

80  Smith JD, Danskine AJ, Rose ML, Yacoub MH (1992) Specificity of lymphocytotoxic antibodies formed after cardiac transplantation and correlation with rejection episodes. *Transplantation* 53: 1358–1362

81   Hosenpud JD, Everett JP, Morris TE, Wagner CR, Shipley GD (1995) Cellular and humoral immunity to vascular endothelium and the development of cardiac allograft vasculopathy. *J Heart Lung Transplant* 14: S185–S187

82   Chow LH, Huh S, Jiang J, Zhong R, Pickering JG (1996) Intimal thickening develops without humoral immunity in a mouse aortic allograft model of chronic vascular rejection. *Circulation* 94: 3079–3082

83   Russell PS, Chase CM, Winn HJ, Colvin RB (1994) Coronary atherosclerosis in transplanted mouse hearts. II. Importance of humoral immunity. *J Immunol* 152: 5135–5141

84   Harris PE, Bian H, Reed EF (1997) Induction of high affinity fibroblast growth factor receptor expression and proliferation in human endothelial cells by anti-HLA antibodies: a possible mechanism for transplant atherosclerosis. *J Immunol* 159: 5697–5704

85   Ravalli S, Albala A, Ming M, Szabolcs M, Barbone A, Michler RE, Cannon PJ (1998) Inducible nitric oxide synthase expression in smooth muscle cells and macrophages of human transplant coronary artery disease. *Circulation* 97: 2338–2345

86   Lafond WA, Chen CL, Augustine S, Wu TC, Hruban RH, Lowenstein CJ (1997) Inducible nitric oxide synthase expression in coronary arteries of transplanted human hearts with accelerated graft arteriosclerosis. *Am J Pathol* 151: 919–925

87   Shears LL, Kawaharada N, Tzeng E, Billiar TR, Watkins SC, Kovesdi I, Lizonova A, Pham SM (1997) Inducible nitric oxide synthase suppresses the development of allograft arteriosclerosis. *J Clin Invest* 100: 2035–2042

88   Russell ME, Wallace AF, Wyner LR, Newell JB, Karnovsky MJ (1995) Upregulation and modulation of inducible nitric oxide synthase in rat cardiac allografts with chronic rejection and transplant arteriosclerosis. *Circulation* 92: 457–464

89   Koglin J, Glysing JT, Mudgett JS, Russell ME (1998) Exacerbated transplant arteriosclerosis in inducible nitric oxide-deficient mice. *Circulation* 97: 2059–2065

90   Garg UC, Hassid A (1989) Nitric oxide-generating vasodilators and 8-bromo-cyclic guanosine monophosphate inhibit mitogenesis and proliferation of cultured rat vascular smooth muscle cells. *J Clin Invest* 83: 1774–1777

91   Lin H, Ignatescu M, Wilson JE, Roberts CR, Horley KJ, Winters GL, Costanzo MR, McManus BM (1996) Prominence of apolipoproteins B, (a), and E in the intimae of coronary arteries in transplanted human hearts: geographic relationship to vessel wall proteoglycans. *J Heart Lung Transplant* 15: 1223–1232

92   Shi C, Lee WS, Russell ME, Zhang D, Fletcher DL, Newell JB, Haber E (1997) Hypercholesterolemia exacerbates transplant arteriosclerosis via increased neointimal smooth muscle cell accumulation: studies in apolipoprotein E knockout mice. *Circulation* 96: 2722–2728

93   Raisanen SA, Tilly KM, Ustinov J, Mennander A, Paavonen T, Tikkanen MJ, Hayry P (1994) Hyperlipidemia accelerates allograft arteriosclerosis (chronic rejection) in the rat. *Arterioscler Thromb* 14: 2032–2042

94   Labarrere CA, Pitts D, Nelson DR, Faulk WP (1995) Vascular tissue plasminogen activator and the development of coronary artery disease in heart-transplant recipients. *N Engl J Med* 333: 1111–1116

95  Faulk WP, Labarrere CA, Nelson DR, Pitts D (1995) Hemostasis, fibrinolysis, and natural anticoagulation in transplant vascular sclerosis. *J Heart Lung Transplant* 14: S158–S164

96  Moons L, Shi C, Ploplis V, Plow E, Haber E, Collen D, Carmeliet P (1998) Reduced transplant arteriosclerosis in plasminogen-deficient mice. *J Clin Invest* 102: 1788–1797

97  Holschermann H, Bohle RM, Zeller H, Schmidt H, Stahl U, Fink L, Grimm H, Tillmanns H, Haberbosch W (1999) *In situ* detection of tissue factor within the coronary intima in rat cardiac allograft vasculopathy. *Am J Pathol* 154: 211–220

98  Fang JC, Kinlay S, Kundsin R, Ganz P (1998) Chlamydia pneumoniae infection is frequent but not associated with coronary arteriosclerosis in cardiac transplant recipients. *Am J Cardiol* 82: 1479–1483

99  Geist LJ, Dai LY (1996) Cytomegalovirus modulates interleukin-6 gene expression. *Transplantation* 62: 653–658

100 Iwamoto GK, Konicek SA (1997) Cytomegalovirus immediate early genes upregulate interleukin-6 gene expression. *J Investig Med* 45: 175–182

101 Humbert M, Devergne O, Cerrina J, Rain B, Simonneau G, Dartevelle P, Duroux P, Galanaud P, Emilie D (1992) Activation of macrophages and cytotoxic cells during cytomegalovirus pneumonia complicating lung transplantations. *Am Rev Respir Dis* 145: 1178–1184

102 Waldman WJ, Knight DA (1996) Cytokine-mediated induction of endothelial adhesion molecule and histocompatibility leukocyte antigen expression by cytomegalovirus-activated T cells. *Am J Pathol* 148: 105–119

103 Burns LJ, Pooley JC, Walsh DJ, Vercellotti GM, Weber ML, Kovacs A (1999) Intercellular adhesion molecule-1 expression in endothelial cells is activated by cytomegalovirus immediate early proteins. *Transplantation* 67: 137–144

104 Streblow DN, Soderberg-Naucler C, Vieira J, Smith P, Wakabayashi E, Ruchti F, Mattison K, Altschuler Y, Nelson JA (1999) The human cytomegalovirus chemokine receptor US28 mediates vascular smooth muscle cell migration. *Cell* 99: 511–520

105 Koskinen P, Lemstrom K, Bruggeman C, Lautenschlager I, Hayry P (1994) Acute cytomegalovirus infection induces a subendothelial inflammation (endothelialitis) in the allograft vascular wall. A possible linkage with enhanced allograft arteriosclerosis. *Am J Pathol* 144: 41–50

106 Lemstrom KB, Bruning JH, Bruggeman CA, Lautenschlager IT, Hayry PJ (1994) Triple drug immunosuppression significantly reduces immune activation and allograft arteriosclerosis in cytomegalovirus-infected rat aortic allografts and induces early latency of viral infection. *Am J Pathol* 144: 1334–1347

107 Lemstrom KB, Aho PT, Bruggeman CA, Hayry PJ (1994) Cytomegalovirus infection enhances mRNA expression of platelet-derived growth factor-BB and transforming growth factor-beta 1 in rat aortic allografts. Possible mechanism for cytomegalovirus-enhanced graft arteriosclerosis. *Arterioscler Thromb* 14: 2043–2052

# Free radicals as mediators of inflammation in atherosclerosis

*Heraldo P. Souza[1,2] and Jay L. Zweier[1]*

[1]Molecular and Cellular Biophysics Laboratories, Department of Medicine, Division of Cardiology and The Electron Paramagnetic Resonance Center, The Johns Hopkins University School of Medicine, 5501 Hopkins Bayview Circle, Baltimore, MD 21224, USA; [2]Disciplina de Emergências Clínicas, Faculdade de Medicina, Universidade de São Paulo, São Paulo, Brazil

## Introduction

Free radicals are chemical species that possess an unpaired electron and are often formed as intermediates in chemical reactions. The presence of the unpaired electron makes these molecules unstable and reactive. Oxygen free radicals are reactive oxygen species (ROS) formed from the incomplete reduction of oxygen and exert a range of important effects in biological cells and tissues. Oxygen radicals and other ROS are produced by normal cellular metabolism and have critical roles in the processes of cellular signaling and injury. The four-electron reduction of molecular oxygen to water, catalyzed by the mitochondrial electron transport chain, accounts for 95% of oxygen consumption in tissues. The remaining 5% proceeds via univalent reduction of oxygen with the production of superoxide anions ($^\bullet O_2^-$), hydrogen peroxide ($H_2O_2$), and hydroxyl radicals ($^\bullet OH$). These reactive products have been documented to cause cell injury. Therefore, cells have evolved several systems that function to avoid or correct damage caused by these oxygen radicals.

Cellular enzymes exist to metabolize and eliminate these toxic forms of reduced oxygen. These include superoxide dismutase which dismutates superoxide to hydrogen peroxide and molecular oxygen, catalase which converts hydrogen peroxide to water and oxygen, glutathione peroxidase which catalyzes the reaction that removes hydrogen peroxide through its reaction with reduced glutathione. In addition, metal-storage and transport proteins such as ferritin and transferrin serve an important role since they minimize the presence of free catalytic metal ions such as ferric or ferrous iron that would otherwise convert weak oxidants such as hydrogen peroxide to highly reactive oxidants such as $^\bullet OH$. Vitamins C and E also serve important roles as radical scavengers, and can prevent or reverse the oxidation of biological macromolecules and terminate lipid peroxidation.

The expression "oxidative stress" corresponds to the situation where production of reactive oxygen species overcome, relatively, the efficiency or acessibility of cellular mechanisms of defense, leading to injury of structures including membranes, proteins and DNA. Oxidative stress can initiate or participate in a series of pathological situations, such as carcinogenesis [1] and neurodegenerative diseases [2] and even in the normal aging process [3]. In the cardiovascular system, reactive oxygen species are described as participants in ischemia-reperfusion injury [4], restenosis after coronary angioplasty [5], hypertension induced by angiotensin II [6] and atherosclerosis.

Our current knowledge about the pathogenesis of atherosclerosis points out that oxygen radicals and other reactive oxygen species are important mediators of this process. ROS can interfere with some of the major processes of vascular and endothelial function and lead to the formation of the atherosclerotic plaque due to: oxidation of lipids, impaired endothelium-dependent vasodilation, increased cellular proliferation and induction of proinflammatory genes. It can also trigger acute vascular events by acting on plaque stability (Fig. 1).

Some of the evidence that links oxidative stress to atherogenesis will be discussed below.

## Reactive oxygen species and modification of lipids

The role of hypercholesterolemia in the pathogenesis of atherosclerosis is based on experimental as well as clinical and epidemiological data [7]. Circulating lipids, mainly low-density lipoprotein (LDL), suffer oxidative modification and are taken up by macrophages inside the vessel wall, in a way that can not be down-regulated. The lipid-laden macrophages, then called "foam-cells", are hallmarks of early atherosclerotic lesion formation [8].

The mechanisms underlying LDL oxidation are still unclear, but some evidence suggests that reactive oxygen species are involved in this process. Phagocytic cells can oxidize LDL *in vitro* and superoxide is required for the initiation of the process as indicated by inhibition of the reaction by early addition of superoxide dismutase [9]. Superoxide dismutase exogenously added to endothelial cell lines decrease the rate of LDL oxidation by four-fold. Overexpression of the enzyme by the same cells has similar but more modest effects [10]. It has also been shown that the increased oxidant stress induced by stretch force can oxidize LDL, being, therefore, one of the potential mechanisms whereby hypertension facilitates atherosclerosis [11]. This matter, however, is still controversial, and some authors advocate that extracellular superoxide generation is required but not sufficient for LDL oxidation by monocytes/macrophages [12].

## Reactive oxygen species and endothelial dysfunction

Among the mechanisms underlying endothelial dysfunction in atherosclerotic vessels [13], impaired nitric oxide (NO) availability seems to be one of the most

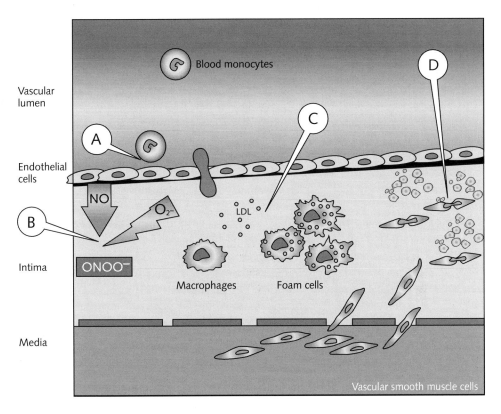

Vascular lumen

Endothelial cells

Intima

Media

*Figure 1*
*Schematic representation of the role of free radicals in the process of atherosclerotic lesion formation*
*(A) Migration of blood monocytes to the vascular wall is a primary feature in atherosclerotic plaque formation. In order to gain access to the vessel intima, monocytes first need to adhere to endothelial cells on the vessel surface. Reactive oxygen species can increase blood monocyte adhesion through stimulating adhesion molecule expression. (B) Superoxide can rapidly react with endothelium-derived nitric oxide, decreasing its availability to promote vasodilation and generating the strong oxidant peroxynitrite, which can cause further tissue damage. Superoxide can be generated by vascular cells and/or macrophages inside the wall of atherosclerotic vessels. (C) Reactive oxygen species generated by vascular cells and/or macrophages can oxydize LDL in* vitro *and probably in* vivo. *Oxidized LDL is taken up by macrophages in the subendothelial layer, thus becoming foam cells. (D) One of the hallmarks of the atherosclerotic lesion is the presence of vascular smooth muscle cells in the subendothelial space, forming the fibrous cap of the atherosclerotic plaque. These vascular smooth muscle cells have their origin in the media. They migrate to the intima and, once there, start proliferating. ROS have been shown, in a series of experimental models (including vascular smooth muscle cells), to be able to stimulate cell proliferation.*

important. There is still controversy about the role of impaired NO synthase function [14], but some studies point to an enhanced catabolism of NO by superoxide as the main cause of decreased NO half-life *in vivo* in this pathological situation [15].

In arteries from hypercholesterolemic rabbits, NO generation has been reported to be enhanced rather than impaired [16] and treatment with polyethylene-glycolated superoxide dismutase (SOD) partially restored endothelium-dependent vascular relaxation [17]. In normal vessels a decrease in active NO was found when SOD was inhibited [18].

The strong oxidant peroxynitrite ($ONOO^-$) is the product of the rapid reaction of NO and superoxide which proceeds nearly at diffusion-limited rates [19]. This reaction, and hence the formation of peroxynitrite is augmented in inflammatory conditions such as ischemia-reperfusion injury when both substrates are present in high concentrations [20]. Nitrotyrosine, the main peroxynitrite-mediated protein modification, can be found bound to beta-VLDL apoproteins in arteries of hypercholesterolemic rabbits [21]. In human vessels with more advanced macrophage-rich lesions, nitrotyrosine residues, characteristic of peroxynitrite-modified proteins, were detected paralleling an increase in inducible nitric oxide synthase (iNOS) expression, implicating peroxynitrite as one of the important mediators of oxidative damage [22].

## Reactive oxygen species and stimulation of cellular growth and proliferation

Smooth muscle cell proliferation and extracellular matrix deposition in the intima are the major processes that convert a fatty streak into a mature fibrofatty atheroma, accounting for the progressive growth of atherosclerotic lesions. There is increasing evidence that superoxide and hydrogen peroxide can stimulate cell proliferation, especially that of vascular smooth muscle cells [23]. In vascular smooth muscle cells, exposure to reactive oxygen species stimulates protooncogene expression and cellular proliferation [24] and hydrogen peroxide seems to be a vital signal-transducing molecule to platelet derived growth factor [25]. Inhibition of the NAD(P)H oxidase-derived superoxide by a $p22^{phox}$ antisense oligonucleotide decreases cell growth and proliferation in vascular smooth muscle cells stimulated with angiotensin-II [26]. Vascular hypertrophy characteristic of hypertensive states is also dependent on secondary intracellular signal transduction mediated by reactive oxygen species [27].

Reactive oxygen species, including $O_2^{-\bullet}$, act also as mediators of Ras-induced cell cycle progression independent of mitogen-activated protein kinase (MAPK) and c-Jun $NH_2$-terminal kinase (JNK) in Ras-transformed fibroblasts, suggesting a possible mechanism for the effects of antioxidants against Ras-induced cellular transformation [28].

Interestingly, expression of p53, which induces programmed cell death, exerts its effects through transcriptional induction of redox-related genes and formation of reactive oxygen species [29].

Therefore, it seems that the complex balance of cell proliferation and apoptosis that takes place in the atherosclerotic lesion is profoundly influenced by reactive oxygen species.

## Reactive oxygen species as mediators of inflammatory injury to vascular tissue

Oxygen free radicals participate in inflammatory processes in several ways. They are generated in large amounts by phagocytic cells, as part of the immune host defense [30] and are also involved in expression of genes and/or proteins that modulate inflammation.

Some of the best characterized examples of free radical action as inflammatory mediators in vessels come from ischemia-reperfusion injury. While timely reperfusion of ischemic tissues such as the heart can reduce the amount of cell death, there is evidence that reperfusion can cause further damage to jeopardized cells [31]. The generation of free radicals has been shown to be an important mechanism of this myocardial reperfusion injury [32].

It has been shown that superoxide and hydroxyl radicals are generated in reoxygenated vascular endothelial cells in sufficient concentrations to cause cellular injury and death [33]. There is evidence indicating that this endothelial radical generation promotes both recruitment of polymorphonuclear leukocytes (PMNs) as well as activation and subsequent endothelial cell-PMN adherence [34, 35].

In previous work from our laboratory [36], flow cytometry experiments on PMNs exposed to $H_2O_2$ demonstrate up-regulation of the adhesion molecules CD18 and CD11b, with a clear shift to the right in the flow cytometry histogram of these cells (Fig. 2). Down-regulation of L-selectin is seen in these cells with a marked shift to the left in the histogram. Increasing concentrations of hydrogen peroxide resulted in a concentration-dependent increase in CD18 and CD11b on the surface of PMNs, while expression of L-selectin is decreased. Exposure of PMNs to a super-oxide generating system also induced expression of the adhesion molecules (Fig. 3). The physiological relevance of this phenomenon is given by the fact that pretreatment of PMNs with oxidants increased adhesion of these cells to monolayers of endothelial cells in a way similar to that obtained by the known activator C5a.

In isolated reperfused hearts, SOD or catalase treatment decreased PMN accumulation and prevented the marked upregulation of CD18 expression seen after reperfusion. These experiments demonstrate that in addition to their direct antioxidative actions, SOD and catalase each decrease PMN adhesion and CD18 expression resulting in marked suppression of PMN-mediated injury in the postischemic

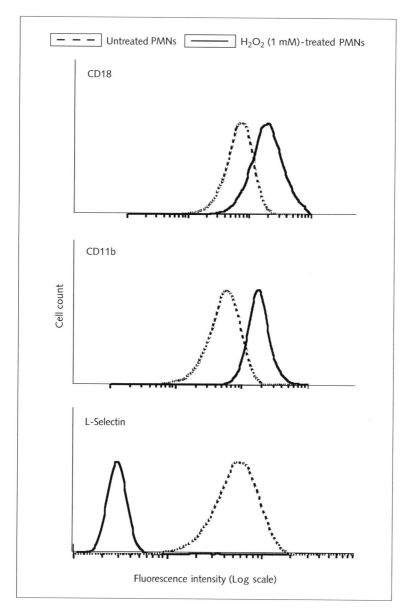

*Figure 2*

*Flow citometry histograms from PMNs stimulated for 30 min with 1.0 mM hydrogen perox-ide, or from untreated PMNs. On the top panel, upregulation of CD18 is seen in $H_2O_2$ treat-ed PMNs, with a rightward shift of the fluorescence intensity histogram. On the center panel, a similar response is seen for CD11b surface expression. On the lower panel, a down regulation of L-selectin expression is noted.*

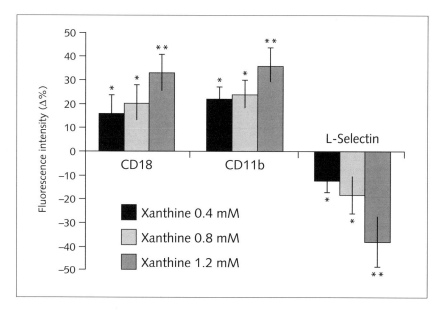

*Figure 3*
*Effect of superoxide on PMN adhesion molecule expression. PMNs were exposed to varying magnitudes of superoxide generation by varying the concentration of the substrate xanthine. CD18, CD11b, and L-selectin surface expression responded to superoxide stimulation in a dose-dependent manner. Values are expresseed in percent changes of mode fluorescence intensity of control, untreated PMNs. Data are plotted as mean ± SEM of 4 experiments and are compared by Student's T-test. $^*p < 0.05$, $^{**}p < 0.01$, untreated versus treated PMNs.*

heart. Thus, endothelium-derived $H_2O_2$ and superoxide further amplify post-ischemic injury by triggering CD18 expression on the surface of PMNs leading to increased PMN adhesion within the heart [37].

Patients with coronary artery disease were shown to have an increase in adhesion molecule expression and a down-regulation of L-selectin [38], findings similar to that obtained by exposing PMNs to free radicals *in vitro*. These features can provide a link between free radical-induced gene expression and inflammatory processes relevant to atherogenesis.

Another way that reactive oxygen species can influence inflammatory repsonse is through promoting gene expression. Nuclear factor-κB (NF-κB) is a ubiquitous transcription factor that can be activated by diverse proatherogenic stimuli such as inflammatory cytokines, lipopolysaccharide, oxidant stress and physical forces [39, 40]. The activated NF-κB has been found in atherosclerotic lesions [41], and it has been involved in the vascular smooth cell dysfunction found in atherosclerosis [42]. As it has been demonstrated that superoxide or hydrogen peroxide can activate NF-κB in endothelial as well as in smooth muscle cells [43], this is another way reactive oxygen species can modulate inflammatory response in vascular tissues, and specifically in atherosclerotic lesions.

## Sources of reactive oxygen species in the vessel wall

All cellular types that form the vessel wall have the ability to generate reactive oxygen species, including endothelial cells, smooth muscle cells and fibroblasts. However, the main cell type or types responsible for vascular free radical production have not yet been unequivocally established .

Xanthine oxidase has been shown to be present in endothelial cells and has been demonstrated to be the major source of oxygen free radical generation in hypoxic and reoxygenated endothelial cells. It has also been shown that radical generation derived from endothelial xanthine oxidase is an important mechanism of oxygen free radical generation in ischemic/reperfused myocardium [44]. In hypercholesterolemic rabbits, it has also been reported that xanthine oxidase can be released into the circulation, and then bind to endothelial cell glycosaminoglycans resulting in increased superoxide generation on the vessel wall [45] .

Endothelial NOS can also generate superoxide (Fig. 4) and this phenomenon is regulated by calcium-calmodulin and tetrahydrobiopterin [46]. Interestingly, it has been reported that endothelial cells exposed to native LDL generate superoxide through eNOS, without a decrease in their NO production, which would likely result in the generation of the strong oxidant peroxynitrite [47].

Another source of superoxide, probably more important in atherosclerotic vessels is inducible NOS (iNOS) [48]. iNOS is present in macrophages and under some circumstances such as the depletion of the substrate L-arginine or the cofactor tetrahydrobiopterin, it can generate superoxide [49]. This finding is very important in atherosclerotic vessels, since activation of metalloproteinases that cause plaque destabilization can be achieved by reative oxygen species generated by macrophages infiltrated in the lesion [50]. Of course, this superoxide generation from iNOS would be in addition to that from the macrophage NADPH oxidase which is normally the major source of macrophage-derived ROS. However, following induction of iNOS we have observed that radical generation from the NADPH oxidase is inhibited [49].

In recent years, a flavoenzyme has been described as the major source of superoxide in the normal vessel wall [51]. The vascular enzyme seems to possess unique features, regarding its structure [52] and function [53]; however, it seems to share some characteristics with the phagocytic NADPH oxidase [54]. An oxidase was cloned recently, which encodes a homologue of the catalytic subunit of the superoxide-generating NADPH oxidase of phagocytes, gp91[phox] [55]. This enzyme is expressed in vascular smooth muscle cells and induces cell proliferation through ROS generation.

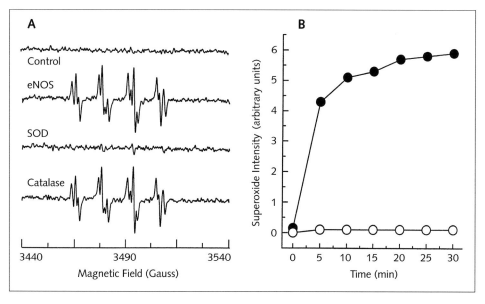

*Figure 4*
*Superoxide formation from endothelial nitric oxide synthase (eNOS). Panel A, electron para-*
*magnetic resonance (EPR) spectra of oxygen free radicals generated by eNOS. The reaction*
*system consists of 0.5 mM NADPH, 0.5 mM Ca²⁺, 10 μg/ml calmodulin, and 50 mM DMPO*
*in 50 mM Tris-HCl buffer, pH 7.4. While no signal was observed in the reaction system with-*
*out enzyme (Control), a prominent spectrum of the DMPO-OOH adduct was seen after*
*adding 15 μg/ml eNOS (eNOS). These signals were totally abolished by SOD (200 units/ml,*
*SOD) but not affected by catalase (300 units/ml, Catalase). Spectra were recorded at room*
*temperature with a microwave frequency of 9.785 GHz, 20 milliwatts of microwave power,*
*and 0.5 G modulation amplitude. Each spectrum is the sum of five 1-min acquisitions. Panel*
*B, time course of $O_2^{-\bullet}$ generation from eNOS in the absence (filled circles) and presence*
*(unfilled circles) of SOD (200 units/ml). Spectra were continuously recorded at every five 1-*
*min acquisitions from the beginning of the reaction until 30 min. Results are the average of*
*three experiments.*

One of the common components of the vascular and phagocytic oxidases, p22$^{phox}$, has been observed to have increased expression in aortas from hypertensive rats [56]. Although an unequivocal role for this enzyme in atherogenesis has not yet been established, the mutation of the potential heme-binding site of the p22$^{phox}$ gene may reduce susceptibility to coronary artery disease [57]. It was also described that in non-atherosclerotic human coronary arteries, examined by immunohistochemistry and Western blotting, p22$^{phox}$ was weakly expressed, mainly in the adventitia. In atherosclerotic coronary arteries, however, intensive immunoreactivity was detected in neointimal and medial smooth muscle cells and infiltrating macrophages in hypercellular regions and at the boundary region. Semiquantitative analysis and Western blotting showed that the expression of p22$^{phox}$ in atherosclerotic coronary arteries was more pronounced than that in non-atherosclerotic arteries. Double staining revealed p22$^{phox}$ expression in adventitial fibroblasts, smooth muscle cells, macrophages in the neointima and media, and endothelial cells. These findings allowed the authors to conclude that as atherosclerosis progressed, the expression of p22$^{phox}$ increased through the vessel wall [58].

## Conclusion

Many of the manifestations of atherosclerosis are likely secondary to the actions of reactive oxygen species. Lipids can be oxidized in the vessel wall by macrophages or endothelial cells through generation of reactive oxygen species. ROS can interfere with endothelium-derived vasodilation through reaction with NO. Increased cellular proliferation, which is an important feature in atheroma formation can be stimulated by ROS. Finally, ROS can modulate the inflammatory response in the vessel wall, a keystone finding in atherogenesis. The source of ROS either in normal or pathological situations are not fully understood with evidence pointing to xanthine oxidase, nitric oxide synthase, leukocyte NAD(P)H oxidase and vascular NAD(P)H oxidase as main contributors to ROS generation in vascular tissue.

*Acknowledgments*
This effort was supported by National Institutes of Health Grants HL38324, HL52315 and HL63744. Heraldo P. Souza is supported by Fundação de Amparo à Pesquisa do Estado de São Paulo - FAPESP - São Paulo - Brazil

## References

1   Schraufstatter I, Hyslop PA, Jackson JH, Cochrane CG (1988) Oxidant induced DNA dmage of target cells. *J Clin Invest* 82: 1040–1050

2   Floyd RA (1999) Antioxidants, oxidative stress, and degenerative neurological disorders. *Proc Soc Exp Biol Med* 222 (3): 236–245

3   Beckman KB, Ames BN (1998) The free radical theory of aging matures. *Physiol Rev* 78 (2): 547–581

4   Wang P, Chen H, Qin H, Sankarapandi S, Becher MW, Wong PC, Zweier JL (1998) Overexpression of human copper, zinc-superoxide dismutase (SOD1) prevents postischemic injury. *Proc Natl Acad Sci USA* 95 (8): 4556–4560

5    Janiszewski M, Pasqualucci CA, Souza LC, Pileggi F, da Luz PL, Laurindo FR (1998) Oxidized thiols markedly amplify the vascular response to balloon injury in rabbits through a redox active metal-dependent pathway. *Cardiovasc Res* 39 (2): 327–338

6    Rajagopalan S, Kurz S, Munzel T, Tarpey M, Freeman BA, Griendling KK, Harrison DG (1996) Angiotensin II-mediated hypertension in the rat increases vascular superoxide production via membrane NADH/NADPH oxidase activation. *J Clin Invest* 97 (8): 1916–1923

7    Gotto AM Jr (1997) Cholesterol management in theory and practice. *Circulation* 96 (12): 4424–4430

8    Steinberg D (1997) Oxidative modification of LDL and atherogenesis. *Circulation* 95 (4): 1062–1071

9    Hiramatsu K, Rosen H, Heinecke JW, Wolfbauer G, Chait A (1987) Superoxide initiates oxidation of low density lipoprotein by human monocytes. *Arteriosclerosis* 7 (1): 55–60

10   Fang X, Weintraub NL, Rios CD, Chappell DA, Zwacka RM, Engelhardt JF, Oberley LW, Yan T, Heistad DD, Spector AA (1998) Overexpression of human superoxide dismutase inhibits oxidation of low-density lipoprotein by endothelial cells. *Circ Res* 82 (12): 1289–1297

11   Inoue N, Kawashima S, Hirata KI, Rikitake Y, Takeshita S, Yamochi W, Akita H, Yokoyama M (1998) Stretch force on vascular smooth muscle cells enhances oxidation of LDL via superoxide production. *Am J Physiol* 274 (6 Pt 2): H1928–H1932

12   Chisolm GM 3rd, Hazen SL, Fox PL, Cathcart MK (1999) The oxidation of lipoproteins by monocytes-macrophages. Biochemical and biological mechanisms. *J Biol Chem* 274 (37): 25959–25962

13   Shimokawa H (1999) Primary endothelial dysfunction: atherosclerosis. *J Mol Cell Cardiol* 31 (1): 23–37

14   Wever RM, Luscher TF, Cosentino F, Rabelink TJ (1998) Atherosclerosis and the two faces of endothelial nitric oxide synthase. *Circulation* 97 (1): 108–112

15   Beckman JS, Koppenol WH (1996) Nitric oxide, superoxide, and peroxynitrite: the good, the bad, and ugly. *Am J Physiol* 271 (5 Pt 1): C1424–C1437

16   Minor RL Jr, Myers PR, Guerra R Jr, Bates JN, Harrison DG (1990) Diet-induced atherosclerosis increases the release of nitrogen oxides from rabbit aorta. *J Clin Invest* 86 (6): 2109–2116

17   Mugge A, Elwell JH, Peterson TE, Hofmeyer TG, Heistad DD, Harrison DG (1991) Chronic treatment with polyethylene-glycolated superoxide dismutase partially restores endothelium-dependent vascular relaxations in cholesterol-fed rabbits. *Circ Res* 69 (5): 1293–1300

18   Mugge A, Elwell JH, Peterson TE, Harrison DG (1991) Release of intact endothelium-derived relaxing factor depends on endothelial superoxide dismutase activity. *Am J Physiol* 260 (2 Pt 1): C219–C225

19   Darley-Usmar V, White R (1997) Disruption of vascular signalling by the reaction of

nitric oxide with superoxide: implications for cardiovascular disease. *Exp Physiol* 82 (2): 305–316

20 Wang P, Zweier JL (1996) Measurement of nitric oxide and peroxynitrite generation in the postischemic heart. Evidence for peroxynitrite-mediated reperfusion injury. *J Biol Chem* 271 (46): 29223–29230

21 Moriel P, Abdalla DS (1997) Nitrotyrosine bound to beta-VLDL-apoproteins: a biomarker of peroxynitrite formation in experimental atherosclerosis. *Biochem Biophys Res Commun* 17 232 (2): 332–335

22 Luoma JS, Stralin P, Marklund SL, Hiltunen TP, Sarkioja T, Yla-Herttuala S (1998) Expression of extracellular SOD and iNOS in macrophages and smooth muscle cells in human and rabbit atherosclerotic lesions: colocalization with epitopes characteristic of oxidized LDL and peroxynitrite-modified proteins. *Arterioscler Thromb Vasc Biol* 18 (2): 157–167

23 Griendling KK, Ushio-Fukai M (1998) Redox control of vascular smooth muscle proliferation. *J Lab Clin Med* 132 (1): 9–15

24 Rao GN, Berk BC (1992) Active oxygen species stimulate vascular smooth muscle cell growth and proto-oncogene expression. *Circ Res* 70: 593–599

25 Sundaresan M, Yu ZX, Ferrans VJ, Irani K, Finkel T (1995) Requirement for generation of $H_2O_2$ for platelet-derived growth factor signal transduction. *Science* 270 (5234): 296–299

26 Ushio-Fukai M, Zafari AM, Fukui T, Ishizaka N, Griendling KK (1996) p22$^{phox}$ is a critical component of the superoxide-generating NADH/NADPH oxidase system and regulates angiotensin II-induced hypertrophy in vascular smooth muscle cells. *J Biol Chem* 271 (38): 23317–23321

27 Zafari AM, Ushio-Fukai M, Akers M, Yin Q, Shah A, Harrison DG, Taylor WR, Griendling KK (1998) Role of NADH/NADPH oxidase-derived $H_2O_2$ in angiotensin II-induced vascular hypertrophy. *Hypertension* 32 (3): 488–495

28 Irani K, Xia Y, Zweier JL, Sollott SJ, Der CJ, Fearon ER, Sundaresan M, Finkel T, Goldschmidt-Clermont PJ (1997) Mitogenic signaling mediated by oxidants in Ras-transformed fibroblasts. *Science* 275 (5306): 1649–1652

29 Polyak K, Xia Y, Zweier JL, Kinzler KW, Vogelstein B (1997) A model for p53-induced apoptosis. *Nature* 389 (6648): 300–305

30 Babior BM (1997) Superoxide: a two-edged sword. *Braz J Med Biol Res* 30 (2): 141–155

31 Theroux P (1999) Protection of the myocardial cell during ischemia. *Am J Cardiol* 83 (10A): 3G–9G

32 Flaherty JT, Zweier JL (1991) Role of oxygen radicals in myocardial reperfusion injury: experimental and clinical evidence. *Klin Wochenschr* 69 (21–23): 1061–1065

33 Zweier JL, Kuppusamy P, Lutty GA (1988) Measurement of endothelial cell free radical generation: evidence for a central mechanism of free radical injury in postischemic tissues. *Proc Natl Acad Sci USA* 85 (11): 4046–4050

34 Petrone WF, English DK, Wong K, McCord JM (1980) Free radicals and inflammation:

superoxide-dependent activation of a neutrophil chemotactic factor in plasma. *Proc Natl Acad Sci USA* 77 (2): 1159–1163

35    Suzuki M, Inauen W, Kvietys PR, Grisham MB, Meininger C, Schelling ME, Granger HJ, Granger DN (1989) Superoxide mediates reperfusion-induced leukocyte-endothelial cell interactions. *Am J Physiol* 257 (5 Pt 2): H1740–H1745

36    Fraticelli A, Serrano CV Jr, Bochner BS, Capogrossi MC, Zweier JL (1996) Hydrogen peroxide and superoxide modulate leukocyte adhesion molecule expression and leukocyte endothelial adhesion. *Biochim Biophys Acta* 1310 (3): 251–259

37    Serrano CV Jr, Mikhail EA, Wang P, Noble B, Kuppusamy P, Zweier JL (1996) Superoxide and hydrogen peroxide induce CD18-mediated adhesion in the postischemic heart. *Biochim Biophys Acta* 1316 (3): 191–202

38    Haught WH, Mansour M, Rothlein R, Kishimoto TK, Mainolfi EA, Hendricks JB, Hendricks C, Mehta JL (1996) Alterations in circulating intercellular adhesion molecule-1 and L-selectin: further evidence for chronic inflammation in ischemic heart disease. *Am Heart J* 132 (1 Pt 1): 1–8

39    Collins T, Read MA, Neish AS, Whitley MZ, Thanos D, Maniatis T (1995) Transcriptional regulation of endothelial cell adhesion molecules: NF-kappa B and cytokine-inducible enhancers. *FASEB J* 9 (10): 899–909

40    Cross SL, Halden NF, Lenardo MJ, Leonard WJ (1989) Functionally distinct NF-kappa B binding sites in the immunoglobulin kappa and IL-2 receptor alpha chain genes. *Science* 244 (4903): 466–469

41    Brand K, Page S, Rogler G, Bartsch A, Brandl R, Knuechel R, Page M, Kaltschmidt C, Baeuerle PA, Neumeier D (1996) Activated transcription factor nuclear factor-kappa B is present in the atherosclerotic lesion. *J Clin Invest* 97 (7): 1715–1722

42    Bourcier T, Sukhova G, Libby P (1997) The nuclear factor kappa-B signaling pathway participates in dysregulation of vascular smooth muscle cells *in vitro* and in human atherosclerosis. *J Biol Chem* 272 (25): 15817–15824

43    Flohe L, Brigelius-Flohe R, Saliou C, Traber MG, Packer L (1997) Redox regulation of NF-kappa B activation. *Free Radic Biol Med* 22 (6): 1115–1126

44    Zweier JL, Broderick R, Kuppusamy P, Thompson-Gorman S, Lutty GA (1994) Determination of the mechanism of free radical generation in human aortic endothelial cells exposed to anoxia and reoxygenation. *J Biol Chem* 269 (39): 24156–24162

45    White CR, Darley-Usmar V, Berrington WR, McAdams M, Gore JZ, Thompson JA, Parks DA, Tarpey MM, Freeman BA (1996) Circulating plasma xanthine oxidase contributes to vascular dysfunction in hypercholesterolemic rabbits. *Proc Natl Acad Sci USA* 93 (16): 8745–8749

46    Xia Y, Tsai AL, Berka V, Zweier JL (1998) Superoxide generation from endothelial nitric-oxide synthase. A $Ca^{2+}$/calmodulin-dependent and tetrahydrobiopterin regulatory process. *J Biol Chem* 273 (40): 25804–25808

47    Pritchard KA Jr, Groszek L, Smalley DM, Sessa WC, Wu M, Villalon P, Wolin MS, Stemerman MB (1995) Native low-density lipoprotein increases endothelial cell nitric oxide synthase generation of superoxide anion. *Circ Res* 77 (3): 510–518

48   Xia Y, Roman LJ, Masters BS, Zweier JL (1998) Inducible nitric-oxide synthase generates superoxide from the reductase domain. *J Biol Chem* 273 (35): 22635–22639

49   Xia Y, Zweier JL (1997) Superoxide and peroxynitrite generation from inducible nitric oxide synthase in macrophages. *Proc Natl Acad Sci USA* 94 (13): 6954–6958

50   Rajagopalan S, Meng XP, Ramasamy S, Harrison DG, Galis ZS (1996) Reactive oxygen species produced by macrophage-derived foam cells regulate the activity of vascular matrix metalloproteinases *in vitro*. *J Clin Invest* 98 (11): 2572–2579

51   Berk BC.(1999) Redox signals that regulate the vascular response to injury. *Thromb Haemost* 82 (2): 810–817

52   Souza HP, Laurindo FRM, Berlowitz CO, Zweier JL (1999) Vascular Superoxide Generation By An Enzymatic System Different From Neutrophil NADPH Oxidase. *Circulation* 100 (18 Suppl I): 362

53   Mohazzab KM, Kaminski PM, Wolin MS (1994) NADH oxidoreductase is a major source of superoxide anion in bovine coronary artery endothelium. *Am J Physiol* 266 (6 Pt 2): H2568–H2572

54   Jones SA, O'Donnell VB, Wood JD, Broughton JP, Hughes EJ, Jones OT (1996) Expression of phagocyte NADPH oxidase components in human endothelial cells. *Am J Physiol* 271 (4 Pt 2): H1626–H1634

55   Suh YA, Arnold RS, Lassegue B, Shi J, Xu X, Sorescu D, Chung AB, Griendling KK, Lambeth JD (1999) Cell transformation by the superoxide-generating oxidase Mox1. *Nature* 401 (6748): 79–81

56   Fukui T, Ishizaka N, Rajagopalan S, Laursen JB, Capers Q 4th, Taylor WR, Harrison DG, de Leon H, Wilcox JN, Griendling KK (1997) p22phox mRNA expression and NADPH oxidase activity are increased in aortas from hypertensive rats. *Circ Res* 80 (1): 45–51

57   Inoue N, Kawashima S, Kanazawa K, Yamada S, Akita H, Yokoyama M (1998) Polymorphism of the NADH/NADPH oxidase p22 phox gene in patients with coronary artery disease. *Circulation* 97 (2): 135–137

58   Azumi H, Inoue N, Takeshita S, Rikitake Y, Kawashima S, Hayashi Y, Itoh H, Yokoyama M (1999) Expression of NADH/NADPH oxidase p22phox in human coronary arteries. *Circulation* 100 (14): 1494–1498

# Myocardial reperfusion: a state of inflammation

*Keith A. Youker, Nikolaos Frangogiannis and Mark L. Entman*

Department of Medicine, Section of Cardiovascular Sciences, Baylor College of Medicine, One Baylor Plaza, M.S. F-602, Houston, TX 77030, USA

## Introduction

Inflammation or reaction to injury is the major mechanism by which the immune system protects the host from invading organisms and remodels injured tissues. The process of inflammation, although aimed at protection and healing, can overwhelm the endogenous protection mechanisms and thereby cause unintentional extension of injury to the host tissues. The inflammatory response can be divided into an acute and a chronic phase with both positive and negative effects to the host tissues in both phases. Many of the cell types involved in inflammatory disease processes are similar although the time course may run from several days (such as in the case of reperfusion injury) to several decades, as occurs in atherosclerosis.

In this chapter, we will focus on our work, which uses a model of reperfusion of occluded myocardium as a model for inflammatory responses and its consequences. Our studies have primarily focused on cytokine and chemokine cascades, which initiate and perpetuate both the initial acute phase as well as the chronic healing phase, and on leukocytes, which participate in the process.

## Reperfusion as a model of inflammation

The normal heart receives oxygen and metabolic substrates from a series of coronary arteries that branch into smaller arterioles that descend into the myocardium and branch into smaller and smaller vessels until they become the capillary network. This network of capillaries supplies oxygen and metabolic substrates to the working cardiac myocyte and supporting tissues and cells. In humans, it has been shown that atherosclerosis begins at birth and continues throughout life, depositing atheromas in many larger cardiac vessels causing a narrowing of the lumen of vessels [1]. Thrombus formation and ulceration of an atherosclerotic plaque can cause partial or complete closure of a portion of the vascular tree particularly in these narrowed regions within the myocardium. Within minutes following a blockage, biochemical changes occur which cause a shift to anaerobic metabolism as demonstrated by Jennings and co-workers [2]. Most of the creatine phosphate in the affected tissues is lost within the first 1–3 min followed by a continuous net decrease in adenosine triphosphate. Ischemia is also attended by structural defects in the plasma membrane, defective cell membrane function and failure of the tissue to maintain high potassium and magnesium levels characteristic of normal myocardium [3, 4]. Ultrastructural studies have shown that within 15 min following coronary occlusion, mitochondrial cristae are broken accompanied by amorphous dense granules, nuclear swelling, distortion and disappearance of sarcomeric units [4].

Recent advances in medicine using procedures such as coronary artery bypass surgery, thrombolytic therapy and angioplasty have allowed the reopening of the coronary vessels and thereby salvage myocardium. Although reperfusion is necessary to resupply the region with oxygen, even short term occlusions (followed by reperfusion) can cause functional abnormalities such as ventricular arrhythmias, contractile dysfunction and vasomotor dysfunction [4–6]. Evidence suggests, however, that these shorter occlusions (less than 20 min) are not accompanied by any lethal injury and the myocardium ultimately recovers. The absence of any leukocyte response in these shorter occlusions also suggests that neutrophil associated extension of injury is only present secondary to lethal tissue injury [7, 8]. Reperfusion of occlusions longer than 20–30 min is associated with influx of neutrophils which have been linked to an extension of injury. Farb and co-workers demonstrated that myocardial infarct extension occurs in a border area during the reperfusion period following occlusion [9]. Their studies showed that while the myocardial cells in the ischemic border area are viable at the beginning of reperfusion, they progress to irreversible injury. This paradox of reperfusion being both detrimental and beneficial led to many studies focusing on the cellular mechanisms that occur upon reperfusion. An early clinical trial attempted to reduce infarct size by administration of the antiinflammatory methylprednisolone at the time of reperfusion in patients with acute myocardial infarction. Unfortunately, this therapeutic strategy led to an increased incidence of cardiac rupture, and frequent malignant ventricular dysrhythmias following multiple doses of the drug [10]. Thus, non-specific anti-inflammatory therapy also appeared to interfere with myocardial healing. This points to the fact that the inflammatory process is critical for repair of the injured myocardium.

Post-reperfusion inflammation in the heart in response to occlusion longer than 30 min shows many of the same characteristics of other types of inflammation, including release of chemical mediators and edema [11], cellular infiltration [12], and a decrease in contractile ability [13]. Many possible mediators have been identified, including lipid derived autacoids [14, 15], complement derived chemotactic factors [16–18] and cytokines [19–21]. A number of studies have addressed the role of leukocytes in acute myocardial injury with many studies now extending into the leukocyte's role in chronic healing of the infarcted myocardium. Substantial evidence now suggests that leukocyte influx into infarcted areas may promote tissue repair [22] by enhancing phagocytic response [23, 24], and by inducing production of cytokines and growth factors, which may modulate scar formation in angiogenesis [25, 26]. We have demonstrated, using a mouse model of occlusion and reperfusion, that even late reperfusion appears to reduce the degree of infarct expansion even under circumstances in which it no longer can alter infarct size. Reperfusion promoted more effective ventricular repair, decreased infarct expansion and allowed significant recovery of ventricular function [27].

## Cytokines and chemokines produced during occlusion

During the occlusion period of a coronary artery and prior to the onset of reperfusion, the classic complement pathway is activated [28, 29]. In an animal model of occlusion, cardiac lymph samples taken at the time of occlusion demonstrate the presence of C5a and C1q binding proteins. The C1q binding proteins have been identified to be of mitochondrial origin and contain cardiolipin, which is capable of activating the entire complement pathway [8]. C5a, resulting from activation of the complement cascade, is a very potent chemotactic factor for both neutrophils and monocytes, and likely plays a role in the immediate activation of leukocytes influxing into the region upon reperfusion.

Recently, we have demonstrated that cardiac mast cells found in the cardiac tissues surrounding arterioles and venules release preformed tumor necrosis factor α (TNFα) and histamine [30, 31]. It is suggested that degranulation of cardiac mast cells occurs, at least in part, before the onset of reperfusion and continues during reperfusion. Mast cell degranulation has been demonstrated in response to both adenosine and C5a, both of which are present in the ischemic myocardium [32, 33]. Histamine is an important inducer of surface expression of P-selectin through its action on Weibel-Palade bodies and P-selectin is considered critical for the margination of leukocytes. All these factors are then present at the time of reperfusion when leukocytes infiltrate the ischemic region (Fig. 1).

## Cytokines, chemokines and leukocytes in early reperfusion

Many of the factors produced during coronary artery occlusion have a direct impact in early reperfusion. Mast cell degranulation continues and is augmented by a response to both adenosine and C5a in addition to the reactive oxygen, all of which are produced during occlusion [32, 33]. Histamine derived from the granules of the mast cells induces the surface expression of P-selectin, increasing leukocyte margination. The release of preformed TNFα from mast cell granules can increase surface expression of adhesion molecules on endothelial cells such as intercellular adhesion molecule-1 (ICAM-1), and may initiate the cytokine cascade which follows by inducing interleukin-6 (IL-6), IL-8 and monocyte chemoattractant protein-1 (MCP-1)

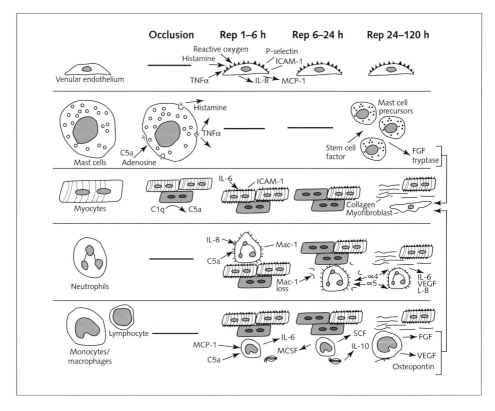

*Figure 1*
*This figure demonstrates some of the cells and factors involved in reperfusion injury and reperfusion-dependent healing of the myocardium at different times.*

expression in endothelial cells and infiltrating mononuclear cells. C5a also activates leukocyte integrins, which control transendothelial and cellular trafficking [16].

During this time there is a rapid cellular infiltration of both neutrophils and monocytic cells primarily into the jeopardized border zone surrounding the myocardial infarction [34]. Intravascular neutrophils migrate into the extracellular spaces and are initially detained in a viable border zone which contains cardiac myocytes expressing ICAM-1 [35], while monocyte migration into the infarct proceeds very rapidly [18]. This migration into the tissues is preceded by the early margination and trapping of the leukocytes within the venules within the first two hours [18, 36]. C5a appears to be the dominant chemotactic factor during these first two hours of reperfusion and is followed by increases in TGFβ$_1$, MCP-1 and IL-8 [16, 18, 37]. These extravascular activated leukocytes further amplify the inflammatory reaction by later production of other cytokines and growth factors.

The activated monocytes in the extravascular space begin to produce IL-6 in the first few hours of reperfusion most likely in response to TNFα release. IL-6 is capable of upregulating adhesion molecules such as ICAM-1 on the surface of viable myocardial cells [21]. Activated neutrophils express macrophage-1 antigen (Mac-1) (CD11b/CD18) and lymphocyte function-related molecule-1 (LFA-1) (CD11a/CD18) on their surface and are capable of binding to these ICAM-1-expressing cells. Adhesion of neutrophils to cardiac myocytes can be cytotoxic to the cardiac myocyte and thus extend the injury [38].

## Cytokines, chemokines and leukocytes following 6–24 h reperfusion

During this time of reperfusion, most leukocytes have begun to enter the infarcted region. The monocytes begin releasing stem cell factor (SCF) and macrophage colony stimulating factor (MCSF) [39, 40]. These cytokines are believed to be involved in the maturation of the monocytes into macrophages and the suppression of the acute response reaction. In addition, IL-10, a cytokine known to downregulate pro-inflammatory cytokine expression, begins being produced by T-lymphocytes in the ischemic and infarcted zones [40]. This may well begin the anti-inflammatory phase of cytokine expression; in addition, IL-10 induces monocyte tissue inhibitor of metalloproteinase-1 (TIMP-1) expression, facilitating scar formation.

The number of newly recruited leukocytes has declined by this time with functional changes of the leukocytes beginning [36]. We have recently demonstrated that Mac-1 is lost on the neutrophils at this stage with increases in other surface integrins [41]. Our studies indicate that after the loss of Mac-1 neutrophils migrate into the necrotic region where they remain for up to five days. We have recently demonstrated that following the loss of Mac-1, the neutrophils begin to express $\beta_1$ integrins including $\beta_1\alpha_4$ (VLA-4) and $\alpha_5\beta_1$ (VLA-5). We hypothesize that these integrins are necessary for the migration of the neutrophils into the necrotic zone. Monocytes, which constitutively express these $\beta_1$ integrins, have already moved into the necrotic zone and begin to shed their $\alpha_5$ integrin. Neutrophils which have reached the necrotic region begin to express IL-6, vascular endothelial growth factor (VEGF) and IL-8 as demonstrated by in situ hybridization for mRNA expression. It appears that integrin expression defines the migration pattern and time of migration of infiltrating leukocytes and these studies demonstrate that neutrophils may also be involved in initiation of the healing process.

## Cytokines, chemokines and leukocytes following 24–120 h reperfusion

Monocytes have fully matured into macrophages and begin production of fibroblast growth factor (FGF), vascular endothelial growth factor (VEGF) and osteopontin [40].

There is a marked increase in mast cells in the infarcted region by 72 h following reperfusion. The mast cell concentration is as high as 12-fold over that of normal myocardium [39]. We have found that this increase in mast cell numbers is a result of tissue infiltration of mast-cell precursors. Studies have shown that stem-cell factor (SCF) is induced in a subset of macrophages found in the infarct and is a potent growth and tactic factor for mast cell precursors. Mast cells are capable of secretion of pre-formed basic fibroblast growth factor (bFGF) and tryptase, which is a very potent mitogen for fibroblasts [42].

## Conclusions

Inflammation is a cascade of events including cellular and cytokine responses ultimately responsible for healing of the injured tissues. A number of factors, including activation of the complement cascade, contribute to the early acute phase as well as the subsequent healing and resolution phases. As discussed, many of the cells intimately involved in healing arrive very early in the acute phase. The interaction of infiltrating and resident cells mediated through inflammatory cytokines and growth factors regulate tissue repair. Our model of reperfusion of the ischemic myocardium allows us to study all these aspects and serves as a good model for understanding the molecular events which occur as we progress from the acute inflammatory phase to healing and tissue repair. While many studies demonstrate negative aspects of the inflammatory response, ultimately, this inflammatory response results in healing, scar formation and remodeling of the infarcted tissues. Non-specific anti-inflammatory therapeutic strategies will most likely negatively affect tissue repair. A better understanding of this process may allow a more targeted therapy for facilitating repair of the infracted and reperfused myocardium.

*Acknowledgements*
This research was funded by HL42550 from the National Institutes of Health, the American Heart Association and the DeBakey Heart Center. The authors wish to acknowledge the editorial assistance of Ms. Sharon Malinowski and Ms. Concepcion Mata.

## References

1    Ross R (1986) The pathogenesis of atherosclerosis-an update. *N Engl J Med* 314: 488–500
2    Jennings RB, Reimer KA (1981) Lethal myocardial ischemic injury. *Am J Pathol* 102: 241–255

3    Jennings RB, Sommers HM, Smyth GA, Flack HA, Limm H (1960) Myocardial necrosis induced by temporary occlusion of a coronary artery in the dog. *A M A Arch Pathol* 70: 68–72

4    Schaper J (1986) Ultrastructural changes of the myocardium in regional ischaemia and infarction. *Eur Heart J* 7: 3–9

5    Hearse DJ, Humphrey SM, Nayler WG, Slade A, Border D (1975) Ultrastructural damage associated with reoxygenation of the anoxic myocardium. *J Mol Cell Cardiol* 7: 315–324

6    Hearse DJ, Bolli R (1993) Reperfusion-induced injury: Manifestations, mechanisms and clinical relevance. *Trends Cardiovasc Med* 1: 233–240

7    Rossen RD, Swain JL, Michael LH, Weakley S, Giannini E, Entman ML (1985) Selective accumulation of the first component of complement and leukocytes in ischemic canine heart muscle: A possible initiator of an extra myocardial mechanism of ischemic injury. *Circ Res* 57: 119–130

8    Rossen RD, Michael LH, Kagiyama A, Savage HE , Hanson G, Reisberg JN, Moake JN, Kim SH, Weakly S, Giannini E et al (1988) Mechanism of complement activation following coronary artery occlusion: Evidence that myocardial ischemia causes release of constituents of myocardial subcellular origin which complex with the first component of complement. *Circ Res* 62: 572–584

9    Farb A, Kolodgie FD, Jenkins M, Virmani R (1993) Myocardial infarct extension during reperfusion after coronary artery occlusion: Pathologic evidence. *J Am Coll Cardiol* 21: 1245–1253

10   Roberts R, DeMello V, Sobel BE (1976) Deleterious effects of methylprednisolone in patients with myocardial infarction. *Circulation* 53 (suppl I): 204–206

11   Reimer KE, Jennings RB (1979) The changing anatomic reference base of evolving myocardial infarction. Underestimation of myocardial collateral blood flow and overestimation of experimental anatomic infarct size due to tissue oedema, haemorrhage and acute inflammation. *Circulation* 60: 866–876

12   Davies RA, Thakur A, Mathew L, Berger HJ, Wackers FJ, Gottschalk A, Zaret BL (1981) Imaging the inflammatory response to acute myocardial infarction in man using indium-111-labeled autologous platelets. *Circulation* 63: 826–832

13   Hillis LD, Braunwald E (1977) Myocardial ischemia. *N Engl J Med* 296: 1093–1096

14   Mullane KM, Salmon JA, Kraemer R (1987) Leukocyte-derived metabolites of arachidonic acid in ischemia-induced myocardial injury. *Fed Proc* 46: 2422–2433

15   Sakai K, Ito T, Ogawa K (1982) Roles of endogenous prostacyclin and thromboxane A2 in the ischemic canine heart. *J Cardio Pharm* 4: 129–135

16   Dreyer WJ, Michael LH, Nguyen T, Smith CW, Anderson DC, Entman ML, Rossen RD (1992) Kinetics of C5a release in cardic lymph of dogs experiencing coronary artery ischemia-reperfusion injury. *Circ Res* 71: 1518–1524

17   Rossen RD, Michael LH, Hawkins HK, Youker K, Dreyer WJ, Baughn RE, Entman ML (1994) Cardiolipin-protein complexes and initiation of complement activation after coronary artery occlusion. *Circ Res* 75: 546–555

18  Birdsall HH, Green DM, Trial J, Youker KA, Burns AR, Mackay CR, LaRosa GJ, Hawkins HK, Smith CW, Michael LH et al (1997) Complement C5a TGF-β1, and MCP-1, in sequence, induce migration of monocytes into ischemic canine myocardium within the first one to five hours after reperfusion. *Circulation* 95: 684–692

19  Elchenholz PW, Elchacker PQ, Hoffman WD, Banks SM, Parrillo JE, Danner RL, Natanson C (1992) Tumor necrosis factor challenges in canines: patterns of cardiovascular dysfunction. *Am J Physiol* 263: H668–H675

20  Frangogiannis NG, Youker KA, Rossen RD, Gwechenberger M, Lindsey ML, Mendoza LH, Michael LH, Ballantyne CM , Smith CW, Entman ML (1998) The microcirculation as a foundation of cardiovascular disease. Cytokines and the microcirculation in ischemia and reperfusion. *J Mol Cell Cardiol* 30: 2567–2576

21  Youker KA, Smith CW, Anderson DC, Miller D , Michael LH, Rossen RD, Entman ML (1992) Neutrophil adherence to isolated adult cardiac myocytes: Induction by cardiac lymph collected during ischemia and reperfusion. *J Clin Invest* 89: 602–609

22  Morita M, Kawashima S, Ueno M, Kubota A, Iwasaki T (1993) Effects of late reperfusion on infarct expansion and infarct healing in conscious rats. *Am J Pathol* 143: 419–430

23  Boyle MP, Weisman HF (1993) Limitation of infarct expansion and ventricular remodeling by late reperfusion. *Circulation* 88: 2872–2883

24  Pierce GF, Mustoe TA, Lingelbach J, Masakowski VR, Griffin GL, Senior RM , Deuel TF (1989) Platelet-derived growth factor and transforming growth factor-β enhance tissue repair activities by unique mechanisms. *J Cell Biol* 109: 429–440

25  Rizzo V, Defoux DO (1996) Mast cell activation accelerates the normal rate of angiogenesis in the chick chorioallantoic membrane. *Microvasc Res* 52: 245–257

26  Gruber BL, Marchese MJ, Kew R (1995) Angiogenic factors stimulate mast-cell migration. *Blood* 86: 2488–2493

27  Michael LH, Ballantyne CM, Zachariah JP, Gould KE, Pocius JS, Taffet GE, Hartley CJ, Pham TT, Daniel SL, Funk E et al (1999) Myocardial infarction and remodeling in mice: Effect of reperfusion. *Am J Physiol* 277: H660–H668

28  Pinckard RN, Olson MS, Kelley RE, Detter DH, Palmer JD, O'Rourke RA, Goldfein S (1973) Antibody-independent activation of human C1 after interaction with heart subcellular membranes. *J Immunol* 110: 1376–1382

29  Rossen RD, Laughter AH, Orson FM, Flagge FP, Cashaw JL, Sumaya CV (1985) Human peripheral blood monocytes release a 30,000 dalton factor (30 Kd MF) that stimulates immunoglobulin production by activated B cells. *J Immunol* 135: 3289–3297

30  Frangogiannis NG, Burns AR, Michael LH, Entman ML (1999) Histochemical and morphological characteristics of canine cardiac mast cell. *Histochem J* 31: 221–229

31  Frangogiannis NG, Lindsey ML, Michael LH, Youker KA, Bressler RB, Mendoza LH, Spengler RN, Smith CW, Entman ML (1998) Resident cardiac mast cells degranulate and release preformed TNF-α initiating the cytokine cascade in myocardial ischemia/reperfusion. *Circ* 98: 699–710

32    Linden J (1994) Cloned adenosine A3 receptors: pharmacological properties, species differences and receptor functions. *Trends in Pharm Sc* 15: 298–306

33    Ito BR, Engler RL, Del Balzo U (1993) Role of cardiac mast cells in complement C5a-induced myocardial ischemia. *Am J Physiol* 264: H1346–H1354

34    Hawkins HK, Entman ML, Zhu JY, Youker KA, Berens K, Dore M, Smith CW (1996) Acute inflammatory reaction after myocardial ischemic injury and reperfusion. Development and use of a neutrophil-specific antibody. *Am J Pathol* 148: 1957–1969

35    Youker KA, Hawkins HK, Kukielka GL, Perrard JL, Michael LH, Ballantyne CM, Smith CW, Entman ML (1994) Molecular evidence for induction of intercellular adhesion molecule-1 in the viable border zone associated with ischemia-reperfusion injury of the dog heart. *Circulation* 89: 2736–2746

36    Dreyer WJ, Michael LH, West MS, Smith CW, Rothlein R, Rossen RD, Anderson DC, Entman ML (1991) Neutrophil accumulation in ischemic canine myocardium: Insights into the time course, distribution, and mechanism of localization during early reperfusion. *Circulation* 84: 400–411

37    Kukielka GL, Smith CW, LaRosa GJ, Manning AM , Mendoza LH, Hughes BJ, Youker KA, Hawkins HK, Michael LH, Rot A et al (1995) Interleukin-8 gene induction in the myocardium following ischemia and reperfusion *in vivo. J Clin Invest* 95: 89–103

38    Entman ML, Youker KA, Shoji T, Kukielka GL, Shappell SB, Taylor AA, Smith CW (1992) Neutrophil induced oxidative injury of cardiac myocytes: A compartmented system requiring CD11b/CD18-ICAM-1 adherence. *J Clin Invest* 90: 1335–1345

39    Frangogiannis NG, Perrard JL, Mendoza LH, Burns AR, Lindsey ML, Ballantyne CM , Michael LH, Smith CW, Entman ML (1998) Stem cell factor induction is associated with mast cell accumulation following myocardial ischemia and reperfusion. *Circ* 98: 687–698

40    Frangogiannis NG, Youker KA, Rossen RD, Gwechenberger M, Lindsey MH, Mendoza LH, Michael LH, Ballantyne CM , Smith CW, Entman ML (1998) Cytokines and the microcirculation in ischemia and reperfusion. *J Mol Cell Cardiol* 30 : 2567–2576

41    Youker KA, Beirne J, Lee J, Michael LH, Smith CW, Entman ML (2000) Time-dependent loss of Mac-1 from infiltrating neutrophils in the reperfused myocardium. *J Immunol* 164: 2752–2758

42    Ruoss SJ, Hartmann T, Caughey GH (1991) Mast cell tryptase is a mitogen for cultured fibroblasts. *J Clin Invest* 88: 493–499

# LOX-1, a potential inflammatory mediator in atherosclerosis

*Mingyi Chen and Tatsuya Sawamura*

National Cardiovascular Center Research Institute, Suita, Osaka 565-8565, Japan

## Introduction

Atherosclerotic lesions contain a significant number of lipid-laden foam cells and are associated with an inflammatory state [1]. Low-density lipoprotein (LDL) modified by oxidation exhibits a variety of proinflammatory potentials. Oxidized LDL (ox-LDL) accumulated in the atherosclerotic lesions is the major culprit in atherogenesis [2]. Ox-LDL induces inflammatory responses in the vessel wall, including endothelial dysfunction, monocyte chemotaxis, and smooth muscle cell proliferation. Specifically, multiple inflammatory cytokines/growth factors are involved in this process [1]. The influence of ox-LDL on cellular properties is mediated by binding to specific receptors, also characterized as "scavenger receptor". Lectin-like oxidized LDL receptor-1 (LOX-1) was initially identified in aortic endothelial cells [3]. Subsequent studies indicated that it is also expressed in macrophages, smooth muscle cells and fibroblast cells , the major cell types in the vessel wall [4–6].

The potential role for LOX-1 in vascular diseases is suggested by three lines of evidence: (a) LOX possesses a strong activity for the binding and internalizing, and proteolytic degradation of oxidized LDL, the chief culprit in atherogenesis; (b) LOX-1 is dynamically upregulated by many pro-atherogenic risk factors; (c) LOX-1 is present on atheroma-derived cells *in vitro* and it accumulates in human and animal atherosclerosis lesions *in vivo* [7–16]. Thus, LOX-1 is a novel molecule expected to be linked to the initiation and progression of atherosclerosis via interaction with oxidized LDL.

## Cloning strategy and characterization

Vascular endothelial cells internalize and degrade ox-LDL through a putative receptor-mediated pathway distinct from macrophage scavenger receptors. To identify the potential gene(s) encoding the endothelial ox-LDL receptors, we transfected mammalian cells with a cDNA expression library derived from bovine aortic

Inflammatory and Infectious Basis of Atherosclerosis, edited by Jay L. Mehta

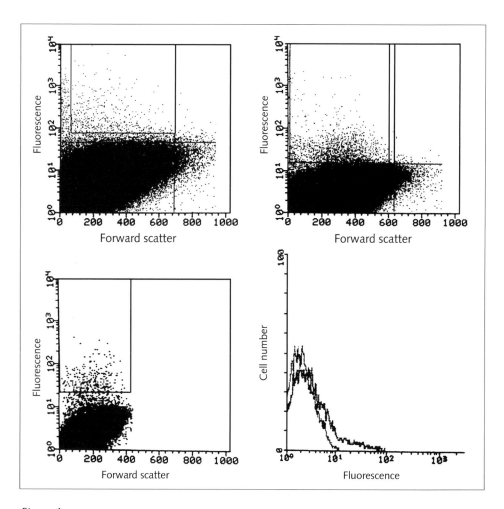

*Figure 1*
*Expression cloning of the endothelial cell specific Ox-LDL receptor, LOX-1. A cDNA library*
*of bovine aortic endothelial cells was constructed in mammalian expression vector pME18s*
*and transfected into COS-7 cells. The cells were incubated with DiI-labelled Ox-LDL, and*
*positive cells were sorted by a FACS Vantage cell sorter (Becton Dickinson). After three*
*rounds of selection, plasmids from a single clone were recovered and individually transfect-*
*ed into COS-7 cells. After sequencing, it was characterized as lectin-like oxidized LDL recep-*
*tor, LOX-1.*

endothelial cells and assayed for the ability to sequester DiI-labeled Ox-LDL. After
multiple rounds of transfection-recovery, we successfully identified a cDNA encoding an endothelial cell-surface receptor for ox-LDL, which was designated as lectin-

like ox-LDL receptor-1, LOX-1 (Fig. 1). It possessed the activity of binding, internalizing, and proteolytic degradation of ox-LDL, and therefore, it might play a critical role in the pathogenesis of atherosclerosis and vascular diseases [17].

The cDNA for LOX-1 cloned from bovine aortic endothelial cells contained an open reading frame of 810 base pairs that encodes a protein of 270 amino acid residues. LOX-1 is a type II membrane protein that structurally belongs to the C-type lectin family. Structure analysis shows that it consists of four functional domains: the cytoplasmic domain; the transmembrane domain; the neck domain; and the extracellular lectin-like domain (from N-terminus to C-terminus). Shortly afterwards, we cloned a cDNA encoding the human homologue of LOX-1 by screening a human lung cDNA library with the bovine LOX-1 cDNA as probe. The cells that express human LOX-1 show uptake of DiI-labeled Ox-LDL. The predicted 273 amino acid residues of human LOX-1 protein are 72% identical to their bovine counterpart [17]. Mouse and rat homologues have also been identified, and found to share similarities with human and bovine LOX-1 except that they possess a longer neck domain encoded by the unique triple-repeat sequences [11, 18]. Recently, the rabbit counterpart of LOX-1 was identified, and characterized as being closely related to human LOX-1 both in sequence and domain structure organization [16]. Notably, sequence analysis indicated that LOX-1 was highly conserved among different species, especially on the six repeats of cysteine in the lectin-like domain. This is consistent with the predicted function as a ligand binding domain (Fig. 2).

Northern blot analysis revealed that human LOX-1 is expressed as a 2.8 kb mRNA in vascular endothelium and vascular-rich organs such as placenta and lung. The extracelluar C-terminal domains of bovine LOX-1 contain four potential N-linked glycosylation sites, therefore, a 50 kDa band was displayed in a non-reducing immnoblot analysis although the calculated Mr was only 30872 Da [17].

Unexpectedly, LOX-1 in endothelium has no homology to any of the known macrophage scavenger receptors. In contrast, it shares significant identity with NK cell receptors, such as CD94 (KLRD1) and NKR-P1 (KLRB1), which are involved in target-cell recognition and NK cell activation. As a new member of the NK cell gene complex, LOX-1 may induce various functional changes in endothelium. In addition, LOX-1 may have some potential (patho)physiological functions in cell-cell interactions as exhibited by NK cell receptors [17].

## Structural organization and chromosomal assignment of the human LOX-1 gene

To advance the knowledge on the genomic organization and the regulation of the cellular expression of the LOX-1 gene, we have determined the structural organization and 5'-proximal flanking region of human LOX-1. The human LOX-1 gene is

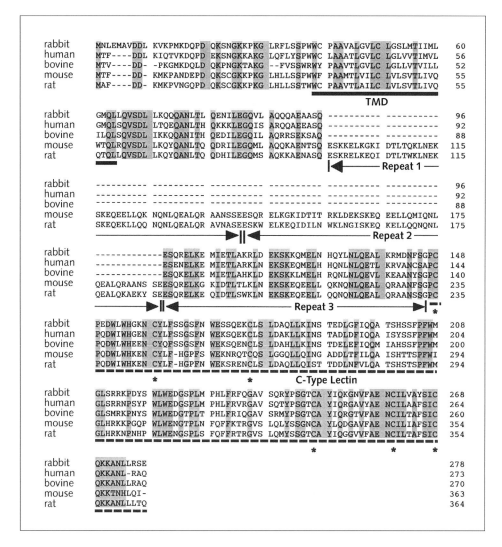

Figure 2

*Alignment of the deduced amino acid sequences of human, bovine, mouse, rat and rabbit LOX-1. The putative transmembrane domain (TMD) is indicated by the bold underline, and the C-type lectin domain is indicated by a dashed line. The conserved six cysteine residues are indicated by asterisks.*

encoded by six exons that span approximately 15 kilobases on the human genome. Typically, the LOX-1 gene structure suggests a relationship between exon/intron architecture and protein structure. Exon 1 encodes the mRNA 5'-untranslated region and the cytoplasmic domain. Exon 2 encodes the remainder of cytoplasmic domain and the transmembrane domain. Exon 3 encodes the neck domain. Exons 4–6 encode the lectin domain, and the 3'-untranslated region. The major transcription initiation site of the human LOX-1 gene is located 29 nucleotides downstream of the TATA box and 60 nucleotides upstream from the translation start codon. Sequence analysis of the proximal 5'-flanking region of the gene reveals the existence of several potential cis-regulatory elements such as GATA-2 and c-ets-1 binding elements, 12-O-tetradecanoylphorbol 13-acetate (TPA)-responsive elements, and a shear-stress element that might contribute to the transcriptional regulation of the LOX-1 gene in an inducible manner. Using fluorescence *in situ* hybridization, the LOX-1 gene was localized to the p12.3–13.2 region of human chromosome 12, where the genes of the natural killer cell receptors cluster. These results demonstrate that the LOX-1 gene is a new member of the lectin-like NK gene complex with a unique expression profile [19, 20].

## Pathophysiology and regulated expression of LOX-1

LOX-1 is expressed *in vivo* in aortic, carotid, thoracic and coronary arteries and veins, and upregulated in pathological conditions of vascular disease such as hypertension and atherosclerosis [10, 14, 17]. Recent investigations have revealed that LOX-1 is transcriptionally upregulated by inflammatory cytokines (tumor necrosis factor (TNF), phorbol 12-myristate 13-acetate (PMA), lipopolysaccharides (LPS), interleukin-1 (IL-1), and transforming growth factor β (TGFβ)), angiotensin II, and shear-stress in a time and dose-dependent manner [7–9, 12, 21]. Interestingly, LOX-1 is also upregulated by both ox-LDL and its atherogenic lipid constituent, LysoPC [19, 22]. In addition to the critical expression in endothelium, LOX-1 has been identified in transformed smooth muscle cells and activated macrophages [4, 9, 14]. All these observations suggest that LOX-1 is dynamically regulated by various pathophysiological stimuli that are closely related to atherogenesis [23]. Specifically, the profound effect of inflammatory mediators might be of great significance. Thus, a vicious cycle of inflammation, upregulation of LOX-1, and further inflammation can be maintained in the affected arteries. Immunostaining studies on human and WHHL rabbit atherosclerotic tissues have shown a characteristic pattern of LOX-1 expression. LOX-1 was most prominently stained in the endothelial cells of early atherosclerotic lesions. The moderate expression in the subendothelial space co-localized with both smooth muscle cells and macrophages. More importantly, LOX-1 was also observed in the endothelium of non-lesion areas of WHHL rabbit aortas, suggesting the upregulation of LOX-1 was a critical early event in atherogenesis [16]. Recently, we have determined that LOX-1 expression was also enhanced by diabetes both *in vitro* and *in vivo*. Therefore, the additive or synergistic effects of the combination of inflammation, hyperlipidemia, hypertension, and diabetes in the

*Table 1 - Multiple ligands of LOX-1.*

Oxidized LDL
Acetylated LDL
Anionic phospholipids
Carrageenan
Poly (I)
Apoptotic cells
Aged red blood cells
Activated platelets

regulation of LOX-1 expression have been suggested. The factors or circumstances which regulate LOX-1 expression are summarized in Table 1.

## Ligand specificity of LOX-1

Although LOX-1 was initially cloned by binding to *in vitro* ox-LDL, the true *in vivo* physiological ligand of LOX-1 is still ambiguous, even the exact ligand epitope for LOX-1 in LDL still remains to be clarified. Preliminary studies show that LOX-1 recognizes the protein moiety of ox-LDL [24]. We have confirmed the presence of multiple ligands for LOX-1, including ox-LDL, acetylated LDL, poly(I), carrageenan, anionic phospholipids, apoptotic/aged cells and activated platelets (Tab. 2) [25]. Therefore, LOX-1 is a multifunctional receptor that binds and internalizes a diverse array of ligands. After binding to its ligand, ox-LDL can be either internalized by phagocytosis, or remain on the cell surface. LOX-1 appears to modulate endothelial cell functions relevant to both physiological and pathological conditions. Under physiological conditions, LOX-1 may serve to scavenge/clean up circulating aged/apoptotic cells and waste materials to maintain homeostasis of the internal environment within the body. However, in the pathological states, LOX-1 recognizes ox-LDL and mediates the various detrimental effects of ox-LDL on endothelial cell activation which is implicated in the initiation and development of atherosclerosis [23–25].

## Potential studies

The identification of the cellular ligand of LOX-1 opens up a new field to investigate the potential physiological roles of LOX-1. During the course of aging and

Table 2 - Regulated expression of LOX-1

| Inducing factors | Inhibition factors | Relevant pathological condition |
|---|---|---|
| TNFα | ACEI | Hypertension |
| IL-1β | HMG-CoA reductase inhibitors | Hyperlipidemia |
| IFNγ | | Atherosclerosis |
| TGFβ | | Diabetes mellitus |
| Shear stress | | |
| Phorbol esters (PMA) | | |
| Lipopolysaccharide (LPS) | | |
| Angiotensin II | | |
| Oxidized LDL | | |
| Lysophosphatidylcholine | | |

ACEI, angiotensin converting enzyme inhibitors; HMG-CoA, 3-hydroxy-3-methylglutaryl coenzyme A

apoptosis, phosphatidylserine (PS) is exposed on the cell surface which can be recognized by LOX-1. This finding prompted us to think about another relevant setting, that of platelet activation, which is also manifested by PS exposition. It was very exciting to find that LOX-1 indeed functioned as an adhesion molecule for platelets. The binding activity of platelets to LOX-1 was greatly enhanced by activation, and competitively blocked by PS-binding protein, annexin V [26]. These data indicate that LOX-1 might be involved in the pathogenesis of thrombosis. Due to its high affinity in binding, internalizing, and degradation of ox-LDL, presently, it may be suggested that the key role of LOX-1 is to recognize oxidative modified LDL in the circulation. The critical issue is how the ox-LDL/LOX-1 system initiates endothelial cell activation or dysfunction. One explanation is that tethering of an oxidizing stimulus (ox-LDL) to endothelium will induce cellular oxidative stress resulting in activation of NF-κB. In addition, we speculate that ox-LDL *via* activation of the endothelial receptor, LOX-1, recruits intracellular signal transduction and regulates the expression of many genes in endothelial cells. In the cytosolic tail of LOX-1, several potential phosphorylation sites are indeed present, suggesting phosphorylation of these sites may transmit biological signals or regulate endothelium function [17]. Taken together, it may be suggested that ox-LDL interacts with endothelial cells mainly *via* LOX-1, making it a more significant risk factor for atherosclerosis.

In conclusion, all the findings support that LOX-1 is a novel pathway linking ox-LDL to atherogenesis. Thus, inhibition of LOX-1 may provide a therapeutic target in atherosclerosis.

# References

1    Ross R (1999) Atherosclerosis – an inflammatory disease. *N Engl J Med* 340: 115–126
2    Steinberg D (1997) Low density lipoprotein oxidation and its pathobiological significance. *J Biol Chem* 272: 20963–20966
3    Steinbrecher UP (1999) Receptors for oxidized low density lipoprotein. *Biochim Biophys Acta* 1436: 279–298
4    Moriwaki H, Kume N, Kataoka H, Murase T, Nishi E, Sawamura T, Masaki T, Kita T (1998) Expression of lectin-like oxidized low density lipoprotein receptor-1 in human and murine macrophages: upregulated expression by TNF-alpha. *FEBS Lett* 440: 29–32
5    Draude G, Hrboticky N, Lorenz RL (1999) The expression of the lectin-like oxidized low-density lipoprotein receptor (LOX-1) on human vascular smooth muscle cells and monocytes and its down-regulation by lovastatin. *Biochem Pharmacol* 57: 383–386
6    Yoshida H, Kondratenko N, Green S, Steinberg D, Quehenberger O (1998) Identification of the lectin-like receptor for oxidized low-density lipoprotein in human macrophages and its potential role as a scavenger receptor. *Biochem J* 334: 9–13
7    Kume N, Murase T, Moriwaki H, Aoyama T, Sawamura T, Masaki T, Kita T (1998) Inducible expression of lectin-like oxidized LDL receptor-1 in vascular endothelial cells. *Circ Res* 83: 322–327
8    Murase T, Kume N, Korenaga R, Ando J, Sawamura T, Masaki T, Kita T (1998) Fluid shear stress transcriptionally induces lectin-like oxidized LDL receptor-1 in vascular endothelial cells. *Circ Res* 83: 328–333
9    Nagase M, Abe J, Takahashi K, Ando J, Hirose S, Fujita T (1998) Genomic organization and regulation of expression of the lectin-like oxidized low-density lipoprotein receptor (LOX-1) gene. *J Biol Chem* 273: 33702–33707
10   Nagase M, Hirose S, Sawamura T, Masaki T, Fujita T (1997) Enhanced expression of endothelial oxidized low-density lipoprotein receptor (LOX-1) in hypertensive rats. *Biochem Biophys Res Commun* 237: 496–498
11   Nagase M, Hirose S, Fujita T (1998) Unique repetitive sequence and unexpected regulation of expression of rat endothelial receptor for oxidized low-density lipoprotein (LOX-1). *Biochem J* 330: 1417–1422
12   Li DY, Zhang YC, Philips MI, Sawamura T, Mehta JL (1999) Upregulation of endothelial receptor for oxidized low-density lipoprotein (LOX-1) in cultured human coronary artery endothelial cells by angiotensin II type 1 receptor activation. *Circ Res* 84: 1043–1049
13   Morawietz H, Rueckschloss U, Niemann B, Duerrschmidt N, Galle J, Hakim K, Zerkowski HR, Sawamura T, Holtz J (1999) Angiotensin II induces LOX-1, the human endothelial receptor for oxidized low-density lipoprotein. *Circulation* 100: 899–902
14   Kataoka H, Kume N, Miyamoto S, Minami M, Moriwaki H, Murase T, Sawamura T, Masaki T, Hashimoto N, Kita T (1999) Expression of lectin-like oxidized low-density lipoprotein receptor-1 in human atherosclerotic lesions. *Circulation* 99: 3110–3117
15   Aoyama T, Sawamura T, Fujiwara H, Masaki T (1999) Induction of lectin-like oxidized

LDL receptor by oxidized LDL and lysophosphatidylcholine in cultured endothelial cells. *J Mol Cell Cardiol* 31: 2101–2114

16  Chen M, Kakutani M, Minami M, Kataoka H, Kume N, Narumiya S, Kita T, Masaki T, Sawamura T (2000) Increased expression of LOX-1 in the initial atherosclerotic lesions of WHHL rabbits. *Arterioscler Thromb Vasc Biol* 20: 1107–1115

17  Sawamura T, Kume N, Aoyama T, Moriwaki H, Hoshikawa H, Aiba Y, Tanaka T, Miwa S, Katsura Y, Kita T et al. (1997) An endothelial receptor for oxidized low-density lipoprotein. *Nature* 386: 73–77

18  Hoshikawa H, Sawamura T, Kakutani M, Aoyama T, Nakamura T, Masaki T (1998) High affinity binding of oxidized LDL to mouse lectin-like oxidized LDL receptor (LOX-1). *Biochem Biophys Res Commun* 245: 841–846

19  Aoyama T, Sawamura T, Furutani Y, Matsuoka R, Yoshida MC, Fujiwara H, Masaki T (1999) Structure and chromosomal assignment of the human lectin-like oxidized low-density-lipoprotein receptor-1 (LOX-1) gene. *Biochem J* 339: 177–184

20  Yamanaka S, Zhang XY, Miura K, Kim S, Iwao H (1998) The human gene encoding the lectin-type oxidized LDL receptor (OLR1) is a novel member of the natural killer gene complex with a unique expression profile. *Genomics* 54: 191–199

21  Minami M, Kume N, Kataoka H, Moriwaki H, Morimoto M, Sawamura T, Masaki T, Kita T (1999) Transforming Growth Factor-β1 increase the expression of lectin-like oxidized LDL receptor-1 (LOX-1) in vascular endothelial cells and smooth muscle cells. *Circulation* 100 (suppl I): I–743. Abstract 3923

22  Mehta JL, Li DY (1998) Identification and autoregulation of receptor for ox-LDL in cultured human coronary artery endothelial cells. *Biochem Biophys Res Commun* 248: 511–514

23  Kita T (1999) LOX-1, a possible clue to the missing link between hypertension and atherogenesis. *Circ Res* 84: 1113–1115

24  Moriwaki H, Kume N, Sawamura T, Aoyama T, Hoshikawa H, Ochi H, Nishi E, Masaki T, Kita T (1998) Ligand Specificity of LOX-1, a novel endothelial receptor for oxidized low density lipoprotein. *Arterioscler Thromb Vasc Biol* 18: 1541–1547

25  Oka K, Sawamura T, Kikuta K, Itokawa S, Kume N, Kita T, Masaki T (1998) Lectin-like oxidized low-density lipoprotein receptor 1 mediates phagocytosis of aged/apoptotic cells in endothelial cells. *Proc Natl Acad Sci USA* 95: 9535–9540

26  Kakutani M, Masaki T, Sawamura T (2000) A novel platelet-endothelium interaction mediated by lectin-like oxidized LDL receptor-1. *Proc Natl Acad Sci USA* 97: 360–364

# Angiotensin II as a mediator of inflammation in atherosclerosis

*M. Ian Phillips, Shuntaro Kagiyama, Hongjiang Chen and Jay L. Mehta*

University of Florida, Departments of Physiology and Medicine, College of Medicine, Box 100274, Gainesville, FL 32610, USA

## Introduction

Atherosclerosis is the result of a complicated cascade of events in blood vessels leading to a reduction in arterial lumen and blockage. The disease may be considered an inflammatory disease, which results from the combined presence of hypercholesterolemia, high blood pressure and an activated renin-angiotensin system (RAS). The progression is through a number of steps involving endothelial cells, monocytes/macrophages and vascular smooth muscle cells (VSMC). The progression to complete blockage of the artery is a slow process taking several decades, but the end result can be sudden death, acute myocardial ischemia, or stroke.

In the initial stages of atherosclerosis, leukocytes (monocytes) passing through the vessel, begin to "roll" instead of passing unhindered over the luminal surface of the blood vessel. The "rolling" is because of vascular cell adhesion molecules (VCAMs) being expressed on the surface of endothelial cells. These include selectins (P & E and cell adhesion molecules (CAMs)), which can be activated by angiotensin II (Ang II). The RAS exists as an endocrine system, resulting in circulating Ang II, and as a paracrine tissue system resulting in local production of Ang II [1, 2]. By "sticking" to the endothelial cells which make up a monolayer around the lumen of blood vessels, the leukocytes adhere to the cell surface and become capable of penetrating between endothelial cells and entering the subendothelial layer. Lipid peroxidation transforms low-density lipoprotein (LDL) into oxidized LDL (ox-LDL) which binds to scavenger receptors on the monocytes. This changes the monocyte to a macrophage, leading to internal vesicles containing ox-LDL and various forms of lipids, plus cholesteryl ester. The monocytes/macrophages, which accumulate under the endothelial cell layer, become "foam cells" because they are full of lipid-rich vesicles. From the lumen, the protrusion of foam cells gives the appearance of "fatty streaks", the first visible sign of atherosclerotic disease. An accumulation of foam cells protrudes into lumen, breaking the protective monolayer of endothelial cells. The ulceration of the endothelium leads to an inflammatory response. Platelets arrive, and release growth factors. Platelets have Ang II receptors and local tissue

Ang II may serve as a vascular marker of injury for platelets. Simultaneous with the formation of foam cells, release of growth factors leads to proliferation and migration of VSMCs to form a neointima of multiplying VSMCs which begin to occlude the arterial lumen. Activation of nuclear factor kappa B (NF-κB) in the VSMCs and macrophages plays a critical role by stimulating chemokines into the neointima. The chemokines attract platelet monocytes, inflammatory cells and macrophages, which in turn attract CD4 T helper cells. The result is an inflamed atherosclerotic plaque filling the blood vessel lumen.

An important link between Ang II and inflammation is the central role of NF-κB, which is stimulated by Ang II [3]. NF-κB activation regulates the gene expression of interleukin-6 (IL-6), interleukin-8 (IL-8), and monocyte chemoattractant protein-1 (MCP-1) [4]. MCP-1 attracts T lymphocytes, and together with growth factors such as platelet derived growth factor β (PDGF-β) stimulates VSMC proliferation so that more cells migrate into the inflamed region. Ang II stimulates collagen I production from the VSMC and fibrosis of the atherosclerotic plaque occurs which can render the plaque stable [5]. Calcification of the plaque may also involve Ang II which stimulates osteopontin, a protein that binds $Ca^{2+}$ [6]. In the last stage of atherosclerosis, the fibrous cap becomes the target of inflammatory cell activity at the vulnerable thinner regions around the shoulder of the cap leading to its rupture. Plaque rupture causes most of the acute complications of atherosclerotic disease including acute myocardial ischemia and stroke [7]. To understand the role of Ang II in this developmental process, we will focus this brief review on the three cellular elements involved. These are the macrophage, or monocyte, the endothelial cells and the VSMC.

## Ang II and the macrophage

Figure 1 shows some of the pathways of macrophages leading to foam cell formation. The formation of foam cells from macrophages is due to accumulation of LDL-cholesterol and is one of the first stages in the developmental stages of atherosclerosis. Ang II increases cholesterol biosynthesis *per se* in macrophages [8]. In addition, Ang II can increase macrophage cholesterol influx indirectly [9]. Ang II acts as an oxidant on the LDL to form ox-LDL on endothelial cells [10]. The scavenger receptors on the monocytes/macrophages are proteoglycous which take up ox-LDL. Ang II also can bind to LDL to form an Ang II-LDL complex, which is also taken up preferentially by macrophages [11]. The uptake of Ang II-LDL complex takes place via scavenger receptors on the cell surface of macrophages. The uptake of ox-LDL may also occur through recently described lectin-like receptors [10]. Synthesis of cholesterol in macrophages has been demonstrated by Keidar et al. [8] to be enhanced by Ang II stimulation through the angiotensin type 1 receptor ($AT_1R$). The conclusion from their study is that $AT_1R$ antagonists, such as losartan, could be ben-

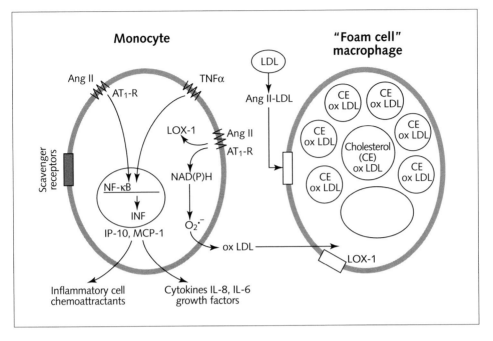

*Figure 1*

*Monocyte/macrophage: Angiotensin II (Ang II) and tumor necrosis factor (TNFα) activate nuclear transcription factor kappa B (NF-κB). NF-κB regulates monocyte stimulating protein (MCP-1), cytokines IL-8 and IL-6, and growth factors. Ang II also stimulates an increase in scavenger receptors. Through the NAD(P)H oxidase pathway, Ang II increases superoxide and reactive oxygen species ($O^-_2$) which oxidize low density lipids (LDL), activate NF-κB, and upregulate lectin-like receptors for ox LDL (LOX-1). The monocyte transforms to macrophage in the subendothelial layer and takes up oxidized LDL to become a "foam cell". Ang II also directly combines to LDL to form Ang II-LDL, which is also taken up in the foam cell. The ox-LDL cholesterol esters (CE) and free cholesterol fill up large vesicles that give the cells their "foam-like" appearance. The accumulation of foam cells raises the subendothelial surface of the lumen to form "fatty streaks". Further amassing of the macrophages disrupts the endothelial cell wall and injures the blood vessel, which triggers an inflammatory response. $AT_1$-R, antiotensin type 1 receptor.*

eficial in reducing the effect of Ang II on increased cholesterol biosynthesis. Further, since macrophages appear to have a complete tissue RAS, including the ecto-enzyme angiotensin converting enzyme (ACE), application of ACE inhibitors would also decrease cholesterol synthesis [12]. The biosynthetic pathway of cholesterol synthesis involves the rate-limiting enzyme, HMG CoA reductase. Ang II increases HMG CoA reductase specific mRNA in a dose-dependent fashion [8]. In the presence of losartan, the stimulatory effects of Ang II can be prevented although the exact path-way for this effect has not been established. While Ang II is known to affect phos-phorylation by the activation of mitogen active protein (MAP) kinase and serine-threonine kinases, which activate nuclear transcription factors, it is not certain that Ang II does this directly. It has been suggested that second messengers from the stim-ulation of the $AT_1R$ must activate a growth factor receptor, such as epidermal growth factor (EGF), or PDGF in order to activate the MAP kinase pathway [11].

A nuclear transcription factor that plays a very central role in Ang II effects is the redox-sensitive NF-κB [3]. Ang II stimulates NF-κB via $AT_1R$ in macrophages. Tumor necrosis factor α (TNFα) also stimulates NF-κB which is a multiprotein com-plex, encoded by different genes that share a homologus DNA binding domain. NF-κB is inactive in cytoplasm where it is bound with inhibitory proteins termed IκB. Cytokines such as TNFα activate NF-κB by uncoupling it from IκB [12]. Without the anchor of IκB, NF-κB is able to enter the nucleus and bind to inducible pro-moters resulting in transcription of cytokines and growth factors. The manner in which Ang II controls NF-κB is not known. It may be through a PKC pathway or through a JAK-STAT pathway. However, the evidence for Ang II stimulating NF-κB in monocytic cells (and not in lymphocytes) is clear [3] and puts both Ang II and NF-κB in a pivotal role in contributing to the chronic inflammation which is the hallmark of atherosclerosis.

NF-κB stimulates the expression of MCP-1, IL-6 and IL-8. The role of MCP-1 is to attract monocytes. Although there are other chemoattractants released from cells, it has recently been shown that JEC-MCP-1 is the predominant chemoattractant from VSMC [13]. JE is one of the "immediate early genes" induced by growth fac-tors and cytokines. JE-MCP-1 protein has been detected in human atheromas [14, 15]. However, since VSMC can produce JE-MCP-1 through NF-κB stimulation, it is not yet established if the MCP-1 from macrophages is a specific chemoattractant [13]. In theoretical terms, reducing the number of monocytes/macrophages to the plaque formation would prevent atherogenesis, rupture of the fibrous cap and for-mation of occlusive thrombosis. The role of Ang II may be important because of the tissue/intravascular RAS. In human atherosclerotic plaques, tissue ACE is increased in areas with inflammatory cells. ACE inhibitors reduce the arterial NF-κB activa-tion in macrophages and VSMC. NF-κB has been demonstrated in the nuclei of macrophages in human atherosclerotic lesions, VSMC and endothelial cells [16].

In summary, the role of Ang II in monocytes/macrophages is critical in the early stage of atherosclerotic disease. Ang II activates the NADPH oxidation pathway to form reactive oxygen species (ROS) which reduce and oxidize (redox) lipids. Macrophage lipid peroxidation through these mechanisms converts native LDL to ox-LDL which is taken up at an increased rate through scavenger receptors on the cell surface of macrophages. This is a key step in the conversion of monocytes to foam cells. Secondly, the Ang II binding to LDL forms the modified-LDL complex, which is also taken up by the scavenger receptors. Thirdly, Ang II increases macrophage cell receptors for the uptake of ox-LDL. Thus, Ang II plays a critical role in the initiation of atherosclerosis through converting monocytes/macrophages to foam cells. In addition, Ang II activates NF-κB to coordinate the expression of inflammatory proteins including the cytokines, chemokines, adhesion molecules, and enzymes. Ang II stimulates HMG-CoA reductase mRNA and activates the enzyme in the biosynthesis of cholesterol. Macrophages form the foam cells that produce the lipid-laden deposits in the artery and macrophages also cluster around the fibrous cap. Ang II activation of NF-κB in macrophages produces cytokines and metalloproteinases which may weaken the cap and cause it to rupture.

## Angiotensin II and endothelial cells

The endothelial cells provide the single cell protective layer over the VSMCs in blood vessels. Therefore, endothelial cells are subject to sheer stresses of blood flow, oxidative stresses, and changes in hormonal levels, including circulating plasma Ang II. In a healthy blood vessel the endothelial cell layer is intact and atherosclerosis does not occur. The beginnings of atherosclerosis involve changes in the endothelial cell biology, which has become known as the syndrome of endothelial dysfunction (ED). ED results from risk factors such as hypertension, hyperlipidemia, smoking, obesity, diabetes, gender and age. Any combination of risk factors exacerbates the risk. ED can be measured by the vascular response to acetylcholine (Ach). In normal vessels, Ach causes vasodilation but ED is associated with absence or diminution of relaxation on nitric oxide (NO) by Ach. NO was discovered in endothelial cells and plays a critical role in maintaining normal endothelial function. Ang II generally opposes the actions of NO and may decrease the NO synthase mRNA. NO is broken down by ROS and Ang II has been shown to increase formation of ROS [17, 18]. Indeed, a number of studies suggest that ROS scavengers restore endothelial function. Risk for ED is increased with higher circulating renin in plasma or tissues, or both.

A key event in the start of atherosclerosis is the expression of vascular cell adhesion molecule-1 (VCAM-1) on the cell surface of endothelial and smooth muscle cells [19, 20]. VCAM-1 causes monocytes to adhere to the surface of endothelial cells *via* interaction with the integrin counter receptor on monocytes. Increased expression of VCAM-1 is characteristic of endothelium in early atherosclerotic lesions. VCAM-1 gene expression can be directly stimulated by Ang II [19]. Rats infused with norepinephrine or Ang II for six days developed similar hypertensive responses, but only in the Ang II-treated group was there a significant rise in VCAM-1 protein and mRNA expression. This was inhibited by losartan treatment. Since Ang II also induces NF-κB activation in endothelial cells, the route of Ang II-mediated VCAM-1 stimulation appears to be via the NF-κB driven VCAM-1 promoter. Ang II also induces E-selectin gene expression in human coronary endothe-

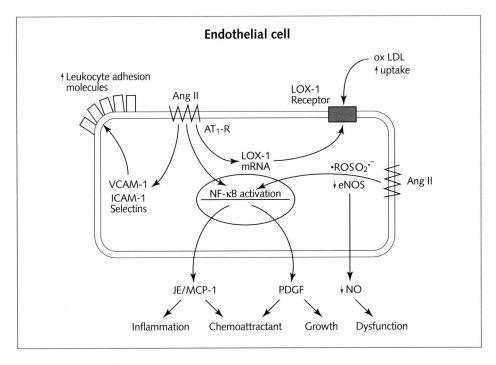

**Figure 2**
*Endothelial cells: Ang II stimulates expression of adhesion molecules including endothelial leukocyte adhesion molecules (selectins) and VCAM-1 and intercellular adhesion molecule-1 (ICAM-1). The expression of these adhesion molecules on the endothelial luminal surface captures leukocytes (monocytes) and begins the process of atherosclerosis. Ang II stimulates LOX-1 mRNA which translates to a lectin-like receptor (LOX-1R) that takes up oxidised LDL (ox-LDL). ROS superoxide ($O^-_2$) decreases available eNOS (endothelial nitric oxide synthase) which is a major factor in endothelial dysfunction. JE/MCP-1, monocyte chemoattractant protein-1.*

lial cells. E-selectin expression induced by Ang II increases leukocyte adhesion by TNFα [20]. Other molecules are no doubt expressed, which together make the endothelial cells "sticky" and dysfunctional. This leads to macrophages "rolling" to openings between endothelial cells thus allowing macrophages to migrate.

Several studies are attempting to define the conditions for the expression of endothelial adhesion molecules. Since normal endothelial function requires NO, the balance between NO and superoxide ($O^-_2$) has been the focus of much attention [21]. Activation of the $AT_1R$ stimulates NAD(P)H-dependent oxidases to form $O^-_2$ in endothelial and vascular cells [17]. $O^-_2$ inactivates NO by reducing NO to peroxinitrate. In cholesterol-fed animals, there is a significant activation of NADH-driven $O^-_2$ production [22]. Animals that were given a $AT_1R$ antagonist, Bay 10-6734, had improved endothelial cells, normalized vascular $O^-_2$ and decreased macrophage infiltration [22]. Hypercholesterolemia is associated with an increased expression of $AT_1R$ [23, 24]. This points to the importance of even low level increases in Ang II, initiating ED by increasing oxidative stress.

Studies in human coronary artery endothelial cells (HCAECs) indicate that Ang II enhances the effect of anoxia-reoxygenation injury, causes apoptosis and necrosis, reduces formation of antioxidant species and enhances ROS formation [25].

Other recent studies have identified the presence of a lectin-like receptor for ox-LDL (LOX-1) in HCAECs. LOX-1 is distinct from macrophage scavenger receptors and binds LDL and facilitates its uptake [10]. Expression and upregulation of LOX-1 causes expression of MCP-1, degradation of IκB, activation of NF-κB and adhesion of monocytes. Ang II upregulates LOX-1 expression in a concentration-dependent manner [10]. These effects of Ang II are mediated by $AT_1R$ activation, since $AT_1R$ antagonists block the upregulation of LOX-1 mRNA and protein, as well as MCP-1 expression [26].

## Ang II and vascular smooth muscle

Figure 3 summarizes some of the known pathways in VSMCs that contribute to the development of lesions. VSMCs undergo hyperplasia i.e. increased numbers of cells by cell division, and hypertrophy i.e. increased cell size and protein content without DNA synthesis or cell division. Hyperplasia of VSMCs is an important characteristic of atherogenesis involving the migration of VSMCs from the media to form neointima which expand into the lumen of the blood vessel. Ang II induces VSMCs hypertrophy and hyperplasia [27, 28]. The signals generated by Ang II stimulation are very similar to those stimulated by PDGF. They involve activation of phospholipase C, the induction of $Na^+$-$H^+$ antiporter and the transcription of several early response genes. Ang II mobilizes intracellular $Ca^+$, stimulates a JAK-STAT pathway and tyrosine phosphorylation [29]. This leads to a rapid increase in c-fos mRNA, which is probably a necessary step in Ang II-induced cell proliferation. Directly or indirectly, Ang II activates mitogen-activated protein kinase (MAPK) which triggers cell mitogenesis. Some data suggest that the activation of MAPK by Ang II and by other GTP-binding protein-coupled receptor (GPCR) agonists such as endothelin-1 (ET-1) and α-thrombin (α-Th), stimulate growth factors including PDGF, basic fibroblast growth factor (bFGF), heparin-binding EGF, transforming growth factor $β_1$ (TGFβ), and insulin-like growth factor 1 (IGF-I) [30–32]. Epiregulin acts as a potent VSMC-derived mitogen through activation of EGF receptor. Taylor et al. [32] have demonstrated that epiregulin expression is regulated by GPCR agonists, including Ang II, ET-1 and α-Thr. Inagami et al. [11, 31] have alternatively sug-

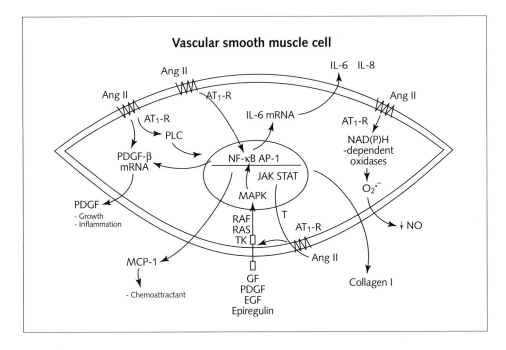

*Figure 3*

*Vascular smooth muscle cell (VSMC). Ang II has several actions on VSMC which are critically important in the development of atherosclerosis. Ang II stimulates PDGF-β, which leads to growth migration of cells and inflammation. Ang II activates phospholipase C (PLC) which activates NF-κB to express MCP-1, a chemoattractant for monocytes, and stimulates proinflammatory of cytokines (IL-6 and IL-8). Ang II also stimulates MAPK (mitrogen activating protein kinase) which acts on the AP-1 nuclear transcription site to promote growth. This action of Ang II is via the JAK-STAT pathway or indirectly through a calcium mediate pathway to activate the tyrosine kinase (TK) of various growth factor receptors. Ang II also stimulates VSMCs to generate collagen-I which makes up a large part of the fibrous cap in a stabilized plaque. Ang II decreases nitric oxide by its oxidative action through NAD(P)H-dependent oxidases. Ang II further stimulates osteopontin which binds calcium and calcifies the plaque. Lastly, Ang II stimulates release of PAI-1 (plasminogen activator inhibitor) and metalloproteinases. This leads to fibrinolysis and thrombosis and the breakdown of the fibrous cap in the final stages of atherosclerosis.GF, growth factor; EGF, epidermal growth factor.*

gested that Ang II acts via stimulation of EGF receptor to activate the mitogenic pathway.

Based on these reports it appears that Ang II, *via* AT$_1$R participates in ion and propagation of VSMC migration and proliferation. The source of Ang II can be local through the tissue RAS. High cholesterol diet is also associated with an upregulation in $AT_1R$ expression in VSMCs [23, 24]. Therefore, even small increases in tissue RAS could activate VSMC proliferation because of upregulation of more $AT_1R$.

As the VSMCs migrate to the intima to form the neointima at the site of tissue injury, monocytes and macrophages are recruited. There are a number of possible chemoattractants that could be released by VSMC, including colony stimulating factors (CSF), granulocyte-macrophage CSF and macrophage CSF, monocyte chemotactic proteins (MCPs), especially JE-MCP-1, TGFβ and PDGF. Poon et al. [13] studied VSMC in culture and found that the secretion of monocyte chemotactic activity by VSMC is surprisingly specific for PDGF-β and was not seen with bFGF, Ang II, IL-1, α-Thr or TNFα. The chemoattractant activity of VSMCs was blocked by an antisense oligonucleotide (AS-ODN) targeted to JE-MCP-1. Thus, they argue that despite a large number of potential chemoattractants, the VSMC-mediated chemotaxis is due predominantly to the highly specific activity of JE-MCP-1.

MCP-1 is expressed when NF-κB is activated. Ang II, working through the $AT_1R$ on VSMC, induces activation of NF-κB which is a redox-sensitive, nuclear transcription factor common to the regulation of many proinflammatory genes including IL-8 and PDGF-β. MCP-1 and IL-8 are implicated in the recruitment of inflammatory cells and PFGF-β is critical for the proliferation and migration of VSMC into the neointima. Hernandez-Presa et al. [33] have reported that the ACE inhibitor, quinapril, reduces the arterial expression of NF-κB in a rabbit model of atherosclerosis. Their report suggests that Ang II, either made locally in tissues such as macrophages and VSMC, or through increased plasma levels, plays a critical role in activating NF-κB. NF-κB is present in human atherosclerotic lesions in the nuclei of VSMC, endothelial cells and macrophages [16]. ACE inhibitors and $AT_1R$ may act not only by the inhibition of Ang II synthesis, but also by promoting NO synthesis by a bradykinin action on NO synthase activity [34]. However, the fact that losartan has similar actions in the atherosclerotic model, as do ACE inhibitors, would indicate that Ang II activation *via* $AT_1R$ is the main activator of IL-8 and MCP-1 expression. NF-κB is also necessary for VSMC proliferation [35]. Therefore, reducing Ang II action on NF-κB will also reduce the number of VSMC proliferating and migrating into the plaque-forming area.

NF-κB is increased in response to a high cholesterol diet. Hernandez-Presa et al. [33] observed that four weeks after a 2% cholesterol diet, the serum cholesterol level had increased about 30-fold over basal values. MCP-1 and IL-8 levels were significantly elevated in femoral arteries of these rabbits. NF-κB was elevated in both macrophages and VSMC, as shown by a double staining procedure. It was also noted that the high cholesterol diet increased vascular ACE activity. Thus, a double danger ensues with hypercholesterolemia with an increase in tissue Ang II generation and increased NF-κB activation. In addition, sensitivity to Ang II is increased by the previously mentioned upregulation of $AT_1R$ in hyperlipidemia [23].

As the plaque develops, it forms a fibrous cap and may remain stable as long as the cap does not rupture. While the lumen is reduced in a stable plaque, blood is still able to flow. Collagen-I and collagen-3 make up 90% of the total collagen in the fibrous cap [36]. Collagen-1 is produced mainly by VSMC. The more VSM cells there are in the area, the more collagen produced; thus contributing to the fibrous nature of the plaque. Because Ang II increases the number of VSMC, it could paradoxically contribute to the stability of the plaque by increased collagen-I expression. The expression of collagen-I is regulated by the transcription factor AP-1 [37]. Morishita et al. [38] have suggested that Ang II can regulate gene expression by the AP-1 binding sequence. Thus, the effect of Ang II on collagen-I appears to be independent of its effect on NF-κB.

Ang II plays a role in the immunological response to the inflammatory condition of the atherosclerosis by inducing IL-6 in VSMC. IL-6 induces B-cell differentiation, T-cell activation, and acute phase protein induction, as well as the production of platelets. IL-6 increases the proliferation of VSMC. It is secreted from macrophages, T-cells, endothelial cells, mesangial cells and VSMC [39]. IL-6 mRNA is overexpressed in the atherosclerotic lesions of Watanabe heritable hyperlipidemic (WHHL) rabbits. Funakoshi et al. [39] have recently demonstrated that Ang II increases IL-6 production in VSMCs in a dose-dependent manner. The effect of Ang II on IL-6 release and mRNA expression was completely blocked by an $AT_1R$ antagonist, CV11974. $AT_2R$ did not appear to be involved. Tyrosine kinase and MAP kinase kinase (MAPKK) inhibition abolished the effect of Ang II on IL-6 production and gene expression. NF-κB is also needed for Ang II-induced IL-6 release [40]. Deletion of the IL-6 gene promoter showed that a cAMP-responsive element (CRE) was essential for the Ang II induction of IL-6 gene expression. IL-6 is important, not only because of the activation of platelets, but also for increasing plasma fibrinogen, which may contribute to the pathological thrombosis in the late stage of plaque instability.

## Implications of the proinflammatory effects of angiotensin II in atherosclerosis

A number of experimental and clinical studies have shown that inhibition of RAS blocks atherosclerosis and related events [33]. A variety of ACE inhibitors decrease atherosclerosis in experimental models. These agents reduce accumulation of inflammatory cells and chemokines reduce arterial expression of NF-κB [33]. Interestingly, there is no reduction in the fibrotic morphology of the plaques. In view of the fact that Ang II is responsible for fibrous cap formation on the plaque, these observations raise the questions as to how quinapril and other ACE inhibitors could selectively inhibit circulation and tissue ACE and subsequent activation of NF-κB, but not of AP-1.

As discussed earlier, most of the proinflammatory and atherosclerotic effects of Ang II are mediated by $AT_1R$ activation. A number of studies have shown that $AT_1R$ blockade with high dose losartan can markedly decrease atherosclerosis. In recent studies, Chen et al. [42] showed a dramatic reduction in intimal proliferation in rabbits on a high cholesterol diet and concurrent administration of losartan (25 mg/kg/ day) for ten weeks. There was also a significant decrease in NF-κB activation with $AT_1R$ blockade. We also examined the expression of matrix metalloproteinase-1 (MMP-1) and its tissue inhibitor (TIMP-2) by immunohistochemistry. Both MMP-1 and TIMP-2 expression increased in the neointimal, as well as in medial and advential layers in hypercholesterolemic animals. Losartan therapy markedly reduced MMP-1 expression, whereas TIMP-2 expression became localized to the intimal region despite hypercholesterolemia. The net effect of these changes would be a firm plaque covered with collagen. This is probably the first demonstration of modulation of collagen formation and inflammatory mediators by $AT_1R$ blockade.

A number of clinical studies have shown that blockade of RAS by ACE inhibitor or specific AT1R antagonists is a very effective and beneficial strategy in the management of hypertension, congestive heart failure and diabetic nephropathy. The recently reported HOPE trial in subjects with vascular disease clearly demonstrated a marked reduction in morbidity and mortality from vascular disease due to treatment with ACE inhibitor [43]. The result of the ELITE study also showed that $AT_1R$ blockers were certainly equally as vasoprotective as the ACE inhibitors [44]. The contribution of inflammation in the genesis of vascular events is uniformly observed in atherosclerosis. As such, a role for modulators of RAS in combating inflammation in relation to the occurrence of vascular events appears to be an important therapeutic approach.


## Is Ang II good or bad

An interesting question is whether the effects of Ang II, summarized here, are all bad or somewhat good. On the one hand, atherosclerosis is characterized by an inflammatory reaction which worsens tissue injury, but on the other hand the inflammatory response is part of a repair process to save tissue from injury. The role of Ang II, therefore, may initially be beneficial. Ang II, whether produced locally or circulating in the plasma, induces adhesion molecules in the endothelium that starts the endothelial dysfunction at the initiation of the atherosclerosis development. Ang II induces hyperplasia and hypertrophy of VSMCs, stimulates the release of reactive oxygen species which oxidizes LDL to the form taken up in cells, but Ang II also stimulates collagen 1 from VSMCs which may be beneficial for the stability of the plaque. At what point an adaptive biological response becomes an uncontrollable pathology is a question yet to be answered.

# References

1   Phillips MI, Speakman EA, Kimura B (1992) Levels of angiotensin and molecular biology of the tissue renin-angiotensin systems. *Regul Pep* 43: 1–20

2   Dzau VJ (1998) Circulating versus local renin-angiotensin system in cardiovascular homeostasis. Circulation 77 (Suppl I): 1–4

3   Kranzhofer R, Browatzki M, Schmidt J, Kubler W (1999) Angiotensin II activates the proinflammatory transcription factor nuclear factor-κB in human monocytes. *Biochem and Biophys Res Commun* 257: 826–828

4   Yia-Herttuala S, Lipton BA, Rosenfeld ME, Sarkloja T, Yoshimura T, Leoanrd EJ, Witztum JL, Steinberg D (1991) Expression of monocyte chemoattractant protein 1 in macrophage rich areas of human and rabbit atherosclerotic lesions. *Proc Natl Acad Sci USA* 88: 5252–5256

5   Liao F, Andalibi A, deBeer FC, Fogelman AM, Lusis AJ (1991) Genetic control of inflammatory gene induction and FT-kappa B-like transcriptional factor activation in response to an atherogenic diet in mice. *J Clin Invest* 91: 2572–2579

6   DeBlois D, Lombardi DM, Su EJ, Clowes AW, Schwartz SM, Giachelli CM (1996) Angiotensin II induction of osteopontin expression and DNA replication in rat arteries. *Hypertension* 28: 1055–1063

7   Mann JM, Davies MJ (1996) Vulnerable plaque. Relation of characteristics to degree of stenosis in human coronary arteries. *Circulation* 94: 928–931

8   Keidar S, Attias J, Heinrich R, Coleman R, Aviram M (1999) Angiotensin II atherogenicity in apolipoprotein E deficient mice is associated with increased cellular cholesterol biosynthesis. *Atherosclerosis* 14: 249–257

9   Keidar S, Kaplan M, Hoffman A, Aviram M (1995) Angiotensin II stimulates macrophage-mediated oxidation of low density lipoproteins. *Atherosclerosis* 115: 201–215

10  Li DY, Zhang YC, Philips MI, Sawamura T, Mehta JL (1999) Upregulation of endothelial receptor for oxidized low-density lipoprotein (LOX-1) in cultured human coronary artery endothelial cells by angiotensin II type 1 receptor activation. *Circ Res* 84: 1043–1049

11  Inagami T, Eguchi S, Numaguchi K, Motley ED, Tang H, Matsumoto T, Yamakawa T (1999) Cross-talk between angiotensin II receptors and the tyrosine kinases and phosphatases. *J Am Soc Nephrol* 10: S57–S61

12  Chabonian AV, Handenschild CC, Nickerson C, Hopes S (1992) Antiatherogenic effect of captopril in Watanabe heritable hyperlipidemic rabbit. *Hypertension* 20: 473–477

13  Poon M, Hsu WC, Bogadanov VY, Taubman MB (1996) Secretion of monocyte chemotactic activity by cultured rat aortic smooth muscle cells in response to PDGF is due predominantly to the induction of JE/MCP-1. *Am J Pathol* 149: 307–317

14  Takeya M, Yoshimura T, Leonard EJ, Takahashi K (1993) Detection of monocyte chemoattractant protein-1 in human atherosclerotic lesions by an anti-monocyte chemoattractant protein-1 monoclonal antibody. *Hum Pathol* 24: 534–539

15  Yu X, Dluz S, Graves DT, Zhang L, Antoniades HN, Hollander W, Prusty S, Valente AJ, Schwartz CJ, Sonenshein GE (1992) Elevated expression of monocyte chemoattractant protein 1 by vascular smooth muscle cells in hypercholesterolemic primates. *Proc Natl Acad Sci USA* 89: 6953–6957

16  Brand K, Page S, Rogler G, Bartsch A, Brandl R, Knuechel R, Page M, Kaltschmidt C, Baeuerle PA, Neumeier D (1996) Activated transcription factor nuclear factor-kappa B is present in the atherosclerotic lesion. *J Clin Invest* 97: 1715–1722

17  Griendling KK, Minieri CA, Ollerenshaw JD, Alexander RW (1994) Angiotensin II stimulates NADH and NADPH oxidase activation in cultured vascular smooth muscle cells. *Circ Res* 74: 1141–1148

18  Li DY, Yang BC, Phillips MI, Mehta JL (1999) Pro-apoptotic effects of angiotensin II in human coronary artery endothelial cells: role of $AT_1$ receptor and PKC activation. *Am J Physiol* 276: H786–H792

19  Tummula PE, Xi-Lin C, Sundell CL, Laursen JB, Hammes CP, Alexander RW, Harrison DG, Medford, RM (1999) Angiotensin II induces vascular cell adhesion molecule-1 expression in rat vasculature. A potential link between the renin-angiotensin system and atherosclerosis. *Circulation* 100: 1223–1229

20  Grafe M, Auch-Schwelk W, Zakrzewicz A, Regitz-Zagrosek V, Bartsch P, Graf K, Loebe M, Gaehtgens P, Fleck E (1997) Angiotensin II-induced leukoycte adhesion of human coronary endothelial cells I mediated by E-selection. *Circ Res* 81: 804–811

21  Abi J-IA, Berk BC (1998) Reactive oxygen species in mediators of signal transduction in cardiovascular disease. *Trends Cardiovasc Med* 8: 59–64

22  Warnholtz A, Nickenig G, Schulz E, Macharzina R, Brasen JH, Skatchkov M, Heitzer T, Stasch JP, Griendling KK, Harrison DG et al (1999) Increased NADH-oxidase-mediated superoxide production in the early stages of atherosclerosis: evidence for involvement of the renin-angiotensin system. *Circulation* 99: 2027–2033

23  Nickenig G, Bohm M (1997) Regulation of the angiotensin $AT_1$ receptor expression by hypercholesterolemia. *Eur J Med Res* 2: 285–289

24  Yang BC, Phillips MI, Mohuczy D, Meng H-B, Shen L, Mehta P, Mehta JL (1998) Increased angiotensin II type 1 receptor expression in hypercholesterolemic atherosclerosis in rabbits. *Arterioscler Thromb Vasc Biol* 18: 1433–1439

25  Li DY, Tomson K, Yang BC, Mehta P, Croker B, Mehta JL (1999) Modulation of constitutive nitric oxide synthase, Bcl-2 and Fas expression in cultured human coronary endothelial cells exposed to anoxia-reoxygenation and angiotensin II: role of AT1 receptor activation. *Cardiovasc Res* 41: 109–115

26  Li DY, Mehta JL (2000) Antisense to LOX-1 inhibited ox-LDL-mediated upregulation of MCP-1 expression and monocyte adhesion to human coronary artery endothelial cells. *Circulation* 101 (25): 2889–2895

27  Geisterfer AAT, Peach MJ, Owens GK (1988) Angiotensin II induces hypertrophy, not hyperplasia, of cultured rat smooth muscle cells. *Circ Res* 62: 749–756

28  Berk BC (1999) Angiotensin II signal transduction in vascular smooth muscle: pathways activated by specific tyrosine kinases. *J Am Soc Nephrol* 10 (Suppl 11): S62–68

29   Shieffer B, Paxton WG, Marrero MB, Bernstein KE (1996) Importance of tyrosine phos-
     phorylation in angiotensin II type 1 receptor signaling. *Hypertension* 27 (2): 476–480

30   Eguici S, Numaguichi K, Iwasaki H, Matsumoto T, Yamakawa T, Utsunomiya H, Mot-
     ley ED, Kawakatsu H, Owada KM, Hirata Y et al (1998) Calcium-dependent epidermal
     growth factor receptor transactivation mediates the angiotensin II-induced mitogen-acti-
     vated protein kinase activation in vascular smooth muscle cells. *J Biol Chem* 15:
     8890–8896

31   Eguchi S, Iwasaki H, Hirata Y, Frank GD, Motley ED, Yamakawa T, Numaguchi K.,
     Inagami T (1999) Epidermal growth factor receptor is indispensable for c-fos expression
     and protein synthesis by angiotensin II. *Eur J Pharmacol* 376: 203–206

32   Taylor DS, Cheng X, Pawlowski JE, Wallace AR, Ferrer P, Molloy CJ (1999) Epiregulin
     is a potent vascular smooth muscle cell-derived mitogen induced by angiotensin II,
     endothelin-1, and thrombin. *Proc Natl Acad Sci USA* 96: 1633–1638

33   Hernandez-Presa MA, Bustos C, Ortego M, Tunon J, Ortega L, Egido J (1998) ACE
     inhibitor quinapril reduces the arterial expression of NF-kappa B-dependent proinflam-
     matory factors but not of collagen I in a rabbit model of atherosclerosis. *Am J Pathol*
     153: 1825–1837

34   Siragyi HM, Carey RM (1997) The subtype 2 (AT$_2$) angiotensin receptor mediates renal
     production of nitric oxide in conscious rats. *J Clin Invest* 100: 264–269

35   Bellas RE, Lee JS, Sonenshein GE (1995) Expression of a constitutive NF-kappa B-like
     activity is essential for proliferation of cultured bovine vascular smooth muscle cells. *J
     Clin Invest* 96: 2521–2527

36   Barnes MJ (1985) Collagens in atherosclerosis. *Coll Relat Res* 5: 65–97

37   Chung KY, Agarwal A, Uitto J, Mauviel A (1996) An AP-1 binding sequence is essential
     for regulation of the human alpha2(I) collagen (COL1A2) promoter activity by trans-
     forming growth factor-beta. *J Biol Chem* 271: 3272–3278

38   Morishita R, Gibbons GH, Horiuchi M, Kaneda Y, Ogihara T, Dzau VJ (1998) Role of
     AP-1 complex in angiotensin II-mediated transforming growth factor-beta expression
     and growth of smooth muscle cells: using decoy approach against AP-1 binding site.
     *Biochem Biphys Res Commun* 243 (2): 361–367

39   Funakoshi Y, Ichiki T, Ito K, Takeshita A (1999) Induction of interleukin-6 expression
     by angiotensin II in rat vascular smooth muscle cells. *Hypertension* 34: 118–125

40   Han Y, Runge MS, Brasier AR (1999) Angiotensin II induces interluekin-6 transcription
     in vascular smooth muscle cells through pleiotropic activation of nuclear factor-kappa
     B transcription factors. *Circ Res* 84: 695–703

41   Chen HJ, Li DY, Shen L, Phillips MI, Mehta JL (2000) Losartan attenuates intimal pro-
     liferation in rabbits on high cholesterol diet despite rise in plasma Ang II levels and per-
     sistently high lipid levels. *JACC; submitted*

42   Mehta JL, Chen, HJ, Li DY (2000) Modulation of matrix metalloproteinase-1, its tissue
     inhibitor (TIMP-2) and NF-κB by losartan in hypercholesterolemic rabbits ATVB; *sub-
     mitted*

43 Kleinert S (1999) HOPE for cardiovascular disease prevention with ACE-inhibitor ramipril. Heart Outcomes Prevention Evaluation. *Lancet* 354–381

44 Pitt B, Segal R, Martinez FA, Meurers G, Cowley AJ, Thomas I, Deedwania PC, New DE, Snavely DB, Chang PI (1997) Randomized trial of losartan versus captopril in patients over 65 with heart failure. *Lancet* 349: 747–752

# Role of interleukins in relation to the renin-angiotensin-system in atherosclerosis

*Bernhard Schieffer and Helmut Drexler*

Abteilung Kardiologie und Angiologie, Medizinische Hochschule Hannover, Carl Neuberg Strasse 1, 30625 Hannover, Germany

## Atherosclerosis: an inflammatory disease

The morphology of human atherosclerotic plaques ranges from a solid fibrous structure to those with substantial lipid cores, covered by only a thin fibrous cap on its luminal aspect [1–4]. Pathological studies have demonstrated that rupture of these coronary atheromas precipitates the formation of the occluding thrombus that causes an acute coronary syndrome, such as unstable angina or myocardial infarction [4]. Plaque-rupture predominantly occurs on the edges of the plaque's fibrous cap, the shoulder region, areas frequently associated with accumulations of monocyte-derived macrophages, T lymphocytes and mast cells in close proximity to vascular smooth muscle cells [1, 4, 5]. These activated macrophages and T lymphocytes stimulate their neighboring cells to erode the collagen and elastin, via the release of inflammatory cytokines, resulting in a decay of the framework which forms the plaque's cap and ultimately leading to the plaque's rupture [1, 5, 6].

The renin-angiotensin-system (RAS) has also been suggested for the past several years to be involved in the development of acute coronary syndromes although the mechanism remained unclear. More recently, evidence emerged that angiotensin II (the effector peptide of the RAS) may stimulate the release of inflammatory markers, so that inflammatory mediators may represent a missing link between the neurohumoral system (the RAS) and the instablity of coronary plaques. Therefore, the focus of the present review delineates the potential interaction and impact of an activated RAS on inflammatory mediators in experimental models of atherosclerosis and patients with coronary artery disease.

## Renin-angiotensin-system and myocardial infarction

The impact of an activated renin-angiotensin system (RAS) on the development of acute myocardial infarction was first demonstrated in epidemiological studies by Aldermann and coworkers [7]. The authors examined, in a long-term study, the relationship between the renin-sodium profile (a surrogate marker of RAS activation) and subsequent myocardial infarction in more than 1700 patients [7]. In the eight-year follow-up phase of this trial, the risk of myocardial infarction was about five-fold higher in patients with a high renin-sodium profile at baseline compared to those with a low profile, although blood pressure reduction was almost identical in both groups. Recent genetic data indicated that the deletion (D/D) polymorphism in the gene that encodes for the angiotensin converting enzyme (ACE) is associated with higher tissue and plasma levels of ACE, whereas the insertion polymorphism ACE-I/I genotype is associated with lower ACE-levels, and the ACE-I/D level with intermediate levels [8]. A retrospective study reported by Cambien et al. [9] reported the prevalence of the ACE-DD genotype in a population with no other significant cardiovascular risk factors to be greater in subjects with a prior myocardial infarction than in those with no previous infarction. In contrast, Ludwig and coworkers reported no difference in the distribution of ACE-genotypes between individuals with and without coronary artery disease, defined as coronary artery stenosis > 60% [10]. Although the results of these studies are difficult to reconcile, it is possible that genetically defined polymorphisms of components of the RAS may be associated with an increased risk of myocardial infarction, particularly at a young age, when other risk factor may not confound the impact of components of the RAS system [11].

The epidemiological, genetic and clinical observations stimulated a diversity of *in vitro* studies investigating the potential mechanisms by which angiotensin II (ANG II) may contribute to the development of ACS. Almost all of these studies pointed to the potential interaction of ANG II with inflammatory cells. ANG II was shown to enhance the migration of monocytes and macrophages into the atherosclerotic vessel area [12], a mechanism which is thought to be essential for both the progression of atherosclerosis and the development of an acute coronary syndrome [6]. Moreover, ANG II stimulates the generation of reactive oxygen species in vascular cells and macrophages [13, 14], which are known activators for signaling cascades, such as nuclear factor kappa B (NF-$\kappa$B), mitogen-activated protein (MAP)-kinases or the janus kinases (JAK) and signal transducers and activators of transcription (STAT) cascade [15]. Together these mechanisms may enhance oxidative stress within the vascular wall and lead to the activation of redox-sensitive genes, such as those for pro-inflammatory cytokines [16, 17]. In this regard, IL-6 transcription was shown to be redox-sensitive [17], so that it is tempting to speculate that ANG II may activate IL-6 transcription and release via redox-sensitive mechanisms.

The results of experimental studies in animal models are consistent with this notion. With the use of ACE-inhibitors, macrophage recruitment into the vessel wall can be abolished in a rabbit model of atherosclerosis as well as apolipoprotein E (apo E)-deficient mice [12, 18]. Keidar and coworkers have also demonstrated that blockade of the AT$_1$ receptor by losartan prevented the accumulation of oxidative reactants and reduced the formation of atherosclerotic lesions in an apo E-deficient mouse model [19]. Thus, the interaction between reactive oxygen species, inflammatory cells and the RAS seems to be crucial not only for the development of acute coronary syndrome (ACS) but also for the progression of atherosclerosis.

With regard to the progression of atherosclerosis, there is also evidence from other experimental animal models that chronic ACE-inhibition can retard the development of atherosclerosis. Animal models, including apo E-deficient mice, Watanabe rabbits and cholesterol-fed monkeys have proven the concept that ACE-inhibition may reduce the extent of vascular lesions [20–22].

Additional mechanisms by which the RAS may enhance the development of atherosclerosis involve the initiation of vasoconstriction (see below) and the activation of thrombosis pathways via plasminogen activator inhibitor-1 (PAI-1) or the stimulation of pro-inflammatory cytokines [23]. Serum PAI-1 levels were investigated by Ridker and coworkers in formerly healthy volunteers of the "Physician Health Study" [24] and were shown to be elevated and associated with a higher risk of myocardial infarction [24].

If ANG II is indeed triggering any or all these mechanisms, one would expect that blockade of the RAS by chronic ACE-inhibition would reduce the risk of myocardial infarction. In fact, retrospective analysis in patients with left ventricular dysfunction, have consistently demonstrated a reduction of myocardial infarction during long-term ACE-inhibition therapy [25, 26]. Nevertheless it was not clear until recently whether or not ACE-inhibitors prevent ischemic cardiovascular events in patients with normal ventricular function. The HOPE trial showed for the first time a reduction of all cardiovascular events when patients with normal left ventricular function were treated long-term with the ACE inhibitor ramipril [27]. Surprisingly, the stroke prevention rate was even better than the reduction of myocardial infarctions [27]. This clinical trial implicates a role for the RAS and its effector peptide ANG II in the progression of atherosclerosis leading to the development of ACS. Moreover, given the central role of inflammatory processes in the atherosclerotic plaque pathophysiology [6], these results raise the possibility that chronic ACE-inhibition may interfere with the inflammatory processes within the atherosclerotic plaque and thereby potentially stabilize these plaques. However, the mechanism of the interaction between the RAS and inflammatory processes in atherosclerotic plaques is still not known.

## Angiotensin II receptors and angiotensin II-signal transduction

In order to understand the potential interacting mechanims of ANG II and pro-inflammatory cytokines, signal transduction events stimulated by the angiotensin II type 1 ($AT_1$) receptor have to be elucidated. As stated above, an important role for ANG II in cell growth and tissue remodeling has also been suggested in experimental models of atherosclerosis and vascular injury [28, 29]. Recent observations suggested that classic G-protein coupled receptors (e.g. the $AT_1$-receptor) stimulate second messenger systems via tyrosine phosphorylation [30]. In many ways, the $AT_1$ receptor resembles cytokine receptors such as the interleukin 2 (IL-2) and interferon $\alpha$ (IFN$\alpha$) receptors, which lack intrinsic tyrosine kinase activity, yet induce tyrosine phosphorylation and mediate cell growth or modulate inflammatory responses [31, 32]. Activation of both $AT_1$ receptors and cytokine receptors leads to a rapid increase in *c-fos* mRNA, an early growth response gene [33, 34]. Although not yet conclusively demonstrated, the induction of *c-fos* is likely an important initial step that participates in a series of molecular events ultimately leading to ANG II-induced cell proliferation and inflammation [30].

The signaling events whereby ANG II induces *c-fos* in vascular smooth muscle cells (VSMC) are not completely explored. However, the ANG II induction of *c-fos* does not require *de novo* protein synthesis and appears to be regulated by post-translational modifications of transcription factors [35, 36]. In this regard, two intracellular pathways have recently been well-defined [36, 37]. The first is a multiple kinase pathway used by a number of growth factors, e.g. platelet derived growth factor (PDGF) and epidermal growth factor (EGF). The second, more direct, signaling pathway is stimulated by cytokines such as IFN$\alpha$ and $\gamma$. Here, ligand binding to a cell surface receptor activates the JAK family of tyrosine kinases. In response to ligand binding these kinases activate downstream signaling molecules, the transcription factors of the STAT family (signal transducers and activators of transcription) [37]. When activated by JAK kinases, STATs form the ISGF3 complex (interferon stimulated growth factor complex 3), translocate to the nucleus and stimulate c-fos transcription by DNA-binding. Thus, the JAK-STAT pathway acts as a direct link between a cell surface receptor and transcriptional events [37]. This was demonstrated in ANG II-stimulated smooth muscle cells [38]. We demonstrated that ANG II stimulates the activation of JAK2 and subsequently STAT1 and STAT2. In addition, observations by Bhat and coworkers demonstrated that activated STAT's bind to specific DNA-binding sites previously known to be exclusive for cytokines [39]. These results suggest that the G protein-coupled $AT_1$ receptors – similar to cytokine receptors – signal directly to the nucleus via signaling cascades previously thought to be exclusive for cytokines and their receptors. These observations represent one pathway by which interactions between ANG II and cytokines may occur.

## Angiotensin II and cytokines

Atherosclerotic plaques are chronic inflammatory lesions composed of dysfunctional endothelium, smooth muscle cells, lipid-laden macrophages, and T lymphocytes [6]. These lipid-laden activated macrophages and T lymphocytes stimulate their neighboring cells to erode the collagen and elastin framework which forms the plaque's cap [4, 5]. This may be induced via the release of pro-inflammatory cytokines, e.g. IL-6. Interestingly, serum-levels of IL-6 are increased in patients with unstable angina [40, 41] and have been implicated in the onset of an ACS [41]. IL-6 is involved in a variety of physiological functions including the stimulation of acute phase protein synthesis ($\alpha$2-macroglobulin and CR-P), the induction of pro-thrombotic factors (e.g. PAI-1) and the stimulation of matrix degrading enzymes, the metalloproteinases, formerly known as collagenases [17, 42].

Diet and coworkers first demonstrated that the ANG II-forming enzyme, ACE, is expressed in human atherosclerotic plaques [43]. The authors demonstrated that in early and intermediate-stage atherosclerotic lesions, ACE was predominantly expressed in lipid-laden macrophages (similar to pro-inflammatory cytokines), whereas in advanced lesions, ACE was predominantly localized throughout the plaque's microvasculature [43]. Potter and coworkers further demonstrated that lipid-laden macrophages contain ANG II in a primate model of atherosclerosis [44]. In humans at least two major enzymes – ACE and chymase – are involved in the conversion of ANG I to ANG II and may contribute to the ANG II formation in coronary arteries. Ohishi and coworkers found that chymase (an ACE-like enzyme) is co-localized with ANG II in normal and atheromatous coronary artery segments of patients dying of malignant diseases [4]. However, only ACE was co-localized with ANG II in the intima of stable atherosclerotic lesions with diffuse intimal thickening whereas immunodouble staining did not show colocalization of ANG II and chymase [45]. These findings suggest that ACE is the primary source of ANG II in atherosclerotic human coronary arteries. Our observations are consistent with the data of Ohishi and collegues. In addition, our analysis of coronary arteries obtained during transplantation revealed that chymase-containing mast cells are consistently seen in the adventitia, but did not stain for ANG II. This analysis from our laboratory can not exclude that chymase secreted by activated mast cells provides an alternative pathway for ANG II-formation, but considering cellular co-localization and abundance of ANG II in macrophage-rich areas, our data suggest that mast-cell derived chymase is not the major contributor to ANG II-formation in human atherosclerotic coronary arteries [46].

In addition, given the recent evidence that pro-inflammatory cytokines are increased in patients with acute coronary syndromes [40] and ANG II and ACE were expressed predominantly in areas of clustered macropages (cells capable of releasing pro-inflammatory cytokines) in atherosclerotic coronary segments [43–45], we hypothesized that both peptides may interact and together may enhance the development of an acute coronary syndrome. Therefore, we investigated whether ANG II induces IL-6 *in vitro*. Results showed that ANG II induced the synthesis and release of IL-6 in smooth muscle cells and human macrophages [46]. *In vivo* experiments further showed that ANG II, the $AT_1$-receptor and ACE are expressed at strategically relevant sites of human coronary atherosclerotic plaques; that is, at the shoulder of macrophage-rich atherosclerotic plaques. Furthermore,

ANG II was detected in close proximity to the potential plaque rupture site in coronary artery sections from patients who died acutely after myocardial infarctions. Co-localization of components of the RAS with IL-6 was observed in stable coronary plaques and atherectomy tissues [46]. These findings suggest that the RAS may contribute to inflammatory processes within the atherosclerotic vascular wall and thereby may contribute to the development of acute coronary syndromes.

## What is the pathophysiogical role of IL-6 in arteriosclerotic plaques, i.e. induced by ANG II?

As a mediator of inflammation, IL-6 stimulates a variety of intracellular signaling mechanisms including the traditional cytokine signaling cascade of the JAK-kinases and STAT transcription factors [17]. *Via* this signaling cascade, IL-6 mediates its physiological functions including macrophage differentiation, B-cell maturation, acute phase protein synthesis and smooth muscle cell proliferation. Moreover, it was shown that cytokine-stimulated smooth muscle cells synthesize and release enzymes for extracellular matrix degradation (matrix metalloproteinases, especially MMP-13), thereby potentially destabilizing the plaque's fibrous cap [42]. The latter implicates a role for pro-inflammatory cytokines, such as IL-6, in the development of an ACS. Finally, IL-6 regulates the expression of adhesion molecules and other cytokines (e.g. IL-1β and TNFα) which together may enhance an inflammatory reaction at the atherosclerotic plaque. Whether or not ANG II induces the synthesis and release of other pro-inflammatoy cytokines, e.g. IL-1β and TNFα, needs further investigation.

Since both ANG II and IL-6 activate, in part, identical signaling events, we investigated whether ANG II induces the release of PAI-1 and CR-P via the activation of the JAK/STAT cascade. Preliminary results demonstrated that PAI-1 and CR-P are released when smooth muscle cells are stimulated with ANG II [47]. Therefore, we here suggest a model in which ANG II and IL-6 together may amplify the development of an ACS via the induction of PAI-1, CR-P and/or other potential atherogenic factors, such as macrophage chemoattractant protein 1 (MCP-1) (Fig. 1).

However, alternative signaling pathways of IL-6 synthesis were reported recently and indicated that IL-6 synthesis by ANG II may also rely on the activation of the nuclear NF-κB [48]. Since the activation of the JAK/STAT cascade and the activation of NF-κB depends on the generation of superoxide anions, further investigation is needed in order to elucidate the intracellular IL-6 activating mechanisms. Griendling and coworkers demonstrated that ANG II is capable of stimulating superoxide anions via the NADH/NADPH oxidase system [13, 14]. Superoxide anions are known activators of JAK2 and of the NF-κB system [15, 49]. Thus it is reasonable to assume, that IL-6 induction by ANG II is redox-sensitive and is stimulated by one of these signaling cascades. In fact, recent observations reported that

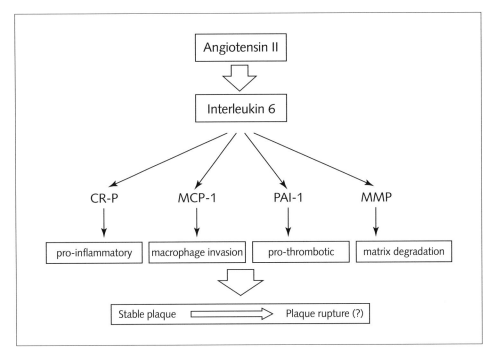

*Figure 1*

*Hypothetical model summarizing the potential interaction of angiotensin II (ANG II) with IL-6 and their impact on plaque stability. ANG II induces IL-6 in smooth muscle cells and macropahges and was shown to mediate, via IL-6, the release of PAI-1 and C-RP. IL-6, independently of ANG II, has been shown to activate MMP's and the synthesis and release of MCP. Together, these observations suggest that ANG II via IL-6 may contribute to the plaque instability via the release of pro-inflammatory, pro-thrombotic and matrix degrading enzymes.*

blockade of the superoxide anion generation by ANG II abolished ANG II-induced IL-6 release *in vitro* [54]. Thus, the generation of superoxide anions *via* the $AT_1$-receptor seems to be a crucial signaling step for the pro-inflammatory potency of ANG II.

## Angiotensin II and mechanical stress

ACE and ANG II are expressed in monkey, rabbit and human stable and unstable coronary arteries [43–46]. Even though one could disagree with the impact of ANG

II on inflammatory effects leading to the development of ACS, ANG II is one of the most powerful vasoconstrictors in mammalians [51]. Biomechanical analysis by Loree and coworkers demonstrated that the shoulder region of the fibrous cap is the predilection site for plaque rupture, since maximal circumferential stress occurs at this location [52, 53]. Therefore it is tempting to speculate that locally secreted ANG II may enhance biomechanical stress at the shoulder region of the plaque and thereby predispose the plaque to rupture [4, 5, 52]. Thus, locally secreted ANG II may induce segmental coronary artery vasoconstriction – beyond its interaction with cytokines – which enhances local circumferential biomechanical stress and ultimately augments the risk of a plaque's rupture.

## Conclusion

Components of an activated RAS are present at the shoulder region of coronary atherosclerotic plaques, areas prone to rupture. *In vitro* observations suggest that ANG II stimulates synthesis and release of IL-6, whose increased serum-concentrations has been consistently observed in unstable angina. This interaction of ANG II and IL-6 may play a role in vessel wall inflammation and possibly contribute to the development of ACS. Whether or not the impact of ANG II is predominantly dependent on its interaction with cytokines or other effects, i.e. biomechanical stress, needs further investigation. Nevertheless, the overall pathophysiological importance of blocking locally-secreted ANG II in atherosclerotic coronary arteries is strongly suggested by the results of recent clinical trials.

*Acknowledgement*
The authors are indebted to Elisabeth Schieffer, M.D., and Denise and Andres Hilfiker, Ph.D., as well as Maren Luchtefeld, B.S.

Studies summarized in this manuscript were supported by DFG-grants Dre 486/8-4 and Schie 386/3-1 as well as by a grant of the DFG-Sonderforschungsbereich 244/C9.

## References

1    Ross R (1993) Pathogenesis of artherosclerosis: a perspective for the 1990s. *Nature* 362: 801–809
2    Alexander RW (1994) Inflammation and coronary artery disease. *N Engl J Med* 331 (7): 468–469
3    Libby P (1995) Molecular bases of the acute coronary syndrome. *Circulation* 21: 2844–2850

4    Davies MJ, Thomas AC (1985) Plaque fissuring: the cause of acute myocardial infarction, sudden ischemic death, and crescendo angina. *Br Heart J* 53: 363–373

5    Van der Waal AC, Becker AE, Loos CM, Das PK (1994) Site of intimal rupture or erosion of thrombosed coronary artherosclerotic plaques is characterized by an inflammatory process irrespective of the dominant plaque morphology. *Circulation* 89: 34–44

6    Ross R (1999) Atherosclerosis – an inflammatory disease. *N Engl J Med* 340 (2): 115–126

7    Aldermann MH, Madhavan S, Ooi WL, Cohen H, Sealy JE, Laragh JH (1991) Association of the renin-sodium profile with the risk of myocardial infarction in patients with hypertension. *N Engl J Med* 324: 1098–1104

8    Cambien F, Poirier O, Lecerf L, Evans A, Cambou JP, Arvelier D, Luc G, Bard JM, Bara R, Richard S et al (1992) Deletion polymorphism in the gene for angiotensin-converting enzyme is a potent risk factor for myocardial infarction. *Nature* 359: 641–644

9    Cambien F, Costerousse O, Tirret L, Poirier O, Lecerf L, Gonzales MF, Evans A, Arveilier D, Cambou JP, Luc G et al (1994) Plasma levels and gene polymorphism of angiotensin converting enzyme in relation to myocardial infarction. *Circulation* 90: 669–676

10   Ludwig E, Corneli PS, Anderson JL, Marshall HW, Lalouel JM, Ward RL (1995) Angiotensin-converting enzyme gene polymorphism is associated with myocardial infarction but not with development of coronary stenosis. *Circulation* 91 (8): 2120–2124

11   Danser AH, Schalekamp MA, Bax WA, van den Brink AM, Saxena PR, Riegger GA, Schunkert H (1995) Angiotensin-converting enzyme in the human heart. Effect of the deletion/insertion polymorphism. *Circulation* 92 (6): 1387–1388

12   Hernandez-Presa M, Bustos C, Ortega M, Tunon J, Renedo G, Ruiz-Ortega M, Egidio J (1997) Angiotensin-converting enzyme inhibition prevents arterial nuclear factor-κB activation, monocyte chemoattactant proetein-1 expression and macrophage infiltration in a rabbit model of early accelerated atherosclerosis. *Circulation* 95: 1532–1541

13   Griendling KK, Alexander RW (1997) Oxidative stress and cardiovascular disease. *Circulation* 96: 3264–3265

14   Griendling KK, Minieri CA, Ollerenshaw JD, Alexander RW (1994) Angiotensin II stimulates NADH and NADPH oxidase activity in cultured vascular smooth muscle cells. *Circ Res* 74 (6): 1141–1148

15   Chakraborti S, Chakraborti T (1998) Oxidant-mediated activation of mitogen-activated protein kinases and nuclear transcription factors in the cardiovascular system: a brief overview. *Cell Signal* 10 (10): 675–683

16   Northermann W, Braciak TA, Hattori M, Lee F, Fey GH (1989) Structure of the rat IL-6 gene and its expression in macrophage-derived cells. *J Biol Chem* 264: 16072–16082

17   Kishimoto T, Akira S, Narazaki M, Taga T (1995) IL-6 family of cytokines and gp130. *Blood* 86: 1243–1254

18   Fuhrman B, Oiknine J, Aviram M (1994) Iron induces lipid peroxidation in cultured

macrophages, increases their ability to oxidatively modify LDL and affect their secretory properties. *Atherosclerosis* 111: 65–78

19  Keidar S, Attias J, Smith J, Breslow JL, Hayek T (1997) The angiotensin II receptor antagonist, losartan, inhibits LDL lipid peroxidation and atherosclerosis in apolipoprotein E deficient mice. *Biochem Biophys Res Commun* 236: 622–625

20  Chobanian AV, Haudenschild CC, Nickerson C, Drago R, (1990) Antiartherogenic effect of captopril in Watanabe herritable hyperlipidemic rabbits. *Hypertension* 15: 327–331

21  Hayek T, Keidar S, Mei-Yi, Oikine J, Breslow J (1995) Effect of angiotensin converting enzyme inhibitors on LDL lipid peroxidation and artherosclerosis progression in apoE deficient mice. *Circulation* 92 (Suppl I): I–625

22  Aberg G, Ferrer P (1990) Effects of Captopril on artherosclerosis in cynomoglus monkeys. *J Cardiovasc Pharmacol* 15 (Suppl I): S65–S72

23  Ridker PM, Gaboury CJL, Conlin PR, Seely EW, Williams GH, Vaughan DE (1993) Stimulation of plasminogen activator inhibitor in vivo by infusion of angiotensin II: evidence of a potential interaction between the renin-angiotensin system and fibrinolytic function. *Circulation* 87: 1969–1973

24  Ridker PM, Vaughan DE (1995) Hemostatic factors and the risk of myocardial infarction. *N Engl J Med* 333 (6): 389–390

25  Pfeffer M, Braunwald E, Moye L, Basta L, Brown EJ, Cuddy TE, Davis BR, Geltmann EM, Goldman S, Flaker GC et al (1992) Effect of captopril on mortality and morbidity in patients with left ventricular dysfunction after myocardial infarction: Results of the survival and ventricular enlargement trial. *N Engl J Med* 327: 669–677

26  The SOLVD Investigators: (1992) Effect of enalapril on mortality and the development of heart failure in asymptomatic patients with reduced left ventricular ejection fraction. *N Engl J Med* 327: 568–574

27  Yusuf N for the investigators of the HOPE Trial (2000) *N Engl J Med* 342: 145–153

28  Daemen MJ, Lombardi DM, Bosman FT, Schwartz SM (1991) Angiotensin II induces smooth muscle cell proliferation in the normal and injured rat arterial wall. *Circ Res* 68: 450–456

29  Powell JS, Clozel JP, Muller RK, Kuhn H, Hefti F, Hosang M, Baumgartner HR (1989) Inhibitors of angiotensin-converting enzyme prevent myointimal proliferation after vascular injury. *Science* 245: 186–188

30  Schieffer B, Paxton WG, Marrero MB, Bernstein KE (1996) Importance of tyrosine phosphorylation in Angiotensin II AT$_1$ receptor mediated signalling. *Hypertension* 27: 476–480

31  Gibbons GH, Pratt RE, Dzau VJ (1992) Vascular smooth muscle cell hypertrophy versus hyperplasia. Autocrine transforming growth factor-beta 1 expression determines growth response to angiotensin II. *J Clin Invest* 90 (2): 456–461

32  Fantl WJ, Johnson DE, Williams LT (1993) Signalling by receptor tyrosine kinases. *Annu Rev Biochem* 62: 453–481

33  Sadoshima J, Izumo S (1993) Signal transduction pathways of angiotensin II induced c-fos gene expression in cardiac myocytes *in vitro. Circ Res* 73: 424–438

34  Naftilan AJ, Pratt RE, Dzau VJ (1989) Induction of platelet-derived growth factor A-chain and c-myc gene expression by angiotensin II in cultured rat vascular smooth muscle cells. *J Clin Invest* 83: 1419–1424

35  Schindler C, Darnell JE (1995) Transcriptional responses to polypeptide ligands: the Jak-Stat pathway. *Annu Rev Biochem* 64: 621–651

36  Van Der Geer, Hunter T, Lindberg RA (1994) Receptor protein tyrosine kinases and their signal transduction. *Annu Rev Cell Biol* 10: 251–338

37  Darnell JE, Kerr IM, Stark GR (1994) JAK-Stat pathways and transcriptional activation in response to IFNs and other extracellular signaling proteins. *Science* 264: 1415–1421

38  Marrero MB, Schieffer B, Paxton WG, Heerdt L, Berk BC, Delafontaine P, Bernstein KE (1995) Direct stimulation of JAK/STAT pathway by the angiotensin II $AT_1$ receptor. *Nature* 375: 247–250

39  Bhat CJ, Thekkumara TJ, Thomas WG, Conrad KM, Baker KM (1994) Angiotensin II stimulates sis-inducing factor-like DNA binding activity. Evidence that the $AT_{1A}$ receptor activates transription factor stat91 and/or a related protein. *J Biol Chem* 269: 31443–31449

40  Biassuci L, Vitelli A, Liuzzo G, Altamura S, Caliguri G, Monaco C, Rebuzzi A, Ciliberto G, Maseri A (1996) Elevated levels of interleukin-6 in unstable angina. *Circulation* 94: 874–877

41  Marx N, Neumann FJ, Ott I, Gawaz M, Koch W, Pikau T, Schömig A (1997) Induction of cytokine expression in leucocytes in acute myocardial infarction. *J Am Coll Cardiol* 30: 165–170

42  Solis-Herruzo JA, Rippe A, Schrum LW, de la Torre P, Immaculada G, Jeffrey J, Munoz-Yague T, Brenner D (1996) Interleukin 6 increases metalloproteinases-13 gene expression through stimulation of activator protein 1 transcription factor in cultured fibroblasts *J Biol Chem* 274 (43): 30919–30926

43  Diet F, Pratt R, Berry GJ, Momose N, Gibbons G, Dzau VJ (1996) Increased accumulation of tissue ACE in human artherosclerotic coronary artery disease. *Circulation* 94: 2756–2767

44  Potter DD, Sobey CG, Tompkins PK, Rossen JD, Heistad DD (1998) Evidence that macrophages in atherosclerotic lesions contain angiotensin II. *Circulation* 98: 800–807

45  Ohishi M, Ueda M, Rakugi H, Naruko T, Kolima A, Okamura A, Higaki J, Ogihara T (1999) Relative localization of angiotensin-converting enzyme, chymase and angiotensin II in human coronary atherosclerotic lesion. *J Hypertens* 17: 547–553

46  Schieffer B, Schieffer E, Hilfiker-Kleiner D, Hilfiker A, Kovanen P, Nussberger J, Harringer W, Drexler H (2000) Expression of angiotensin II in human coronary atherosclerotic plaques – Potential implications for inflammtation and plaque instability. *Circulation* 101 (12): 1372–1378

47  Moreno PR, Falk E, Palaicos IF, Newell JB, Fuster V, Fallon JT (1994) Macrophage infil-

tration in acute coronary syndromes. Implications for plaque rupture. *Circulation* 90: 775–778

48  Han Y, Runge M, Brasier A (1999) Angiotensin II induces interleukin-6 transcription in vascular smooth muscle cells through pleiotropic activation of nuclear factor-κB transcription factor. *Circ Res* 84: 695–703

49  Pagano PJ, Clark JK, Cifuentes-Pagano ME, Clark SM, Callis GM, Quinn MT (1997) Localization of a constitutively active, phagocyte-like NADPH oxidase in rabbit aortic adventitia: enhancement by angiotensin II. *Proc Natl Acad Sci USA* 94 (26): 14483–14488

50  Schieffer B, Kowert A, Brauer N, Wengler A, Schieffer E, Gutzke S, Harringer W, Haverich A, Drexler H (1998) Irbesartan inhibits angiotensin II-induced pro-inflammatory and prothrombotic factors in human coronary arteries: Role of the Jak/STAT cascade. *Europ Heart J* (Suppl II) P322

51  Skeggs LT, Dorer FE, Kahn JR, Lentz KE, Levin M (1981) Experimental renal hypertension: The discovery of the renin-angiotensin system. In: RL Soffer (ed): *Biochemical regulation of blood pressure.* Wiley, New York, NY, 3–38

52  Loree HM, Kamm RD, Stringfellow RG, Lee RT (1992) Effects of fibrous cap thickness on peak circumferential stress in model artherosclerotic vessels. *Circ Res* 71: 850–858

53  Richardson PD, Davies MJ, Born GV (1989) Influence of plaque configuration and stress distribution on fissuring of coronary atherosclerotic plaques. *Lancet* 21; 2 (8669): 941–944

54  Schieffer B, Wagner M, Hilfiker-Kleiner D, Hilfiker A, Drexler H (1999) NADPH-oxidase dependent activation of Jak/STAT cascade by angiotensin II: Role of p47phox. *Circulation* (Suppl II) P–355 (Abstract)

# Heme oxygenase-1, inflammation and atherosclerosis

Anupam Agarwal[1], Nathalie Hill-Kapturczak[1] and Harry S. Nick[2]

[1]Department of Medicine, Division of Nephrology, Hypertension and Transplantation, and
[2]Department of Neuroscience, University of Florida, Box 100224 JHMHC, 1600 SW Archer Road, Gainesville, FL 32610, USA

## Introduction

Cell injury and inflammation evoke several adaptive responses that are beneficial and protective. Many of these cellular responses occur due to inflammatory stimuli such as cytokines, endotoxin, growth factors (e.g. transforming growth factor-β), lipid derivatives (e.g. oxidized LDL) and a diverse array of oxidants [1, 2]. One such cellular response in cells and tissues exposed to these stimuli is the induction of heme oxygenase-1 (HO-1), a ~ 32 kDa microsomal enzyme [3–9]. HO-1 catalyzes the rate limiting step in heme degradation resulting in the liberation of equimolar quantities of biliverdin, iron and carbon monoxide (CO) as shown below. Biliverdin is subsequently converted to bilirubin. Heme is derived from ubiquitously distributed heme proteins such as cytochromes, peroxidases, respiratory burst oxidases, pyrrolases, catalase, nitric oxide synthases, hemoglobin and myoglobin; all crucial in the maintenance of normal cellular functions [6]. Recent attention has focussed on the by product(s) of this reaction which possess important antioxidant, anti-inflammatory, anti-apoptotic and possible immune modulatory functions [10–17].

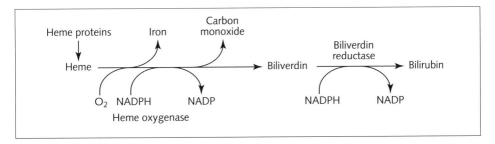

Two isoforms of heme oxygenase, expressed in the vasculature, have been extensively characterized: an inducible enzyme (HO-1, Hmox1) and a constitutive isoform (HO-2, Hmox2) [6]. Recently, a third isoform (HO-3) sharing ~ 90% amino acid homology with HO-2 has been identified [18], however, there is no evidence to

*Table 1 - Characteristics of the different heme oxygenase isoforms*

| Properties | Heme oxygenase-1 | Heme oxygenase-2 | Heme oxygenase-3 |
|---|---|---|---|
| Cellular localization | Microsomes | Mitochondria | ? |
| Chromosomal localization | 22q12 | 16p13.3 | ? |
| Molecular weight | ~32 kDa | ~36 kDa | ~33 kDa |
| Tissue distribution | Liver, spleen, pancreas, intestine, kidney, heart, retina, prostate, vascular smooth muscle cells, endothelium, lung, skin, brain and spinal cord | Brain and spinal cord, testes, liver, vascular smooth muscle cells, endothelium, pancreas, intestine | Liver, spleen, kidney, heart prostate, thymus, brain, testes |
| Regulation | Heme, hydrogen peroxide, cytokines, endotoxin, heavy metals, UV radiation, nitric oxide and nitric oxide donors, oxidized LDL, shear stress, hyperoxia, hypoxia, growth factors (PDGF, TGF-β) | Glucocorticoids | ? |

*PDGF, platelet-derived growth factor; TGF-β, transforming growth factor-β*

date that HO-3 is expressed in the vasculature. Furthermore, HO-3 has very low heme degrading activity [18]. Table 1 summarizes some of the important features of the different isoforms of heme oxygenase. The isozymes of heme oxygenase are products of different genes, with HO-1 and HO-2 sharing only roughly 40% amino acid homology [19]. HO-1 and HO-2 differ in regulation and tissue distribution. While HO-1 is ubiquitously distributed in mammalian tissues, HO-2 is expressed in the brain, testes, endothelium, liver (hepatocytes and sinusoidal endothelial cells) and myenteric plexus of the gastrointestinal tract [6, 20, 21]. Bilirubin, from activation of HO-2 is neuroprotective [22] and CO, derived from HO-2 enzyme activ-

*Table 2 - Effects of carbon monoxide*

Inhibits platelet function
Vasodilator
Enhances neutrophil migration
Inhibits iron-sulphur centers of enzymes
Putative neurotransmitter
Binds to hemoglobin and impairs oxygen delivery
Stimulates mitochondrial generation of free radicals

ity, plays a role in male reproductive behaviour; mice deficient in HO-2 demonstrate decreased reflex activity of the bulbospongiosus muscle and ejaculatory abnormalities [23]. It has been suggested that HO-2 may function as a physiological regulator of cellular function and HO-1 plays a role in modulating tissue responses to injury in pathophysiological states [24].

HO-1 is induced by a variety of stimuli which provoke oxidant stress, including heme, hydrogen peroxide, ultraviolet radiation, heavy metals, hypoxia, hyperoxia, shear stress, endotoxins, cytokines, nitric oxide and nitric oxide donors, growth factors and oxidized LDL [4, 5, 8, 25–38]. Induction of HO-1 is considered to be an adaptive and beneficial response to oxidative stress in a wide variety of cells [3-9]. Beneficial effects of HO-1 induction include degradation of the toxic heme moiety and generation of bilirubin, an antioxidant capable of scavenging peroxy radicals and inhibiting lipid peroxidation [39–42]. Ferritin, an intracellular repository for iron, is co-induced with HO-1 allowing safe sequestering of the unbound iron liberated during the degradation of heme [43]. Finally, CO has received considerable attention as a signaling molecule similar to nitric oxide (NO) in the nervous system [44, 45]. The vasodilatory effects of CO, mediated via cGMP, may be beneficial in an abnormal atherosclerotic vessel [11]. The biological effects of CO are summarized in Table 2.

## Atherosclerosis and heme oxygenase-1

There is considerable evidence that oxidized LDL contributes to the pathogenesis of atherosclerosis [46–48]. Oxidized LDL is directly cytotoxic, stimulates the release of a variety of cytokines and autacoids, as well as promoting and sustaining mononuclear cell infiltration in the vessel wall. Potential mechanisms by which oxidized LDL may be atherogenic include enhanced uptake by macrophages, cytotoxicity, alteration of gene expression (e.g. monocyte chemotactic protein-1 and leukocyte adhesion molecules), immunogenic effects, alteration of coagulation pathways and adverse effects on vasomotor properties of vessels [46–48]. Oxidation of LDL can be induced by prolonged incubation with cells in culture or by incubation with trace metal ions such as copper [46–48]. Furthermore, heme, an iron containing porphyrinic compound found in hemoglobin and other heme proteins (e.g. inducible nitric oxide synthase (iNOS), soluble guanylyl cyclase) and myeloperoxidase have also been demonstrated to initiate LDL oxidation [49, 50].

The oxidant stress generated by developing atherosclerotic lesions influences vascular cell gene expression, resulting in the induction of antioxidant defense mechanisms to counteract and prevent further oxidative damage [51]. HO-1 induction is one such antioxidant defense mechanism. It has been demonstrated that HO-1 is induced by several pro-atherogenic agents including lipid metabolites [11, 29, 30, 52], pro-inflammatory cytokines [31–33], peroxynitrite [34, 35] and heme [53]. Oxidized LDL, prepared by *in vitro* oxidation with either copper, hemin or cellular modification, has been shown to upregulate the HO-1 gene in endothelial cells and vascular smooth muscle cells, while native LDL does not result in gene induction [28, 30, 36, 52]. Other modifications of LDL, such as glycation and glyco-oxidation, have also been shown to induce HO-1 [54]. The *in vivo* relevance of HO-1 induction is suggested by the identification of an abundance of HO-1 mRNA and protein in animal and human atherosclerotic plaques [55]. Wang et al. [55] demonstrated the presence of HO-1 mRNA by *in situ* hybridization in a human atherosclerotic plaque in endothelial cells, macrophages and smooth muscle cells in conjunction with increased expression of ferritin [56]. Ferritin upregulation occurs following induction of HO-1 and may represent a mechanism to safely sequester the iron released from the HO-1 catalyzed reaction [43].

## Functional significance of HO-1 in atherosclerosis

The expression of HO-1 by oxidized LDL is important in the pathogenesis of atherosclerosis and is functionally significant. Induction of HO-1 inhibits monocyte chemotaxis induced by mildly oxidized LDL [52]. Ishikawa et al. [52] used co-cultures of aortic endothelial cells and smooth muscle cells and demonstrated that induction of HO-1 by hemin significantly reduced oxidized LDL-mediated monocyte chemotaxis. Hemin pretreatment resulted in augmentation of oxidized LDL-mediated induction of HO-1 in endothelial cells and not in smooth muscle cells suggesting that endothelial cells are responsible for the effects on monocyte migration after hemin pretreatment. Inhibition of heme oxygenase activity with tin protoporphyrin increased monocyte chemotaxis while pretreatment with either biliverdin or bilirubin reduced chemotaxis. The effects of CO on monocyte chemotaxis were not examined in this study. These authors suggest that the induction of HO-1 by mildly oxidized LDL may protect against the inflammatory responses in atherosclerotic vessels through the production of biliverdin and bilirubin. Bilirubin and biliverdin have potent antioxidant activity *in vitro* and *in vivo*. Bilirubin blocks the oxidation of linoleic acid and LDL by free radicals, and inhibits peroxidation of phospholipids, triglycerides and cholesterol esters.

In addition to bilirubin formation, CO, a potent vasodilator, is generated during heme degradation by HO-1. CO causes smooth muscle cell relaxation by a mechanism similar to that of nitric oxide. Endothelium-derived CO diffuses to adjacent smooth muscle cells and binds to the heme-iron of soluble guanylyl cyclase, causing a conformational change and activation of the catalytic site, resulting in an increase in intracellular cGMP [57, 58], leading to smooth muscle relaxation. Whereas CO is generated in response to atherogenic stimuli, atherosclerotic arteries are associated with diminished NO generation and activity [59, 60]. Therefore, an atherosclerotic blood vessel may depend on the vasodilator actions of CO in order to maintain vascular tone.

The expression of HO-1 in atherosclerosis is an important adaptive mechanism with several possible cytoprotective and antioxidant actions. A model proposed for the functional relevance of HO-1 expression in atherosclerosis is shown in Figure 1. An increase in plasma LDL leads to the adherence of circulating monocytes to arterial endothelial cells and influx of LDL into the arterial wall. LDL is then oxidatively modified by endothelial cells, smooth muscle cells and/or macrophages. The site of LDL oxidation is not entirely known, but is presumed to be in the subintimal space. Oxidized LDL has several pro-atherogenic effects, which include platelet aggregation, smooth muscle cell proliferation, gene activation and cell injury. The release of heme proteins from necrotic and damaged cells in the vicinity of atherosclerotic plaques increases the levels of heme, a potent inducer of HO-1. Heme is also a prooxidant that exhibits acute cytotoxicity [34]. Increased heme leads to further oxidation of LDL [49], another inducer of HO-1, further propagating vascular injury. Induction of HO-1 with the concomitant induction of the iron-sequestering enzyme, ferritin, within the vascular cells increases the production of antioxidants (bilirubin) decreases prooxidants (heme) as well as removes free iron. It has been reported that bilirubin, *in vitro*, inhibits oxidation of LDL [61, 62], a critical event in atherogenesis [63, 64]. Furthermore, induction of HO-1 inhibits monocyte chemotaxis [52]. Finally, it has been demonstrated that pre-exposure to oxidants or overexpression of HO-1 protects cultured vascular endothelial cells from damage from additional oxidative stress [40, 65]. Therefore, HO-1 induction and the subsequent production of bilirubin in early atherosclerotic lesions could reduce further oxidative reactions and attenuate the progression of plaques.

## Functional significance of HO-1 in inflammation

In addition to the pathogenesis of atherosclerosis, HO-1 plays an important role in the inflammatory response [10]. Willis et al. [10] reported the beneficial effects of heme oxygenase upregulation in a model of pleural inflammation. Inhibition of

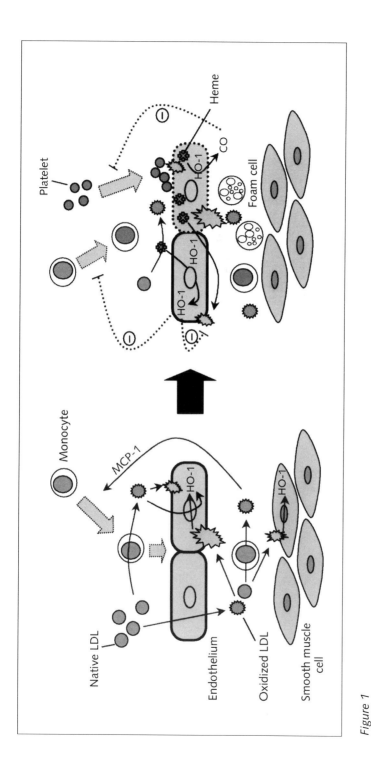

*Figure 1*

Schematic of the pro-atherogenic effects of oxidized LDL and the cytoprotective effects of HO-1.

Native LDL undergoes oxidative modification in the subintimal space and alters endothelial, monocyte (via monocyte chemotactic protein-1 (MCP-1)) and smooth muscle cell function. Oxidized LDL also results in the upregulation of several genes including HO-1 (left panel). Oxidized LDL-induced cell injury leads to an increased level of heme from damaged and necrotic cells, further propagating cell injury. Heme and oxidized LDL are potent inducers of HO-1 enzyme activity. The cytoprotective effects of increased HO-1 activity are due to the formation of biliverdin and bilirubin (antioxidants) and CO (vasodilator). CO also inhibits platelet aggregation. Furthermore, induction of HO-1 inhibits oxidized LDL-mediated monocyte chemotaxis (right panel).

*Table 3 - Inflammatory conditions associated with heme oxygenase-1*

| |
|---|
| Atherosclerosis |
| Transplant rejection |
| Sepsis and endotoxemia |
| Acute glomerulonephritis |
| Acute pancreatitis |
| Acquired immunodeficiency syndrome |
| Hyperoxia-induced lung injury |
| Pleuritis |
| Asthma |
| Keratitis |

HO-1 using tin protoporphyrin significantly worsened inflammatory exudate and cell number, while prior induction with iron protoporphyrin showed a significant reduction in inflammatory cell infiltration and exudate suggesting that HO-1 activity would serve as a novel target to modulate the inflammatory response. Similar findings have been reported in other models of inflammation as well [12, 66]. Vogt et al. [66] demonstrated a novel phenomenon of acquired resistance to renal tubular injury in acute glomerular inflammation that was dependent on the induction of HO-1 in renal tubules. Induction of HO-1 occurs in immune-mediated renal injury, as demonstrated by the expression of this protein in infiltrating macrophages in acute renal transplant rejection [12].

Studies in HO-1 knockout mice further corroborate these observations in that mice lacking HO-1 develop a progressive inflammatory disease characterized by splenomegaly, lymphadenopathy, leukocytosis, hepatic periportal inflammation and glomerulonephritis [67]. These mice show evidence of iron accumulation and are more sensitive to oxidant injury [14, 67]. Expression of HO-1 has been shown to be important in xenograft rejection, since hearts transplanted from homozygote mice lacking HO-1 were rejected in three days compared to hearts transplanted from wild or heterozygote mice which survived up to 60 days [13]. More recently, the first known case of human HO-1 deficiency was reported [68]. Several phenotypical features observed in the mouse HO-1 knockout model were reported in this patient, most notably, enhanced endothelial injury and hyperlipidemia. HO-1 has also been implicated in several clinically relevant disease states including atherosclerosis [52, 55], hypertension [38], acute renal injury [69], toxic nephropathy [70], transplant rejection [12, 13, 15], endotoxic shock [33] and Alzheimer's disease [71] as well as others [72]. A list of inflammatory diseases associated with heme oxygenase is shown in Table 3.

Overexpression of HO-1 or prior induction of HO-1 is cytoprotective in both *in vitro* and *in vivo* models of injury [65]. Abraham and coworkers [65] employing transfection studies resulting in the overexpression of HO-1 in coronary microvascular endothelial cells demonstrated cytoprotective effects against heme and hemoglobin toxicity. Vile et al. [73] have demonstrated a beneficial role of HO-1 in ultraviolet A radiation-induced cell injury. Inhibition of HO-1 activity by tin protoporphyrin, an enzymatic inhibitor, or by antisense oligonucleotides abolished the protective effect of pre-irradiation, implicating HO-1 in the mechanism of cellular protection. Expression of HO-1 is also protective in hyperoxia-induced lung injury [74]. The generation of CO seems to be the mechanism involved in this model since exogenous administration of CO protects against hyperoxia-induced lung injury, results similar to gene delivery studies with HO-1. We have also demonstrated that HO-1 gene expression modulates cisplatin-mediated apoptosis both *in vivo* and *in vitro* [75]. Overexpression of HO-1 also provides protection in oxidized LDL-mediated cell injury (unpublished observations).

## Induction of HO-1 by constituents of oxidized LDL

Oxidized LDL is a complex structure consisting of several chemically distinct prooxidant components including fatty acid hydroperoxides, oxidized phospholipids, oxidized sterols and modified apolipoprotein B [76, 77]. Fatty acid hydroperoxides, such as linoleyl hydroperoxide (LAox or 13-HPODE), and phospholipids, such as lysophosphatidylcholine (lyso-PC), are abundant components of oxidized LDL, and act as specific redox signals in the expression of cell adhesion molecules and growth factors in endothelial cells [76–79]. Studies using antibodies to LAox, have demonstrated the presence of fatty acid hydroperoxides in oxidized LDL as well as in human atherosclerotic plaques [80, 81].

To determine whether these chemical constituents of oxidized LDL were responsible for HO-1 gene induction, we exposed confluent monolayers of human aortic endothelial cells (HAECs) to media containing PBS (control), lyso-PC (25 µM), LAox (25 µM) or ethanol (EtOH 0.5%) (Fig. 2) [30]. Cells were exposed to lyso-PC for 8 h and LAox for 4 h, time points at which maximal induction of HO-1 was seen. As shown in Figure 2, incubation with lyso-PC (25 µM) resulted in a ~ 2.6-fold increase in HO-1 mRNA whereas exposure to LAox (25 µM) resulted in a much higher induction (~ 16 fold) of HO-1 mRNA. The parent phospholipid compound, PC (25 µM), did not induce HO-1 mRNA (Fig. 2, lower panel). Thus, LAox mediates significant induction of HO-1 mRNA in HAECs. We also performed experiments in which HAECs were incubated with media containing PBS (control), LAox (1, 10 and 25 µM), unoxidized linoleic acid (LA 25 µM), or lipoxygenase alone (Lip 100 U) for 4 h (Fig. 3). These concentrations of LAox are approximately equivalent to their abundance in 100 µg/ml oxidized LDL [77]. As shown in Fig. 3, significant induction of HO-1 mRNA and protein occurred with LAox in HAECs, while linoleic acid and lipoxygenase alone did not induce HO-1 expression. Preliminary studies

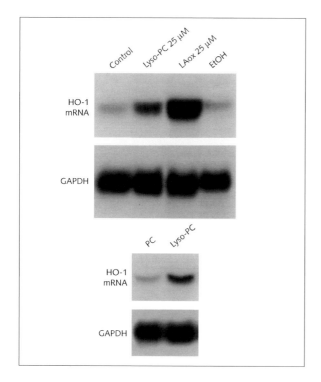

*Figure 2*
*Differential induction of HO-1 mRNA with lysophosphatidylcholine (lyso-PC) and linoleyl hydroperoxide (LAox).*
*Confluent monolayers of human aortic endothelial cells (HAECs) were incubated with media containing PBS (control), lyso-PC 25 μM for 8 h, LAox 25 μM for 4 h or carrier (EtOH 0.5%) as indicated. In separate experiments, cells were exposed to PC (25 μM) or lyso-PC (25 μM) for 8 h (lower panel). RNA was isolated, electrophoresed, transfered to a nylon membrane and hybridized with a ³²P-labeled human HO-1 cDNA probe. The membrane was stripped and reprobed with a human GAPDH cDNA probe to control for loading and transfer. The results are representative of several experiments performed in duplicate. Reprinted with permission from [30].*

demonstrate a ~2 h half-life for HO-1 mRNA in response to LAox in human endothelial and smooth muscle cells.

Our findings that LAox results in significantly higher HO-1 induction than lyso-PC demonstrates the differential effects of the components of oxidized LDL [30]. With regards to oxidized LDL, previous studies report induction of adhesion molecules such as intercellular cell adhesion molecule-1, vascular cell adhesion molecule-

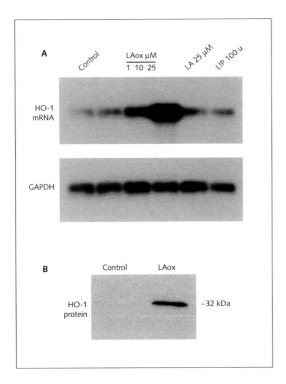

*Figure 3*
*Induction of HO-1 in HAECs with LAox.*
*Confluent monolayers of HAECs were incubated with media containing PBS (control), LAox, unoxidized linoleic acid (LA) or lipoxygenase (Lip) for 4 h in serum free media. RNA was isolated, electrophoresed, transfered to a nylon membrane and hybridized with a $^{32}$P-labeled human HO-1 cDNA probe. The membrane was stripped and reprobed with a human GAPDH cDNA probe to control for loading and transfer. (B) Confluent monolayers of HAECs were incubated with media containing PBS (control), or linoleyl hydroperoxide (LAox 25 µM) for 4 h and then replaced with media alone for an additional 8 h. Western blot analysis was performed using a polyclonal anti-HO-1 antibody (Stressgen, Canada) as described in [30]. HO-1 is identified as a 32 kDa size protein. Reprinted with permission from [30].*

1, growth factors, endothelial nitric oxide synthase and cyclooxygenase-2 by LAox and/or lyso-PC [30, 77, 82]. Oxidized arachidonic acid containing phospholipids also induce HO-1 but to a much lesser extent than oxidized LDL or LAox [52]. Our results indicate that LAox, an oxidized C:18 fatty acid, is the major component of oxidized LDL that induces HO-1 and may serve as a critical cellular signal for HO-1 gene induction during the progression of atherosclerosis [30].

## Molecular regulation of HO-1 by oxidized LDL

The regulatory elements that control LAox-mediated HO-1 induction are not known. Consensus binding sites for NF-κB, activator protein-2 (AP-2) and interleukin-6 (IL-6) responsive elements as well as other transcription factors have been reported in the promoter region of the HO-1 gene [83] suggesting a potential role for these trans-acting factors in modulating HO-1 gene expression. We have reported that the induction of HO-1 by LAox occurs *via* transcriptional mechanisms, since treatment with actinomycin D (4 μM), a transcriptional inhibitor, as well as nuclear run-on assays demonstrated that LAox-mediated HO-1 gene induction is dependent on *de novo* transcription. Interestingly, no significant response was observed with a ~ 4.5 kb human HO-1 promoter fragment as assessed by both reporter gene mRNA or protein expression [30], implying that upregulation of HO-1 by LAox requires sequences outside of this 4.5 kb promoter fragment.

Regarding the cis-acting elements which modulate HO-1 gene expression, a potential cadmium response element has been identified 5' to the transcriptional initiation site of the human HO-1 gene, between – 4.5 and – 4 kb [84]. We have shown that this 4.5 kb human HO-1 gene promoter fragment, which responds to known inducers of the gene such as heme and cadmium, does not completely recapitulate the induction of the gene seen by steady state northern analysis and also lacks the cis-acting elements necessary for LAox-dependent gene induction [30]. Our findings of the absence of a response with this promoter fragment to LAox is further corroborated by the failure of this fragment to respond to other stimuli that directly increase *de novo* HO-1 gene transcription, i.e. hyperoxia and iron/hyperoxia [85].

In contrast, in the mouse HO-1 gene, Alam et al. [86] have described two distal enhancers, one at – 4.0 and another at – 10 kb, that are required for induction of HO-1 in response to heme, heavy metals, hydrogen peroxide and sodium arsenite. It is possible, therefore, that the human HO-1 gene also requires distal enhancer element(s) similar to the mouse HO-1 gene for induction with LAox. Further experiments using additional promoter transfections, chromatin structure analysis and *in vivo* footprinting are currently underway in our laboratory to delineate the region of the HO-1 gene that controls oxidized lipid-mediated induction as well as the sites for other mediators.

## Iron and HO-1 gene expression

The role of iron in regulating expression and the effects of HO-1 have been well documented. We have previously demonstrated that deferoxamine (DFO) blocks oxidized LDL-mediated cytotoxicity in endothelial and renal epithelial cells. DFO blocks oxidized LDL-mediated HO-1 induction as well [36]. Most interestingly, iron potentiates hyperoxia-mediated transcriptional activation of HO-1 [85]. The HO-1 knock-out mouse develops a chronic inflammatory disease with tissue iron accumulation in the liver and kidney, thus presenting with a disorder of iron reutilization [67]. Ferris et al. [87] have recently provided a link between intracellular iron levels and attenuation of cell death by serum deprivation, staurosporine and etoposide. Incubation with either bilirubin or a cGMP analogue to mimic the production of carbon monoxide failed to protect against serum deprivation-induced cell death suggesting that, at least in this model of cell injury, by-products of heme oxygenase activity were not cytoprotective.

## Conclusions

In summary, the induction of HO-1 plays an important role in atherogenesis and several inflammatory disorders. Identification of the molecular mechanisms that control HO-1 expression by inflammatory mediators, including oxidized LDL and its constituents will provide insight into the pathogenesis of atherosclerosis.

*Acknowledgments*
This work was supported by grants from the National Institutes of Health, K08 DK02446 (to A. Agarwal), HL39593 (to H.S. Nick). Dr. Hill-Kapturczak is supported by an NIH Postdoctoral training grant to the Division of Nephrology, University of Florida.

## References

1   Yu BP (1994) Cellular defenses against damage from reactive oxygen species. *Phys Rev* 74: 139–162

2   Janssen YMW, Van Houten B, Borm PJA, Mossman BT (1993) Cell and tissue responses to oxidative damage. *Lab Invest* 69: 261–274

3   Nath KA (1994) The functional significance of the induction of heme oxygenase by oxidative stress. *J Lab Clin Med* 123: 461–463

4   Stocker R (1990) Induction of haem oxygenase as a defence against oxidative stress. *Free Rad Res Comm* 9: 101–112

5   Keyse SM, Tyrrell RM (1989) Heme oxygenase is the major 32-kDa stress protein induced in skin fibroblasts by UVA radiation, hydrogen peroxide and sodium arsenite. *Proc Natl Acad Sci USA* 86: 99–103

6   Maines MD (1997) The heme oxygenase system: A regulator of second messenger gases. *Annu Rev Pharmacol Toxicol* 37: 517–554

7   Platt JL, Nath KA (1998) Heme oxygenase: protective gene or Trojan horse. *Nat Med* 4: 1364–1365

8    Choi AMK, Alam J (1996) Heme oxygenase-1: Function, regulation, and implication of a novel stress-inducible protein in oxidant-induced lung injury. *Am J Respir Cell Mol Biol* 15: 9–19

9    Elbirt KK, Bonkovsky HL (1999) Heme oxygenase: Recent advances in understanding its regulation and role. *Proc Assoc Am Phys* 111: 438–447

10   Willis D, Moore AR, Frederick R, Willoughby DA (1996) Heme oxygenase: A novel target for the modulation of the inflammatory response. *Nat Med* 2: 87–90

11   Siow RCM, Sato H, Mann GE (1999) Heme oxygenase-carbon monoxide signalling pathway in atherosclerosis: Anti-atherogenic actions of bilirubin and carbon monoxide? *Cardiovasc Res* 41: 385–394

12   Agarwal A, Kim Y, Matas AJ, Alam J, Nath KA (1996) Gas-generating systems in acute renal allograft rejection in the rat: Co-induction of heme oxygenase and nitric oxide synthase. *Transplantation* 61: 93–98

13   Soares MP, Lin Y, Anrather J, Csizmadia E, Takigami K, Sato K, Grey ST, Colvin RB, Choi AM, Poss KD et al (1998) Expression of heme oxygenase-1 can determine cardiac xenograft survival. *Nature Med* 4: 1073–1077

14   Poss KD, Tonegawa S (1997) Reduced stress defense in heme oxygenase-1 deficient cells. *Proc Natl Acad Sci USA* 94: 10925–10930

15   Hancock WW, Buelow R, Sayegh MH, Turka LA (1998) Antibody-induced transplant arteriosclerosis is prevented by graft expression of anti-oxidant and anti-apoptotic genes. *Nat Med* 4: 1392–1396

16   Otterbein LE, Mantell LL, Choi AMK (1999) Carbon monoxide provides protection against hyperoxic lung injury. *Am J Physiol* (*Lung Cell Mol Physiol* 20) 276: L688–L694

17   Nath KA (1999) Heme oxygenase-1: a redoubtable response that limits reperfusion injury in the transplanted adipose liver. *J Clin Invest* 104: 1485–1486

18   McCoubrey WK, Huang TJ, and Maines MD (1997) Isolation and characterization of a cDNA from the rat brain that encodes hemoprotein heme oxygenase-3. *Eur J Biochem* 247: 725–732

19   Kutty RK, Kutty G, Rodriguez IR, Chader CJ, Wiggert B (1994) Chromosomal localization of the human heme oxygenase genes: Heme oxygenase-1 (Hmox1) maps to chromosome 22q12 and heme oxygenase-2 (Hmox2) maps to chromosome 16p13.3. *Genomics* 20: 513–516

20   Suematsu M, Ishimura Y (2000) The heme oxygenase-carbon monoxide system: A regulator of hepatobiliary function. *Hepatology* 31: 3–6

21   Zakhary R, Gaine SP, Dinerman JL, Ruat M, Flavahan NA, Snyder SH (1996) Heme oxygenase 2: Endothelial and neuronal localization and role in endothelium-dependent relaxation. *Proc Natl Acad Sci USA* 93: 795–798

22   Dore S, Takahashi M, Ferris CD, Hester LD, Guastella D, Snyder SH (1999) Bilirubin, formed by activation of heme oxygenase-2, protects neurons against oxidative stress injury. *Proc Natl Acad Sci USA* 96: 2445–2450

23   Burnett AL, Johns DG, Kriegsfeld LJ, Klein SL, Calvin DC, Demas GE, Schramm LP,

Tonegawa S, Nelson RJ, Snyder SH et al (1998) Ejaculatory abnormalities in mice with targeted disruption of the gene for heme oxygenase-2. *Nat Med* 4: 84–87

24  Wagener FA, da Silva JL, Farley T, de Witte T, Kappas A, Abraham NG (1999) Differential effects of heme oxygenase isoforms on heme mediation of endothelial intracellular adhesion molecule 1 expression. *J Pharmacol Exp Ther* 291: 416–423

25  Rizzardini M, Terao M, Falciani F, Cantoni L (1993) Cytokine induction of haem oxygenase mRNA in mouse liver: Interleukin 1 transcriptionally activates the haem oxygenase gene. *Biochem J* 290: 343–347

26  Wagner CT, Durante W, Christodoulides N, Hellums JD, Schafer AI (1997) Hemodynamic forces induce the expression of heme oxygenase in cultured vascular smooth muscle cells. *J Clin Invest* 100: 589–596

27  Kutty RK, Nagineni CM, Kutty G, Hooks JJ, Chader GJ, Wiggert B (1994) Increased expression of heme oxygenase-1 in human retinal pigment epithelial cells by transforming growth factor-β. *J Cellular Physiol* 159: 371–378

28  Siow RC, Ishii T, Sato H, Taketani S, Leake DS, Sweiry JH, Peason JD, Bannai S, Mann GE (1995) Induction of the antioxidant stress proteins heme oxygenase-1 and MSP23 by stress agents and oxidized LDL in cultured vascular smooth muscle cells. *FEBS Lett* 368: 239–242

29  BasuModak S, Luscher P, Tyrrell RM (1996) Lipid metabolite involvement in the activation of the human heme oxygenase-1 gene. *Free Rad Biol Med* 20: 887–897

30  Agarwal A, Shiraishi F, Visner GA, Nick HS (1998) Linoleyl hydroperoxide transcriptionally upregulates heme oxygenase-1 gene expression in human renal epithelial and aortic endothelial cells. *J Am Soc Nephrol* 9: 1990–1997

31  Terry CM, Clikeman JA, Hoidal JR, Callahan KS (1998) Effect of tumor necrosis factor α and interleukin-1 α on heme oxygenase-1 expression in human endothelial cells. *Am J Physiol* 274: H883–H891

32  Durante W, Kroll MH, Christodoulides N, Peyton KJ, Schafer AI (1997) Nitric oxide induces heme oxygenase-1 gene expression and carbon monoxide production in vascular smooth muscle cells. *Circ Res* 80: 557–564

33  Yet SF, Pellacani A, Patterson C, Tan L, Folta SC, Foster L, Lee WS, Hsieh CM, Perrella MA (1997) Induction of heme oxygense-1 expression in vascular smooth muscle cells. A link to endotoxic shock. *J Biol Chem* 272: 4295–4301

34  Foresti R, Clark JE, Green CJ, Motterlini R (1997) Thiol compounds interact with nitric oxide in regulating heme oxygenase-1 induction in endothelial cells. Involvement of superoxide and peroxynitrite anions. *J Biol Chem* 272: 18411–18417

35  Foresti R, Sarathchandra P, Clark JE, Green CJ, Motterlini R (1999) Peroxynitrite induces haem oxygenase-1 in vascular endothelial cells: a link to apoptosis. *Biochem J* 339: 729–736

36  Agarwal A, Balla J, Balla G, Croatt AJ, Vercellotti GM, Nath KA (1996) Renal tubular epithelial cells mimic endothelial cells upon exposure to oxidized LDL. *Am J Physiol (Renal, Fluid and Electrolyte 40)* 271: F814–F823

37  Durante W, Peyton KJ, Schafer AI (1999) Platelet-derived growth factor stimulates heme

oxygenase-1 gene expression and carbon monoxide production in vascular smooth muscle cells. *Arterioscler Thromb Vasc Biol* 19: 2666–2672

38    Ishizaka N, Leon HD, Laursen JB, Fukui T, Wilcox JN, Keulenaer GD, Griendling KK, Alexander RW (1997) Angiotensin II-induced hypertension increases heme oxygenase-1 expression in rat aorta. *Circulation* 96: 1923–1929

39    Balla G, Vercellotti GM, Muller-Eberhard U, Eaton JW, Jacob HS (1991) Exposure of endothelial cells to free heme potentiates damage mediated by granulocytes and toxic oxygen species. *Lab Invest* 64: 648–655

40    Balla, J, Jacob HS, Balla G, Nath KA, Eaton JW, Vercellotti GM (1993) Endothelial cell heme uptake from heme proteins: Sensitization and desensitization to oxdiant damage. *Proc Natl Acad Sci USA* 90: 9285–9289

41    Stocker R, Yamamoto Y, McDonagh AF, Glazer AN, Ames BN (1987) Bilirubin is an antioxidant of possible physiologic significance. *Science* 235: 1043–1046

42    Dore S, Takahashi M, Ferris CD, Hester LD, Guastella D, Snyder SH (1999) Bilirubin, formed by activation of heme oxygenase-1, protects neurons against oxidative stress injury. *Proc Natl Acad Sci USA* 96: 2445–2450

43    Balla G, Jacob HS, Balla J, Rosenberg M, Nath KA, Apple F, Eaton JW, Vercellotti GM (1992) Ferritin: A cytoprotective antioxidant strategem of endothelium. *J Biol Chem* 267: 18148–18153

44    Marks GS, Brien JF, Nakatsu K, McLaughlin BE (1991) Does carbon monoxide have a physiological function? *Trends Pharm Sci* 12: 185–188

45    Dawson TM, Snyder SH (1994) Gases as biological messengers: Nitric oxide and carbon monoxide in the brain. *J Neuroscience* 14: 5147–5159

46    Witztum JL, Steinberg D (1991) Role of oxidized low density lipoprotein in atherogenesis. *J Clin Invest* 88: 1785–1792

47    Steinberg D, Parthasarathy S, Carew TE, Khoo JC, Witztum JL (1989) Beyond cholesterol. Modifications of Low density lipoprotein that increase its atherogenicity. *N Engl J Med* 320: 915–924

48    Steinberg D (1997) Low density lipoprotein oxidation and its pathobiological significance. *J Biol Chem* 272: 20963–20966

49    Balla G, Jacob HS, Eaton JW, Belcher JD, Vercellotti GM (1991) Hemin: A possible physiological mediator of low density lipoprotein oxidation and endothelial injury. *Arterioscler Thromb* 11: 1700–1711

50    Daugherty A, Dunn JL, Rateri DL, Heinecke JW (1994) Myeloperoxidase, a catalyst for lipoprotein oxidation, is expressed in human atherosclerotic lesions. *J Clin Invest* 94: 437–444

51    Sen C, Packer L (1996) Antioxidant and redox regulation of gene-transcription. *FASEB J* 10: 709–720

52    Ishikawa K, Navab M, Leitinger N, Fogelman AM, Lusis AJ (1997) Induction of heme oxygenase-1 inhibits monocyte transmigration induced by mildly oxidized LDL. *J Clin Invest* 100: 1209–1216

53    Vigne P, Feolde E, Ladoux A, Duval D, Frelin C (1995) Contributions of NO synthase

and heme oxygenase to cGMP formation by cytokine and hemin treated brain capillary endothelial cells. *Biochem Biophys Res Commun* 214: 1–5

54    Agarwal A, Shiraishi F, Truong L, Nick HS, Joyce K, Lyons TJ, Jenkins A (1998) Glycated LDL imposes oxidant stress in renal proximal tubule cells: Implications in diabetic nephropathy (DN). *J Am Soc Nephrol* 9: 627A

55    Wang LJ, Lee TS, Lee FY, Pai RC, Chau LY (1998) Expression of heme oxygenase-1 in atherosclerotic lesions. *Am J Pathol* 152(3): 711–720

56    Pang JH, Jiang MJ, Chen YL, Wang FW, Wang DL, Chu SH, Chau LY (1996) Increased ferritin gene expression in atherosclerotic lesions. *J Clin Invest* 97: 2204–2212

57    Morita T, Kourembanas S (1995) Endothelial cell expression of vasoconstrictors and growth factors is regulated by smooth muscle cell-derived carbon monoxide. *J Clin Invest* 96: 2676–2682

58    Morita T, Mitsialis SA, Koike H, Liu YX, Kourembanas S (1997) Carbon monoxide controls the proliferation of hypoxic vascular smooth muscle cells. *J Biol Chem.* 272: 32804–32809

59    Cox DA, Cohen ML (1996) Effects of oxidized low-density lipoprotein on vascular contraction and relaxation: Clinical and pharmacological implication in atherosclerosis. *Pharmacol Rev* 48: 3–19

60    Jay MT, Chirico S, Siow RCM, Bruckdorfer KR, Jacobs M, Leake DS, Pearson JD, Mann GE (1997) Modulation of vascular tone by low density lipoproteins: Effects on L-arginine transport and nitric oxide synthesis. *Exp Physiol* 82: 349–360

61    Neuzil J, Stocker R (1994) Free and albumin-bound bilirubin are efficient co-antioxidants for α-tocopherol, inhibiting plasma and low density lipoprotein lipid peroxidation. *J Biol Chem* 269: 16712–16719

62    Wu TW, Fung KP, Wu J, Yang CC, Weisel RD (1996) Antioxidation of human low density lipoprotein by unconjugated and conjugated bilirubins. *Biochem Pharmacol* 51: 859–862

63    Ross R (1993) The pathogenesis of atherosclerosis: a perspective for the 1990's. *Nature* 362: 801–809

64    Berliner JA, Navab M, Fogelman AM, Frank JS, Demer LL, Edward PA, Watson AD, Lusis AJ (1995) Atherosclerosis: basic mechanisms, oxidation inflammation, and genetics. *Cirulation* 91: 2488–2496

65    Abraham NG, Lavrovsky Y, Schwartzman ML, Stoltz RA, Levere RD, Gerritsen ME, Shibahara S, Kappas A (1995) Transfection of the human heme oxygenase gene into rabbit coronary microvessel endothelial cells: protective effect against heme and hemoglobin toxicity. *Proc Natl Acad Sci USA* 92: 6798–6802

66    Vogt BA, Shanley TP, Croatt A, Alam J, Johnson KJ, Nath KA (1996) Glomerular inflammation induces resistance to tubular injury in the rat. A novel form of acquired, heme oxygenase-dependent resistance to renal injury. *J Clin Invest* 98: 2139–2145

67    Poss KD, Tonegawa S (1997) Heme oxygenase-1 is required for mammalian iron reutilization. *Proc Natl Acad Sci USA* 94: 10919–10924

68    Yachie A, Niida Y, Wada T, Igarashi N, Kaneda H, Toma T, Ohta K, Kasahara Y, Koizu-

mi S (1999) Oxidative stress causes enhanced endothelial cell injury in human heme oxy-genase-1 deficiency. *J Clin Invest* 103: 129–135

69    Nath KA, Balla G, Vercellotti GM, Balla J, Jacob HS, Levitt MD, Rosenberg ME (1992) Induction of heme oxygenase is a rapid, protective response in rhabdomyolysis in the rat. *J Clin Invest* 90: 267–270

70    Agarwal A, Balla J, Alam J, Croatt AJ, Nath KA (1995) Induction of heme oxygenase in toxic renal injury: A protective role in cisplatin nephrotoxicity in the rat. *Kidney Int* 48: 1298–1307

71    Smith MA, Kutty RK, Richey PL, Yan SD, Stern D, Hader GJ, Wiggert B, Petersen RB, Perry G (1994) Heme oxygenase-1 is associated with the neurofibrillary pathology of Alzheimer's disease. *Am J Pathol* 145: 42–47

72    Levere RD, Staudinger R, Loewy G, Kappas A, Shibahara S, Abraham NG (1993) Ele-vated levels of heme oxygenase-1 activity and mRNA in peripheral blood adherent cells of acquired immunodeficiency syndrome patients. *Am J Hematol* 43: 19–23

73    Vile GF, Basu-Modak C, Waltner C, Tyrrell RM (1994) Heme oxygenase-1 mediates an adaptive response to oxidative stress in human skin fibroblasts. *Proc Natl Acad Sci USA* 91: 2607–2610

74    Otterbein LE, Kolls JK, Mantell LL, Cook JL, Alam J, Choi AM (1999) Exogenous administration of heme oxygenase-1 by gene transfer provides protection against hyper-oxia-induced lung injury. *J Clin Invest* 103: 1047–1054

75    Shiraishi F, Curtis LM, Truong L, Poss K, Visner GA, Madsen KM, Nick HS, Agarwal A (2000) Heme oxygenase-1 gene ablation or overexpression modulates cisplatin-induced renal tubular apoptosis and necrosis. *Am J Physiol (Renal)* 278: F726–F736

76    Fruebis J, Parthasarathy S, Steinberg D (1992) Evidence for a concerted reaction between lipid hydroperoxides and polypeptides. *Proc Natl Acad Sci USA* 89: 10588–10592

77    Khan BV, Parthasarathy SS, Alexander RW, Medford RM (1995) Modified low density lipoprotein and its constituents augment cytokine-activated vascular cell adhesion mol-ecule-1 gene expression in human vascular endothelial cells. *J Clin Invest* 95: 1262–1270

78    Kume N, Gimbrone MA (1994) Lysophosphatidylcholine transcriptionally induces growth factor gene expression in cultured human endothelial cells. *J Clin Invest* 93: 907–911

79    Fang X, Gibson S, Flowers M, Furui T, Bast RC, Mills GB (1997) Lysophosphatidyl-choline stimulates activator protein-1 and the c-Jun N-terminal kinase activity. *J Biol Chem* 272: 13683–13689

80    Kato Y, Makino Y, Osawa T (1997) Characterization of a specific polyclonal antibody against 13-hydroperoxyoctadecadienoic acid-modified protein: formation of lipid hydroperoxide-modified apoB-100 in oxidized LDL. *J Lipid Res* 38: 1334–1346

81    Kim JG, Sabbagh F, Santanam N, Wilcox JN, Medford RM, Parthasarathy S (1997) Generation of a polyclonal antibody against lipid peroxide-modified proteins. *Free Rad Biol Med* 23: 251–259

82 Ramasamy S, Parthasarathy S, Harrison DG (1998) Regulation of endothelial nitric oxide synthase gene expression by oxidized linoleic acid. *J Lipid Res* 39: 268–276

83 Lavrovsky Y, Schwartzman ML, Levere RD, Kappas A, Abraham NG (1994) Identification of binding sites for transcription factors NF-κB and AP-2 in the promoter region of the human heme oxygenase 1 gene. *Proc Natl Acad Sci USA* 91: 5987–5991

84 Takeda K, Ishizawa S, Sato M, Yoshida T, Shibahara S (1994) Identification of a cis-acting element that is responsible for cadmium-mediated induction of the human heme oxygenase gene. *J Biol Chem* 269: 22858–22867

85 Fogg S, Agarwal A, Nick HS, Visner GA (1999) Iron regulates hyperoxia-dependent human heme oxygenase-1 gene expression in pulmonary endothelial cells. *Am J Respir Cell Mol Biol* 20: 797–804

86 Alam J, Camhi S, Choi AMK (1995) Identification of a second 5' distal region that functions as a basal and inducer-dependent transcriptional enhancer of the mouse heme oxygenase-1 gene. *J Biol Chem* 270: 11977–11984

87 Ferris CD, Jaffrey SR, Sawa A, Takahashi M, Brady SD, Barrow RK, Tysoe SA, Wolosker H, Baranano DE, Dore S et al (1999) Haem oxygenase-1 prevents cell death by regulating cellular iron. *Nat Cell Biol* 1: 152–157

# Lymphocyte activation in acute coronary syndromes

*Stefano De Servi and Antonino Mazzone*

Unità di Cardiologia, Medicina Generale II, Ospedale Civile di Legnano, Via Candiani 2, 20025 Legnano (Milan), Italy

## Introduction to the immune system

The immune system has evolved to protect us from pathogens [1]. A great number of infectious microbes, viruses, bacteria, fungi, protozoa and multicellular parasites are present in our environment. The cells which mediate immunity include lymphocytes and phagocytes. Lymphocytes recognize antigens on pathogens. Phagocytes internalize the pathogens and degrade them. Any immune response involves, first, a recognition of the pathogen or other foreign material, and second, a reaction to eliminate it (Fig. 1). Different types of immune responses fall into two categories: innate (or non-adaptive) immune responses, and adaptive immune response. Specificity and memory are two essential features of adaptive immune responses. Lymphocytes have specialized functions. B cells make antibodies [2]; cytotoxic T (CD8)-cells kill virally infected cells; helper T cells subdivided into Th1 and Th2 coordinate the immune response by directing cell-cell interactions and the release of cytokines, which help B cells to make antibodies [3]. Antigens are molecules which are recognized by receptors on lymphocytes [4]. B lymphocytes usually recognize intact antigen molecules, while T lymphocytes recognize antigen fragments on the surface of other cells. Clonal selection involves recognition of antigen by particular lymphocytes; this leads to clonal expansion and differentiation to effector and memory cells. The immune system may break down. This can lead to immunodeficiency or hypersensitivity diseases or to autoimmune diseases.

## Cells involved in the immune response

Physiologically, leukocytes migrate through all tissues of the body [5]. All types of cells have particular patterns of migrations. This pattern also depends on the state of cell differentiation and activation:

- Phagocytes, including neutrophils and monocytes, leave the bone marrow and migrate to peripheral tissues, particularly at sites of infection or inflammation [1].

Inflammatory and Infectious Basis of Atherosclerosis, edited by Jay L. Mehta
© 2001 Birkhäuser Verlag Basel/Switzerland

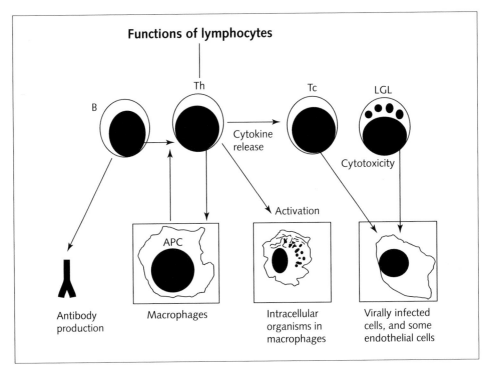

*Figure 1*
*There are several different types of lymphocytes and they have a variety of functions. B-lymphocytes produce antibodies. Th cells are stimulated by antigen-presenting cells (APC), B, T lymphocytes and macrophages to produce cytokines, which control immune responses. Macrophages are activated to kill intracellular microorganisms. Cytotoxic T (Tc) cells and large granular lymphocytes (LGL) can recognize and kill target host cells.*

Neutrophils make a one way trip, but monocytes differentiate into macrophages and may re-circulate back to the secondary lymphoid tissues to act as antigen presenting cells (APCs) [4].

- Lymphocytes migrate from the thymus and bone marrow to the secondary lymphoid tissues. After activation by antigen, activated T cells tend to move to sites of inflammation while B cells and memory T cells seed other lymphoid tissues [4].
- Dendritic cells, such as the Langherans cells of the skin, are originally derived from bone-marrow stem cells which colonize various organs. After taking up antigen, they may migrate to local lymph nodes to present antigen to CD4+ cells [6].

Inflammation is a response that brings leukocytes and plasma molecules to sites of infection or tissue damage. The principal effects are an increase in blood supply, an increase in vascular permeability to large serum molecules, and enhanced migration of leukocytes across the local vascular endothelium and in the direction of the inflammation site. The migration of cells is a complex process that depends on which populations of cells are involved, their state of activation and how they interact with endothelium in different vascular beds throughout the body [2]. Cell activation partly determines the pattern of migration. Resting or naive lymphocytes tend to migrate across high endothelial venules into lymphatic tissues, whereas activated lymphocytes tend to migrate to inflammatory sites. Adhesion molecules that control leukocyte migration fall into families that are structurally related: the cell adhesion molecules (CAMs) of the immunoglobulin supergene family, the selectins and their carbohydrate ligands, and the integrins [8]. Endothelial adhesion molecules are induced by cytokines [9, 10]. The expression of leukocyte adhesion molecules is determined by the cell population involved and by the cell's state of differentiation. Chemotactic molecules are important both in directing cell migration and in triggering leukocytes at the endothelial surface to initiate their migration [11]. Inflammatory mediators released by mast cells, platelets and leukocytes in immune reactions, or following tissue damage, act in concert with molecules released by the plasma enzyme system to control vascular permeability and blood supply.

## Interaction between lymphocytes and endothelium

According to the current hypothesis of atherogenesis the circulating lymphocytes must attach to the endothelium to enter the intimal space [12]. The endothelial cells respond to both mechanical and chemical stress and may do so by an alteration in adhesion proteins [12]. During injury, leukocyte-endothelial interactions may be invoked [11].

There are three types of interactions between the lymphocytes and the endothelium that are facilitated by the adhesion molecules [13–15]. The interactions begin with rolling of the leukocyte over the endothelium due to the formation and breakage of adhesive bonds, primarily through L-,E-, and P-selectins located on leukocytes and endothelial cells, respectively [16]. The conversion of rolling from the second stage of firm attachment is mediated by signals from the endothelial cell surface or the intra/extravascular space [17] (Fig. 2). These signals include the selectins and immunoglobulin adhesion molecules (ICAM-1, 2, VCAM-1) as well as cytokines such as interleukin-1 (IL-1) and tumor necrosis factor (TNF), which are often secreted from the injured endothelium itself and may stimulate selectin ligand synthesis [18–20]. The movement of the leukocytes beyond the endothelial monolayer characterizes the third stage and appears to involve ICAM-1 as it is found both on the apical and basal surfaces of the endothelium. All three of these stages appear to involve adhesion molecules which can therefore be implicated in atherogenesis. In an immunohistochemical study, the expression of VCAM-1, ICAM-1 and E-selectin were found to be higher on

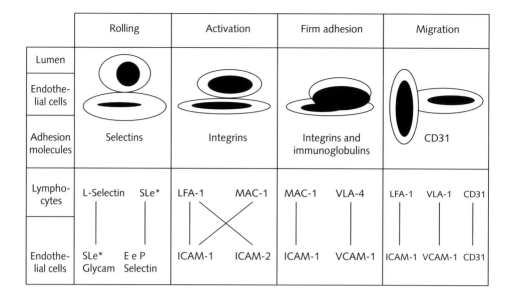

| | Rolling | Activation | Firm adhesion | Migration |
|---|---|---|---|---|
| Lumen | | | | |
| Endothe-lial cells | | | | |
| Adhesion molecules | Selectins | Integrins | Integrins and immunoglobulins | CD31 |
| Lympho-cytes | L-Selectin   SLe* | LFA-1        MAC-1 | MAC-1     VLA-4 | LFA-1   VLA-1   CD31 |
| Endothe-lial cells | SLe*      E e P Glycam   Selectin | ICAM-1     ICAM-2 | ICAM-1     VCAM-1 | ICAM-1 VCAM-1 CD31 |

*Figure 2*

*Interactions between lymphocytes and endothelium. Lymphocyte recruitment is a funda-mental component of atherogenesis. The first step is mediated by selectins while in subse-quent interactions integrins play a prominent role. These adhesion molecules cause lym-phocytes and monocytes to adhere to endothelium and to insert the pseudopodia in the endothelial cells so that they can pass out the basal membrane. LFA1, leukocyte function antigen-1; ICAM-1, intercellular adhesion molecule-1; MAC-1, monocyte activation com-plex-1; VLA-4, very late antigen 4; CD31, cluster designation 31.*

the intimal neovasculature than on the arterial luminal surface of arterial plaques, suggesting that this may provide a route for lymphocyte recruitment, lipid deposition, and or activation in atherosclerosis. There are several risk factors for atherosclerosis that have been well documented in epidemiological studies, including hypertension, hypercholesterolemia, smoking and diabetes. Several investigations have been under-taken to see if the correlation between these risk factors and atherosclerosis may be mediated by alterations in adhesion molecule expression [21–26].

## B-lymphocyte and antibody production

About 5–15% of the circulating lymphocytes in blood are B cells defined by their surface immunoglobulins [1]. These are constitutively produced and are inserted into the cell-surface membrane, where they act as specific antigen receptors. The majority of human B cells in peripheral blood express two immunoglobulin isotypes on their surface: IgM and IgD. On any B cell, the antigen-binding sites of these isotypes are identical. Fewer than 10% of the B lymphocytes in the circulation express IgG, IgA or IgE although these are present in larger numbers in specific locations of the body, for example IgA-bearing cells in the intestinal mucosa. The majority of B cells carry MHC class II antigens which are important for cooperative interactions with T lymphocytes. Complement receptors for C3b (CR1, CD35) and C3d (CR2, CD21) are commonly found on B cells and are associated with activation and, possibly, 'homing' of the cells. CD19, CD20 and CD22 are the main markers currently used to identify human B cells [1].

After lymphocyte activation by mitogens or antigens, distinctive differentiation features are observed at the ultrastructural level. Ultimately, many B-cell blasts mature into antibody-forming cells (AFCs), which progress *in vivo* to terminally differentiated plasma cells. These cells are infrequent in the blood, comprising less than 0.1% of the circulating lymphoid cells. Plasma cells have a short life span, survive for only a few days, and die from apoptosis.

## T lymphocytes

The definitive T-cell lineage marker is the T-cell antigen receptor (TCR) (Fig. 3). There are two defined types of TCR: one is a heterodimer of two disulphide-linked polypeptides ($\alpha$ and $\beta$); the other is structurally similar, but consists of $\gamma$ and $\delta$ polypeptides. Both receptors are associated with a set of five polypeptides, the CD3 complex, and together form the T-cell receptor complex. Approximately 90–95% of blood T cells are $\alpha\beta$ cells and the remaining 5–10% are $\gamma\delta$ T cells [1]. $\alpha\beta$ T lymphocytes are subdivided into two distinct non-overlapping populations: a subset which carries the CD4 marker and mainly 'helps' or induces immune response (Th), and a subset which carries the CD8 marker and is predominantly cytotoxic (Tc) [3] (Fig. 4). CD4+ T lymphocytes recognize their specific antigens in association with MHC class II molecules, whereas CD8+ T lymphocytes recognize antigens in association with MHC class I molecules (Fig. 5). Thus, the presence of CD4 or CD8 limits the type of cell with which the T cells can interact.

## CD4+ (Th1 and Th2 lymphocytes)

CD4+ T lymphocytes can be classified on the basis of cytokine production. In the last few years, it has been shown that both murine and human CD4+ T-helper (Th) cells represent a functionally heterogeneous population, including at least three distinct types of Th lymphocytes termed Th1, Th2, and Th0 cells on the basis of their secretion profile [1, 27].

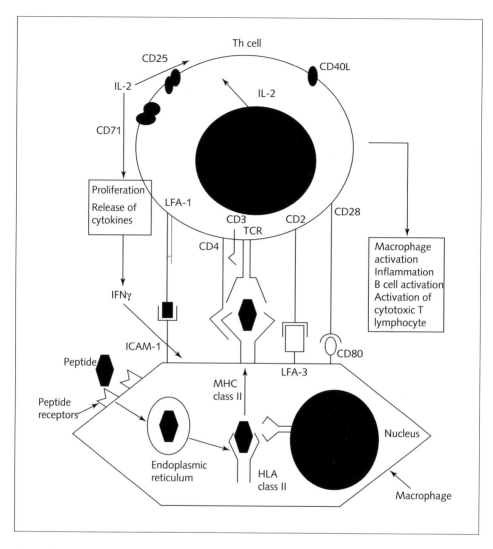

*Figure 3*

*Activation of CD4⁺ T lymphocytes. Antigen presenting cells (Macrophage) present processed antigen to helper (Th) cells, which recognize particular epitopes and select them as targets. Antigen processing involves degrading the antigen into peptide fragments. Th lymphocytes recognize a distinct peptide from that antigen, depending on the ability of a particular peptide to bind to a particular MHC class II. The peptide-HLA class II complex is transported to the cell surface, where it can be detected by CD4⁺ T Lymphocytes. Several other receptors on the CD4⁺ lymphocytes and the macrophage cell stabilize the cell-cell interaction. Cytokines and IFNγ are secreted and activate macrophages, B cells and cytotoxic T cells, initiating inflammatory reactions and regulating the immune response.*

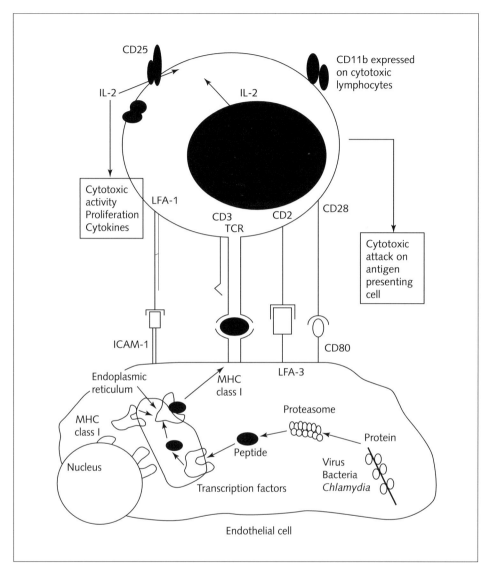

*Figure 4*
*Activation of CD8 lymphocytes. The most important role of CD8⁺ cytotoxic T lymphocytes is the elimination of cells infected with viruses. Nearly all nucleated cells express MHC class I molecules and if they become infected they can present antigen to CD8⁺ lymphocytes. Cellular molecules that have been partly degraded by proteasomes are transported to the endoplasmic reticulum to become associated with MHC class I molecules and are transported to the cell surface. Additional interactions may be required to stabilize the bond between the CD8⁺ cytotoxic lymphocytes and the target adhesion receptors on both cells.*

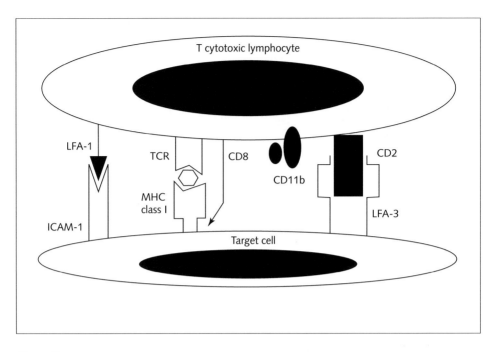

*Figure 5*

*Cytotoxic T lymphocytes recognize processed antigen presented on the target cell by MHC molecules using their T-cell receptor (TCR). Most cytotoxic lymphocytes are CD8+ and recognize antigen presented by MHC class I. They use a number of different receptors to positively identify their targets, including LFA-1, CD2, TCR, CD11b.*

Th1 cells produce IL-2 [28], interferon-γ (IFNγ) and TNFβ [19] and promote both macrophage activation (resulting in delayed-type hypersensitivity) and production of complement-fixing and opsonizing antibodies. Th2 cells secrete IL-4, IL-5, IL-6, IL-10 and IL-13 [3, 4, 29, 30] provide optimal help for antibody production, and promote both mast cell growth and eosinophil differentiation and activation [31–34] (Fig. 6). Clonal analysis of murine CD4+ Th cells has revealed that the ability to produce procoagulant inducing factor and to drive monocyte procoagulant response is a peculiar function of both Th1 and Th0, but not Th2 clones [35].

## NK cells

Natural killer (NK) cells account for up 15% of blood lymphocytes and express neither T-cell nor B-cell antigen receptors. Most surface antigens detectable on NK cells

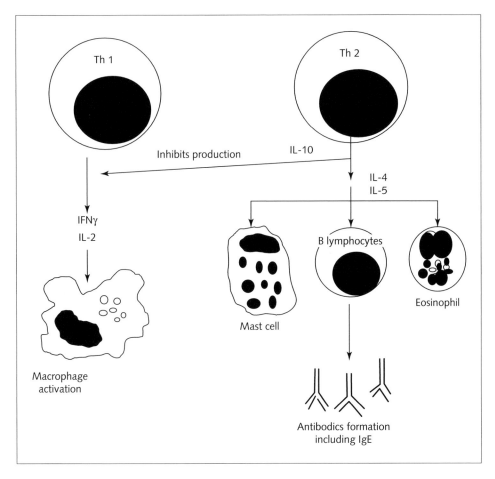

*Figure 6*
*Selection of effector mechanisms by Th1 and Th2 cells. CD4+ Th lymphocytes have two dif-*
*ferent profiles of cytokine production (Th1 and Th2). Typical human Th1 cytokines include*
*IFNγ, TNFβ, IL-2. In contrast, Th2 cells are typified by the production of IL-4 ,IL-5, IL-6, IL-*
*9, IL-10 and IL-13. Th2 cytokines are associated with regulation of strong antibody and aller-*
*gic responses. Cytokines from Th1 lymphocytes inhibit the actions of Th2 cells and* vice
versa.

by monoclonal antibodies are shared with T cells or monocytes/macrophages. Monoclonal antibodies to CD16 (FcγRIII) are commonly used to identify NK cells in purified lymphocyte populations. The CD56 molecule, a homophilic adhesion molecule of the Ig super-family (N-CAM), is another important marker of NK cells. The absence of CD3, (specific marker of T lymphocytes), but the presence of

CD56, CD16 or both, is currently the most reliable marker for NK cells in humans. The function of NK cells is to recognize and kill certain tumor cells and virus-infected cells.

## Antigen presentation

A normal immune response starts when T lymphocytes recognize a foreign antigen [1, 12]. Following antigen presentation, T-cell receptor (TCR) signaling is the next decisive factor in the initiation of the specific immune response [4]. T cells can kill target cells, promote antibody production by B cells and activate macrophages. The activation of the T lymphocytes is the key to most immune reactions. Antigen recognition by T lymphocytes is central to the generation and regulation of an effective immune response. The cells that process antigen in this way may be either specialized antigen-presenting cells (APCs), which are capable of stimulating T-lymphocyte division, or may be virally infected cells within the body which than become a target for T lymphocytes. T lymphocytes recognize cell-bound antigen in association with MHC class I or class II molecules. Peptide fragments from processed antigen bind to grooves in MHC molecules. MHC class I and class II molecules present peptides derived, respectively, from endogenous and exogenous antigens. This is reflected by the intracellular site at which the processed antigen accesses and binds to the MHC molecules. Peptides that bind to MHC class I molecules are produced in the cytoplasm, by the activity of an intracellular organelle called a "proteasome" (Fig. 4). Peptides that bind to class II molecules are derived from endocytosed exogenous antigen which has been processed in an endosomal/lysosomal compartment. Peptide/MHC molecule complexes on the cell surface can be recognized by a specific T-lymphocyte receptor. However, a variety of additional interactions involving accessory molecules are required for T-cell activation. Antigen presentation is not a unidirectional process. T cells, as they become activated, release cytokines such as IFNγ and granulocyte-macrophages colony stimulating factor (GM-CSF), in addition to surface signals such as CD40 ligand, which enhance the function of antigen presentation. Lymphocytes in human atherosclerotic lesions express the immune mediator CD40 and its ligand CD40L (also known as CD154) [36, 37].

## Role of T lymphocytes in the evolution of atherosclerotic lesions

The precursor stage of atherosclerotic plaques is represented by the "fatty streaks" that may revert to normal or progress to more advanced stages of the disease [38]. Modified (e.g. oxidized) low-density lipoprotein (LDL) is taken up by endothelial cells and is internalized by macrophages by means of the scavenger receptors, leading to the formation of lipid peroxides, facilitating the accumulation of cholesterol esters resulting in the formation of the foam cells [60]. Modified LDL is chemotactic for other monocytes and can up-regulate the expression of genes for monocyte-chemotactic protein 1 derived from endothelial cells. Moreover, the presence of modified LDL induces the production of inflammatory cytokines, such as IL-1, expanding the inflammatory response [38].

The evolution of atherosclerotic lesions involves an interaction between endothelial cells, smooth muscle cells, macrophages and lymphocytes (Fig. 7). Immunohistochemical studies have localized T lymphocytes in human atherosclerotic plaques [39, 40]. Several laboratories have provided evidence for the presence of various cytokines, like interleukins (IL) and IFNγ during different phases of atherogenesis [13]. mRNA for all these cytokines has been detected in human atherosclerotic lesions and IFNγ has been detected in areas surrounding T lymphocytes as well as intracellularly. Both IFNγ and IL-4-producing T lymphocytes have been cloned from human atherosclerotic plaques [41].

T lymphocytes are among the earliest cells infiltrating the arterial intima in the initial stages of atherosclerosis. They are commonly found in fatty streaks together with monocytes-macrophages. T cells in early lesions are outnumbered by macrophages and are predominantly composed of CD8+ cells [39]. In contrast, in advanced lesions CD4+ cells dominate over CD8+ cells, suggesting the occurrence of a switch from a response driven by HLA-class I to HLA-class II-restricted antigens during the evolution of the fatty streak into a mature plaque lesion. The expression of MCH class II by smooth muscle cells, macropahges and endothelial cells confirms that the above-mentioned cytokines modulate an inflammatory response in the lesion environment [42].

The role of the potent immunostimulatory cytokine IFNγ in the atherosclerotic process is controversial [41]. On one hand, IFNγ stimulates the expression of adhesion molecules on endothelial cells, and MHC-class II on macrophages and smooth muscle cells, all potentially proatherogenic properties. On the other hand, IFNγ decreases lipoprotein receptor expression on macrophages, decreases collagen synthesis in smooth muscle cells and blocks smooth muscle cells proliferation, all potentially antiatherogenic effects. Moreover, IFNγ is able to inhibit LDL oxidation by activated monocytes, whereas pretreatment of monocytes with other cytokines, such as IL-4 and IL-13, significantly enhances the ability of activated human monocytes to oxidize LDL. In a recent work, Gupta et al. [41] studied the evolution of atherosclerotic plaques in IFNγ receptor-deficient mice which provide a unique opportunity to directly examine the role of IFNγ in atherosclerosis. When compared to apo-E-deficient mice, which are hypercholesterolemic and atherosclerosis-prone, lesions in IFNγ receptor-deficient mice crossed with apo-E-deficient mice were smaller, with a 60% decrease in lipid content. These observations support a model where IFNγ potentiates an immune response, which in turn promotes atherogenesis.

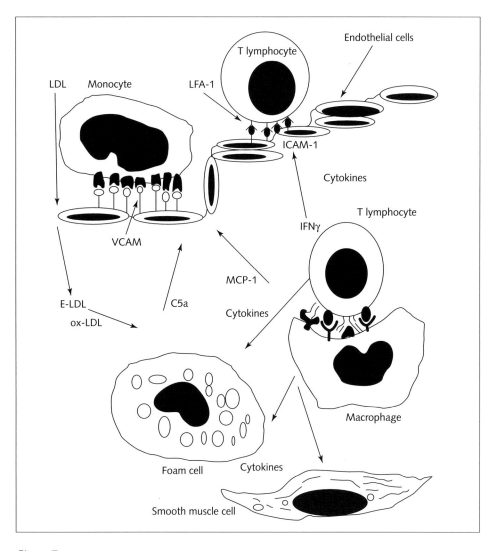

*Figure 7*

*Lymphocytes and atherosclerosis. The atherosclerotic lesion contains large numbers of macrophages and T lymphocytes. Endothelial cells in the early event of atherosclerosis express VCAM-1 induced by E-LDL and ox-LDL in the intima. Monocytes and T lymphocytes adhere to endothelial VCAM and other adhesion molecules. The production from monocytes of IFNγ and MCP-1 and activation of complement (C5a) induce the transmigration of these cells in to the intima. Antigen-specific T lymphocytes are activated in the atherosclerotic lesion. Lymphocytes, macrophages, endothelial cells and smooth muscle cells produce cytokines to regulate adhesion molecule expression, cell migration, chemotaxis, procoagulant activity, proliferation, contractility and cholesterol uptake.*

Lesion evolution is importantly affected by the CD40 signaling, that is, the interaction between CD40 ligand (expressed by CD4+ T lymphocytes, smooth muscle cells, macrophages, endothelial cells) and CD40 receptor (expressed by monocytes macrophages, endothelial cells and smooth muscle cells). Anti-CD40 ligand treatment significantly limited atherosclerotic lesion formation compared with a control group in hyperlipidemic mice. Examination of the aortic arch, as well as of the abdominal aorta showed a marked decrease in atherosclerotic lesion progression and aortic lipid deposition in mice treated with the anti-CD40 ligand antibody. Moreover, atheroma of mice treated with anti-CD40 ligand antibody exhibited a 64% decrease in macrophages, contained 70% fewer lymphocytes and showed a markedly reduced expression of vascular cell adhesion molecule-1 (VCAM-1) in atherosclerotic lesions compared to controls [36, 37]. Therefore, interruption of the CD40 signaling may identify a new potentially promising therapeutic target in atherosclerosis.

## T lymphocytes and plaque destabilization

Libby and coworkers [43] investigated whether cytokines or growth factors would regulate the synthesis of the interstitial forms of collagen that preserve the integrity of the fibrous cap. In this context, an important role is played by IFNγ, a cytokine secreted only by activated T lymphocytes. Production of IFNγ within atherosclerotic plaques was demonstrated by Hansson et al. [39]. This cytokine inhibits collagen synthesis in vulnerable regions of the fibrous cap, which becomes weak and prone to rupture. Moreover, IFNγ can inhibit smooth muscle cell proliferation, activating their apoptosis program. These data explain the relative paucity of smooth muscle cells in vulnerable regions of human atherosclerotic plaques. Moreover, IFNγ is able to activate macrophage functions related to plaque disruption. Activated macrophages have the capacity to synthesize matrix-degrading neutral metalloproteinases, including interstitial collagenase, gelatinase A, B and stromelysin [44]. This family of enzymes can digest all the structural matrix components of the fibrous cap. These enzymes are usually localized to rupture-prone shoulder regions and to sites of enhanced circumferential stress. They require activation from proenzyme precursors to attain enzymatic activity and their degradation is regulated by tissue inhibitors which are co-secreted with metalloproteinases, rendering them inactive under basal conditions. However, inflammatory cytokines, like IL-1 and TNF induce the release of stromelysin and gelatinase B, without affecting the production of tissue inhibitors. Therefore, exposure to inflammatory mediators, elaborated by T cells, can trigger the proteolytic cascade, promoting the capacity of macrophages and smooth muscle cells to degrade the extracellular matrix and favouring plaque rupture.

In a recent study positive immunostaining for gelatinase B was present in 82% of coronary atherectomy specimens from both unstable and stable angina patients

[44]. However, intracellular localization of the enzyme, indicating active synthesis, was found in 10 out of 10 positively stained specimens from patients with unstable angina, compared with 3 out of 10 positively stained specimens from patients with stable angina.

Although IL-1 and TNFγ can elicit gelatinase production by macrophages, the exact knowledge of the mechanisms generating the expression of interstitial collagenase and stromelysin in plaques was elusive. Recent data from the Libby group however have elucidated the signals that elicit the expression of interstitial collagenase and stromelysin, as well as the production of tissue factor, a potent procoagulant, by macrophages [43]. As mentioned above, activated T lymphocytes can express on their surface the CD40 ligand, a TNF-like molecule, whereas smooth muscle cells and monocytes-macrophages express both the ligand and its receptor, CD40, *in vitro* as well as in atherosclerotic plaques in humans [36]. In an elegant experimental study, these authors showed that stimulation of human monocytes-macrophages by either membranes from activated CD4+ T cells or recombinant CD40 ligand induced expression of interstitial collagenase, stromelysin and tissue factor protein and activity. Neutralization with anti-CD40 ligand antibody inhibited these effects of both T-cell membranes and recombinant CD40 ligand. Activated T cells also secrete, together with stimulatory mediators such as IL-1 and TNFγ, IFNγ which is able to suppress the release of metalloproteinases induced by recombinant CD40 ligand. However, this inhibition *in vivo* may be outweighed by the stimulation induced by other cell types, such as smooth muscle cells and macrophages which also express the CD40 ligand [37].

## Antigen presentation and immune activation in atherosclerotic plaques

Expression of activation markers on T lymphocytes suggests antigenic stimulation during atherogenesis [12, 45]. The multifactorial determinants that are involved in the development and progression of atherosclerosis have received increasing attention in recent years (Tab. 1). Accordingly, the role of autoimmune factors has attracted intensive research aimed at defining the autoantigenic materials expressed within plaques that may influence the fate of lesions. Candidate proteins that have been mentioned include modified forms of LDL. Enzymatically degraded LDL (E-LDL) being more active than oxidized LDL (ox-LDL) whereas native LDL produced only minor adhesive effects. Both E-LDL and ox-LDL enhance transmigration of monocytes and of T lymphocytes in the plaque [46–48]. In endothelial cells E-LDL was more potent than ox-LDL in stimulating upregulation of ICAM-1, platelet endothelial cell adhesion molecule-1 (PECAM-1), P-selectin and E-selectin with distinct kinetics [7, 8]. E-LDL also upregulated expression of ICAM-1 in human aortic smooth muscle cells, and this correlated with increased adhesion of T lymphocytes. E-LDL is thus able to promote the selective adhesion of monocytes and T lym-

Table 1 - Interaction between candidate antigens for stimulating immunity in atherosclerotic plaques and their immune response

| Antigen | Lymphocyte response |
| --- | --- |
| Modified lipoproteins Ox-LDL E-LDL | B-cell response, antibody production |
| Heat-shock-protein HSP 60 HSP 70 | B-cell response, antibody production, expression of adhesion molecules, proinflammatory and immune-regulating cytokines |
| β2GPI | B-cell response, antibody production, CD4+ Th1 cell activation |
| Virus-infected endothelial cells | Cytotoxic CD8+ T cells |
| Cytokine-induced surface antigens | NK, CD4+, CD8+ |

phocytes to the endothelium, stimulate transmigration of these cells, and foster their retention in the vessel wall by increasing their adherence to smooth muscle cells. These observations underline the potential immunogenetic significance of E-LDL in the pathogenesis of atherosclerosis [47].

Stress or heat shock proteins (Hsp) are part of a tightly regulated and phylogenetically old biological system that enables organisms to respond adequately to detrimental environmental factors. Hsp has been repeatedly incriminated to be involved in various autoimmune conditions as well as in atherogenesis [49]. Heat shock proteins are a family of approximately 24 proteins, whose expression is induced by various forms of stress, like high temperature, infection, free radicals, cytokines and heavy metals. They function as "chaperonins" that stabilize cellular proteins from denaturation by environmental injuries. Rabbits immunized with HSP65 develop atherosclerotic lesions which contain T cells, macrophages and smooth muscle cells, but no foam cells. Additional feeding with a cholesterol-rich diet significantly increased the areas of atherosclerotic lesions that also included abundant foam cells [50]. Interestingly, the presence of antibodies to HSP65 in the sera of a large number of clinically healthy individuals correlated with the presence of ultrasonographically demonstrable atherosclerotic lesions in the carotid arteries [51].

$\beta_2$-Glycoprotein I ($\beta$2GPI) is a highly glycosylated plasma protein with an approximate molecular weight of 50 kDa that has received recent attention because it serves as a major antigenic target of thrombosis-associated antiphosphilipid antibodies (aPL) [52, 53]. The physiological role of $\beta$2GPI is still obscure, yet it possesses several properties that may bear relevance to progression of human athero-sclerotic plaques. It binds activated platelets and apoptotic cells on exposure to inner-membrane phosphatydilserine; it inhibits the intrinsic blood coagulation path-way and ADP-dependent platelet aggregation; it serves a requisite role in the acti-vation of endothelial cells induced by aPL; and it may assist in mediating clearance of senescent cells and foreign particles from the circulation. Immunization of LDL receptor-deficient mice with β2GPI results in acceleration of aortic fatty streak for-mation.

Antigens of herpes virus type I and cytomegalovirus have also been found in ath-erosclerotic arterial walls. *Chlamydia pneumoniae* has also been identified in atheromatous lesions in coronary arteries and in other organs obtained at autopsy (see the chapter by Romeo et al. in this volume). Increased titers of antibodies to these organisms have been shown to be predictors of adverse events in patients with prior myocardial infarction. However, no direct evidence has been provided that these organisms cause the lesions of atherosclerosis [38].

## Pathological observations in acute coronary syndromes: role of T lymphocytes

Several studies have shown that acute coronary syndromes result from coronary thrombosis occurring at sites of plaque rupture or superficial erosion [54]. Plaques prone to rupture are characterized by (1) a large lipid core; (2) a thin fibrous cap containing a reduced amount of collagen, glycosaminoglycans and smooth muscle cells; and (3) an active inflammatory cell infiltrate, particularly located underneath disrupted portions of the cap. This infiltrate is formed by monocyte-derived macrophages and by increased numbers of activated T lymphocytes and mast-cells.

The cellular characteristics of the fibrous cap at the immediate site of rupture were studied by van der Wal et al. in 20 patients who had died of acute myocardial infarction [55]. A deep rupture extending into the lipid core was observed in 12 plaques, whereas in eight cases superficial erosion was found. Macrophages and T cells were the dominant cell type at the site of plaque rupture or erosion. These inflammatory cells were characterized by a strong expression of HLA-DR antigens, indicating activation of these cells. Smooth muscle cells were almost completely absent at sites of rupture or erosion, but HLA-DR positive smooth muscle cells also occurred, albeit limited to sites immediately adjacent to inflammatory infiltrates [56].

The presence and phenotype of inflammatory infiltrates and their possible role in thrombotic events were studied by Arbustini et al. [57] in a large series of cases. Samples were taken during coronary artery bypass graft surgery in patients with sta-ble and unstable angina and from autopsies in cases of acute myocardial infarction or sudden death. Adventitial and plaque infiltrates were evaluated separately, because of their possibly different pathogenetic role. In adventitia, inflammatory cells, largely composed of T and B lymphocytes with rare macrophages, were found clustered around nerves or vascular structures. Within plaques, infiltrates either scattered or grouped together were predominantly composed of macrophages with the presence of T and B lymphocytes. No difference was observed between samples with or without thrombus [58].

The role of neovasculature, consisting of small vessels arising primarily from adventitial vasa vasorum, in the pathogenesis of atherosclerosis was investigated by O'Brien et al. [59] in 99 coronary artery segments, of which 65 had atheroscleric plaques, obtained from 15 hearts explanted at the time of cardiac transplantation. These authors found that the prevalence of adhesion molecules (like E-selectin, ICAM-1 and VCAM-1) was two-fold higher than their prevalence on arterial luminal endothelium. Increased plaque intimal T-lymphocyte density was associated with the presence of both ICAM-1 and VCAM-1 on neovasculature [24]. These data raise the possibility that intimal neovasculature is a potential route for leukocyte recruitment into atherosclerotic plaques.

Immunohistochemical methods and Western blotting techniques were also used by Arbustini et al. [57] to detect the presence of inflammatory cytokines within plaques. TNFγ was predominantly found in lipid-rich plaques without correlation with the presence of thrombus. Smooth muscle cells, monocyte-macrophages and intimal cells were TNFγ immunoreactive. Barath et al. [60] observed that TNFγ was expressed by intimal smooth muscle cells, whereas, it was not expressed by media cells. The other TNFγ immunoreactive population is represented by macrophages, probably activated by lymphocytes and complement activation products. The presence of IL-2 was also revealed in a high percentage of plaques. Lymphocyte-induced macrophage activation occurs, at least partially, through release of IL-2, which is a marker of activated T cells, activates monocyte-macrophages, promotes growth of NK cells as well as of activated B and T cells.

In a recent study, van der Wal et al. [56] studied 71 patients who underwent directional coronary atherectomy. Patients were clinically classified as stable angina, refractory unstable angina, stabilized unstable angina and acute myocardial infarction. The expression of IL-2 receptors on T lymphocytes was used as a marker of T-cell activation. Since IL-2 receptors on T lymphocytes are expressed shortly after stimulation and persist for only a few days, their presence indicates recent T cell activation in a tissue immune response. The amount of lesions containing IL-2 receptor-positive cells increased with severity of the ischemic coronary syndrome (from 52% in stable angina to about 90% in refractory unstable angina and acute myocardial infarction). Also the percentage of activated T cells with respect to the global T-cell population increased from stable angina (2.2%) to acute myocardial infarction (18.5%) (Fig. 8). These data indicate that in acute coronary syndromes recent stimulation of T lymphocytes takes place within the culprit coronary plaque. The authors speculate that a causal role for the local burst of inflammatory activity and the onset of acute coronary syndromes seems likely, because inflammatory sub-

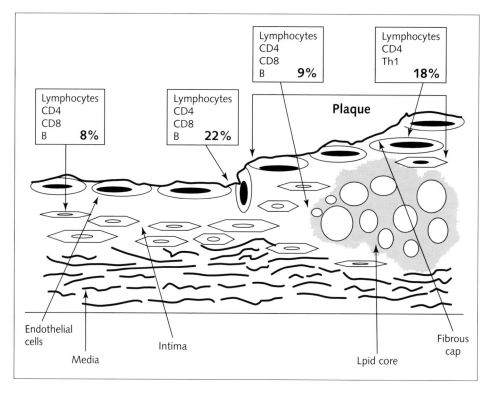

*Figure 8*

*Atherosclerosis can be viewed as a chronic inflammatory disease induced and perturbed by lipid accumulation. T lymphocytes and monocyte-derived macrophages infiltrate the arterial intima at various stages of atherosclerotic plaque evolution. Values are expressed as percentages of total cells in different regions obtained from various studies [12, 13, 39, 40, 45, 48, 55, 56]. An increased number of Th1 lymphocytes in the plaque shoulder underlines the role of these cells in plaque rupture.*

stances secreted during the amplification of the immune response may have a destabilizing effect on the plaque.

## T-lymphocyte activation in ischemic heart disease

In 1992 Neri Serneri et al. published a pioneering paper [61] entitled "Transient intermittent lymphocyte activation is responsible for the instability of angina", in which they stated that the increased thrombin formation in unstable angina patients is due to the expression of tissue-factor like activity by activated monocytes. Such monocyte activation was believed to be a part of a lymphocyte cell-instructed response intermittently triggered by unknown factors. To reach these conclusions they studied 31 consecutive patients with Braunwald class IIB and IIIB unstable angina, 23 with stable exertional angina and 35 age-matched healthy controls. Monocytes and lymphocytes were separated from other blood cell components and monocyte procoagulant activity was assessed. Monocytes from unstable angina patients expressed significantly increased procoagulant activity, which was triggered by a direct contact with lymphocytes of the same patients. In cross-mixing experiments, only lymphocytes from patients with unstable angina induced the expression of procoagulant activity by monocytes from both control and patient groups. Moreover, patients with unstable angina had higher fibrinopeptide A plasma levels, indicating increased thrombin formation, than stable angina patients or control subjects. Interestingly, these observations were limited to the acute phase of unstable angina, since these data were not reproducible in the same patients studied 8–12 weeks after their clinical presentation. In the revolutionary pathogenetic hypothesis supported by these data, a central role is played by lymphocytes, whose activation by unknown factors triggers a series of reactions finally leading to thrombus formation.

Recently the same authors [62] further expanded their previous observations by investigating T-lymphocyte receptor expression in patients with unstable angina, as well as in stable angina patients and healthy control subjects. Unstable angina was characterized by an increased expression of HLA-DR positive cells, both CD4+ (10.5%) and CD8+ (9.7%) T lymphocytes which were significantly higher than those expressed by the same cells in stable angina patients or in normal controls. Although the IL-2α receptor was shown in similar percentages by T lymphocytes in the three groups, the soluble form of this receptor was found to be significantly increased in the serum of unstable angina patients. Both the incidence of HLA-DR positive cells and soluble IL-2 receptor levels were higher in those patients who needed revascularization procedures because of refractory unstable angina, indicating a relation between the intensity of the immunological reaction and clinical outcome.

These data however were not confirmed by other studies [63–67]. Caligiuri et al. [63] correlated the time course of immune system activation with disease progression in 35 patients with unstable angina by measuring the prevalence of activated T lymphocytes (HLA-DR positive T cells) and serum levels of IL-2, as markers of cell-mediated immunity [64]. A group of 35 patients with stable angina was also studied as controls. Blood samples were taken on admission, after 7–15 days and after 6 months. No difference was found in IL-2 and percentages of HLA-DR positive cells on admission between unstable and stable angina patients. An increase in IL-2 levels as well as of circulating HLA-DR positive cells was only observed in unstable patients with a favorable outcome, leading the authors to speculate that the immune response might actually favor the waning of instability. This observation is in contrast to the data reported by Neri Serneri et al. [61] who found that clinical outcome was related to the intensity of the immunological reaction.

We recently observed increased plasma levels of IFNγ in patients with unstable angina, as compared to stable angina patients [65]. However, IFNγ concentrations were markedly elevated only in those patients who had increased values of troponin-T, a marker of an active thrombotic process with distal embolization of platelet thrombi originating from the culprit lesion. Since only a single blood sample was taken before cardiac catheterization in all patients, it's impossible to establish if the increased concentrations of IFNγ shared the same pathogenetic mechanism as well as the prognostic value of increased Troponin-T.

Data from several laboratories have shown that T-cell activation is present in patients with coronary artery disease, irrespective of their clinical presentation [60–63, 66, 67]. In a recent study from our group, IL-2 levels were higher in patients with ischemic heart disease than in age-matched control subjects, without differences between stable and unstable angina groups [65]. Blum et al. [68] studied 24 patients with stable exertional angina who underwent coronary angioplasty (PTCA). Soluble IL-2 receptor levels were high in eleven patients at the time of the procedure, but concentrations reverted progressively to normal in the 2-month follow-up. Interestingly, soluble IL-2 levels remained elevated in two patients who had either an unsuccessful PTCA or an early restenosis. The authors concluded that T lymphocytes are activated in about half the patients with stable angina and that soluble IL-2 receptor levels may be a reliable marker for follow-up of patients undergoing PTCA. They also speculated that in the development of atherosclerotic plaques some stages demonstrate active T-cell involvement, while others are immunologically silent.

Vaddi et al. measured kinetics and secretion of TNFα and IFNγ by isolated mononuclear leukocytes from eight control subjects, ten patients with stable angina pectoris and ten patients with unstable angina pectoris [69]. Secretion of both TNFα and IFNγ was consistently higher in patients compared to control subjects, but a similar increase in cytokine secretion was observed in stable and unstable patients. It was concluded that similar increases in cytokine secretion by mononuclear leukocytes in stable or unstable angina indicate that such release is a nonspecific inflammatory response in acute myocardial ischemia and is possibly related to progression of atherosclerosis.

## T-lymphocyte phenotypes in patients with ischemic heart disease

Only a few studies have dealt with the phenotypic characterization of T lymphocytes in patients with ischemic heart disease. Nevertheless, data reported so far are often conflicting, the reasons for such discrepancies being obscure. Neri Serneri et al. [62] found that CD4 and CD8 receptors were equally expressed in patients with stable and unstable angina. Similar percentages of positive cells were also observed for the transferrin receptor (CD71), and the IL-2 receptor (CD25), which can be upregulated in the case of T-cell activation. We also found no difference in CD4+ and CD8+ cells in three groups of patients with stable angina, unstable angina and control subjects [65]. Contrary to these observations, Caligiuri et al. [63] observed increased percentages of CD4+ cells in unstable angina than in stable angina patients. In a recent study, we found that patients with ischemic heart disease had a significantly increased expression of cytotoxic CD8+ CD11b+ T lymphocytes as compared to healthy control subjects. Although the exact nature of this finding is unclear, a potential mechanism by which cytotoxic lymphocytes are increased may be represented by the stimulus of vascular endothelium injury caused by chronic infections [70–73].

Finally, Liuzzo et al. [74] recently reported that patients with ischemic heart disease have increased frequencies of CD4+ T lymphocytes characterized by defective cell surface expression of CD28, a major co-stimulatory molecule, critically involved in determining the outcome of antigen recognition by T lymphocytes. Patients with unstable angina had these cells more frequently than patients with stable angina. Moreover, in a six-month follow-up of 32 patients, such a T-cell phenotype was a predictor of in-hospital and long-term outcome, independent of other risk factors and clinical variables.

## Conclusions

The data reported so far do not permit definite conclusions. Nevertheless it seems reasonable to state that T-cell activation is present in a sizable proportion of patients with stable and unstable angina [75]. In the former group, increased concentrations of IL-2 or of its soluble receptor may reflect an accelerated atherosclerotic process or a greater propensity to restenosis after PTCA. In unstable angina, T-lymphocyte activation can be detected during the course of the disease, but its clinical significance as well as its pathogenetic role is uncertain. In particular, further studies should assess if the immune response, transiently observed in some patients, may have favorable or unfavorable effects on their short or long-term outcome.

## References

1    Roitt I, Brostoff J, Male D (eds) (1998) *Immunology*, 5th edition, London, Mosby
2    Banchereau J, Rousset F (1992) Human B-lymphocytes: phenotype, proliferation and differentiation. *Adv Rev Immunol* 52: 125–162
3    Robey E, Fowlkes BJ (1994) Selective events in T cell development. *Annu Rev Immunol* 12: 675–705

4   Brodsky FM, Guagliardi LE (1991) The cell biology of antigen processing and presentation. *Annu Rev Immunol* 9: 707–744

5   Springer TA (1994) Traffic signals for lymphocyte recirculation and leukocyte emigration:the multistep paradigm. *Cell* 76: 301–314

6   Pober JS, Collins T, Gimbrone MA (1983) Lymphocytes recognize human vascular endothelial and dermal fibroblast Ia antigens induced by recombinant immune interferon. *Nature* 305: 726–729

7   Frenette PS, Wagner DD (1996) Adhesion molecules part I. *N Engl J Med* 334: 1526–1529

8   Frenette PS, Wagner DD (1996) Adhesion molecules part II. *N Engl J Med* 335: 43–45

9   Pober JS, Cotran RS (1990) Cytokines and endothelial cell biology. *Physiol Rev* 70: 427–456

10  Paul WE (1989) Pleiotropy and redundancy of T cell derived lymphokines in the immune responses. *Cell* 57: 521–524

11  Stemme S, Rymo L, Hansson GK (1991) Polyclonal origin of T -Lymphocytes in human atherosclerotic plaques. *Lab Invest* 6: 654–660

12  Van der Wal AC, Das PK, Bentz van de Berg D, Van der Loos CM, Becker AE (1989) Atherosclerotic lesions in humans: *in situ* immunophenotypic analysis suggesting an immune mediated response. *Lab Invest* 61: 166–170

13  Hansson GK, Libby P (1996) The role of the lymphocytes. In: V Fuster, EJ Topol (eds): *Atherosclerosis and coronary artery disease*. Lippincott-Raven Publishers, Philadelphia, 557–568

14  Alexander RW (1994) Inflammation and coronary artery disease. *N Engl J Med* 331: 468–469

15  Ross R (1986) The pathogenesis of atherosclerosis: an update. *N Engl J Med* 314: 488–500

16  Cybulsky MI, Gimbrone MA Jr (1991) Endothelial expression of a mononuclear leukocyte adhesion molecule during atherogenesis. *Science* 251: 788–791

17  Li H, Cybulsky MI, Gimbrone MA Jr (1993) An atherogenic diet rapidly induces ICAM-1, a cytokine regulatable mononuclear leukocyte adhesion molecule, in rabbit aortic endothelium. *Arterioscler Thromb* 3: 197–204

18  Dinarello CA (1994) The biological properties of interleukin-1. *Eur Cyt Network* 5: 517–531

19  Vassalli P (1992) The pathophysiology of tumor necrosis factors. *Annu Rev Immunol* 10: 411–520

20  Farrar MA, Schreiber RD (1993) The molecular cell biology of interferon-γ and its receptor. *Annu Rev Immunol* 11: 571–611

21  Blann AD, McCollum CN (1994) Circulating endothelial cell/leukocyte adhesion molecules in atherosclerosis. *Thromb Haemost* 72: 151–154

22  Chia MC (1998) The role of adhesion molecules in atherosclerosis *Clin Lab Sci* 35: 573–602

23  Poston RN, Haskard DO, Coucher JR (1992) Expression of intercellular adhesion molecule-1 in atherosclerotic plaques. *Am J Pathol* 140: 665–673

24  Sheridan FM, Cole PG, Ramage D (1996) Leukocyte adhesion to the coronary microvasculature during ischemia and reperfusion in an *in vivo* canine model. *Circulation* 93: 1784–1787

25  Villanueva FS, Jankpwski RJ, Klibanov S, Pina ML, Alber SM, Watkins SC, Brandenburger GH, Wagner WR (1998) Microbubbles targeted to intercellular adhesion molecule-1 bind to activated coronary artery endothelial cells. *Circulation* 98: 1–5

26  Jang Y, Lincoff M, Plow EF, Topol EJ (1994) Cell adhesion molecules in coronary artery disease. *J Am Coll Cardiol* 24:1591–1601

27  Mosmann TR,Cherwinski H, Bond MW (1986) Two types of murine helper T-cell clone. Definition according to profiles of lymphokine activities and secreted proteins. *J Immunol* 136: 2348–2357

28  Smith KA (1988) Interleukin-2: inception, impact and implications. *Science* 240: 1169–1176

29  Van Snick J (1991) Interleukin-6: an overview. *Annu Rev Immunol* 8: 253–278

30  Paul WE (1991) Interleukin-4: a prototypic immunoregulatory lymphokine. *Blood* 77: 1627–1652

31  Boehm U, Klamp T, Groot M (1997) Cellular responses to interferon-γ. *Annu Rev Immunol* 15: 749–795

32  Wang HM, Smith KA (1987) The interleukin-2 receptor. Functional consequences of its bimolecular structure. *J Exp Med* 166: 1055–1069

33  Arai K, Lee F, Miyajima A (1990) Cytokines: coordinators of immune and inflammatory responses. *Annu Rev Biochem* 59: 783–836

34  Sad S, Mosmann T (1994) Single IL-2 secreting precursor CD4 T cell can develop into either Th1 or Th2 cytokine secretion phenotype. *J Immunol* 153: 3514–3519

35  Del Prete G, De Carli M, Lammel RM, D'Elios MM, Daniel KC, Giusti B, Abbate R, Romagnani S (1995) Th1 and Th2-Helper cells exert opposite regulatory effects on procoagulant activity and tissue factor production by human monocytes. *Blood* 86: 250–257

36  Mach F, Schonbeck U, Bonnefoy JY, Pober JS, Libby P (1997) Activation of monocyte/macrophage functions related to acute atheroma complication by ligation of CD40. *Circulation* 96: 396–399

37  Mach F, Schonbeck U, Sukhova GK, Atkinson E, Libby P (1998) Reduction of atherosclerosis in mice by inhibition of CD40 signaling. *Nature* 394: 200–203

38  Ross R (1999) Mechanisms of disease: Atherosclerosis an inflammatory disease *N Engl J Med* 340: 115–126

39  Hansson GK, Holm J, Jonasson L (1989) Detection of activated T-lymphocytes in the human atherosclerotic plaque. *Am J Pathol* 135: 169–175

40  Gown AM, Tsukada T, Ross R (1986) Human atherosclerosis: Immunocytochemical analysis of the cellular composition of human atherosclerotic lesions. *Am J Pathol* 125: 191–196

41    Gupta S, Pablo AM, Jiang XC, Wang N, Tall AR, Schindler C (1997) IFN-γ potentiates atherosclerosis in APO-E knock-out mice. *J Clin Invest* 99: 2752–2761

42    Folcik VA, Azamir R, Cathcart MK (1997) Cytokine modulation of LDL oxidation by activated human monocytes. *Arterioscler Vasc Biol* 17: 1954–1961

43    Libby P (1995) Molecular bases of the acute coronary syndromes. *Circulation* 91: 2844–2850

44    Brown DL, Hibbs MS, Kearney M, Loushin C, Isner JM (1995) Identification of 92-kD gelatinase in human coronary atherosclerotic lesions. Association of active enzyme synthesis with unstable angina. *Circulation* 91: 2125–2131

45    Wick G, Schett G, Amberger A, Kleindienst R, Xu Q (1995) Is the atherosclerosis an immunologically mediated disease? *Immunology Today* 16: 27–33

46    Mehta A, Yang B, Khan S, Hendricks JB, Stephen C, Mehta JL (1995) Oxidized low-density lipoproteins facilitate leukocyte adhesion to aortic intima without affecting endothelium-dependent relaxation: role of P-selectin. *Arterioscler Thromb Vasc Biol* 15: 2076–2083

47    Klouche M, May AE, Hemmes M, Meßner M, Kanse SM, Preissner KT, Bhakdi S (1999) Enzymatically modified, nonoxidized LDL induces selective adhesion and transmigration of monocytes and T-lymphocytes through human endothelial cell monolayers. *Arterioscler Thromb Vasc Biol* 9: 784–793

48    Stemme S, Faber B, Holm J (1995) T-lymphocytes from human atherosclerotic plaques recognize oxidized low-density lipoprotein. *Proc Natl Acad Sci USA* 92: 3893–3897

49    Schett G, Redlich K, Xu Q, Bizan P, Groger M, Tohidast-Akrad M, Klener H, Smolen J, Steiner G (1998) Enhanced expression of heat shock protein 70 (hsp 70) and heat shock factor 1 (HSF1). Activation in rheumatoid arthritis synovial tissue. *J Clin Invest* 102: 302–311

50    Xu Q, Luef G, Weimann S, Gupta RS, Wolf H, Wick G (1993) Staining of endothelial cells and macrophages in atherosclerotic lesions with human heat-shock protein-reactive antisera. *Arterioscler Thromb* 13: 1763–1769

51    Xu Q, Willeit J, Marosi M, Kleindienst R, Oberhollenzer F, Kiechl S, Stulning T, Luef G, Wick G (1993) Association of serum antibodies to heat-shock protein 65 with carotid atherosclerosis. *Lancet* 341: 255–259

52    George J, Harats D, Gilburd B, Afek A, Levy Y, Schneidermann J, Barshack I, Kopolovic J, Shoenfeld Y (1999) Immunolocalization of β2-glycoprotein I (Apolipoprotein H) to human atherosclerotic plaques. *Circulation* 99: 2227–2230

53    George J, Afek A, Gilburd B, Aron-Maor A, Shaish A, Levkovitz H, Blank M, Harats D, Shoenfeld Y (1998) Induction of early atherosclerosis in LDL receptor deficient mice immunized with β2 glycoprotein I. *Circulation* 15: 1108–1115

54    Shah PK (1997) New insights into the pathogenesis and prevention of acute coronary syndromes. *Am J Cardiol* 79: 17–23

55    Van der Wal AC, Beker AE, Van der Loos CM, Das PK (1994) Site of intimal rupture or erosion of thrombosed coronary atherosclerotic plaques is characterized by an inflammatory process irrespective of the dominant plaque morphology. *Circulation* 89: 36–44

56   Van der Wal AC, Pick JJ, de Boer OJ, Koch KT, Teeling P, Van der Loos CM, Becher AE (1998) Recent activation of the plaque immune response in coronary lesions underlying acute coronary syndromes. *Heart* 80: 14–18

57   Arbustini E, Grasso M, Diegoli M, Pucci A, Bramerio M, Ardissino D, Angoli L, de Servi S, Bramucci E, Mussini A et al (1991) Coronary atherosclerotic plaques with and without thrombus in ischemic heart syndromes: a morphologic, immunohistochemical, and biochemical study. *Am J Cardiol* 68: 36B–50B

58   Mann JM, Davies MJ (1996) Vulnerable plaque: Relation of characteristics to degree of stenosis in human coronary arteries. *Circulation* 94: 928–931

59   O'Brien K, McDonald TO, Chait A, Allen MD, Alpers CE (1996) Neovascular expression of E-selectin, intracellular adhesion molecule-1 in human atherosclerosis and their relation to intimal leukocyte content. *Circulation* 93: 672–682

60   Barath P, Fishbein MC, Cao J, Berenson J, Helefant RH, Forrester JS (1990) Tumor necrosis factor gene expression in human vascular intimal smooth muscle cells detected by *in situ* hybridization. *Am J Pathol* 137: 503–509

61   Neri Serneri GG, Abbate R, Gori AM, Attanasio M, Martini F, Giusti B, Dabizzi P, Poggesi L, Modesti PA, Trotta F et al (1992) Transient intermittent lymphocyte activation is responsible for the instability of angina. *Circulation* 86: 790–797

62   Neri Serneri GG, Prisco D, Martini F, Gori AM, Brunelli T, Poggesi L, Rostagno C, Gensini GF, Abbate R (1997) Acute T-cell activation is detectable in unstable angina. *Circulation* 95: 1806–1812

63   Caligiuri G, Liuzzo G, Biasucci LM, Maseri A (1998) Immune system activation follows inflammation in unstable angina: pathogenetic implications. *J Am Coll Cardiol* 32: 1295–1304

64   Nath N, Bian H, Reed EF, Chellappan SP (1999) HLA Class I-mediated induction of cell proliferation involves cyclin E-mediated inactivation of Rb function and induction of E2F activity. *J Immunol* 162: 5351–5358

65   Mazzone A, De Servi S, Mazzucchelli I, Vezzoli M, Fossati G, Gritti D, Ottini E, Mussini A, Specchia G (1999) Plasma levels of interleukin 2,6,10 and phenotypic characterization of circulating T-lymphocytes in ischemic heart disease. *Atherosclerosis* 145: 369–374

66   Mazzone A, De Servi S, Ricevuti G, Mazzucchelli J, Fossati G, Pasotti D, Bramucci E, Angoli L, Specchia G, Notario A (1993) Increased expression of neutrophil and monocyte adhesion molecules in unstable coronary artery disease. *Circulation* 88: 358–363

67   De Servi S, Mazzone A, Ricevuti G, Mazzucchelli J, Fossati G, Gritti D, Angoli L, Specchia G (1995) Clinical and angiographic correlates of leukocyte activation in unstable angina. *J Am Coll Cardiol* 26: 1146–1150

68   Blum A, Sclarovsky S, Shohat B (1995) T-lymphocyte activation in stable angina pectoris and after percutaneous transluminal coronary angioplasty. *Circulation* 91: 20–22

69   Vaddi K, Nicolini FA, Mehta P, Mehta JL (1994) Increased secretion of tumor necrosis factor alpha and interferon gamma by mononuclear leukocytes in patients with ischemic heart disease: relevance in superoxide anion generation. *Circulation* 90: 694–699

70  Gupta S, Leatham EW, carrington D, Mendall MA,Kaski JC, Camm J (1997) Elevated *Chlamydia pneumoniae* antibodies, cardiovascular events and azithromycin in male survivors of myocardial infarction. *Circulation* 96: 404–407

71  Reddehase MJ, Mutter W, Munch K, Buhring HJ, Koszinowsky UH (1987) CD8 positive T-lymphocytes specific for murine cytomegalovirus immediate early-antigens mediate protective immunity. *J Virol* 61: 3102–3108

72  Larsen HS, Feng MF, Horohow DW, Moore RN, Rouse BT (1984) Role of T-lymphocytes subsets in recovery from herpes simplex virus infection. *J Virol* 50: 56–59

73  Riddell SR, Gilbert MJ, Greenberg PD (1993) CD8$^+$ cytotoxic T-cell therapy of cytomegalovirus and HIV infection. *Curr Opin Immunol* 5: 484–491

74  Liuzzo G, Kopecky SL, Cornwell K, Frye RL, Goronzy JJ, Weyand CM (1999) Expansion of unusual CD4$^+$ lymphocytes as a prognostic indicator of short and long-term outcome in ischemic heart disease. *J Am Coll Cardiol (*Suppl) 362A: 1127

75  Mehta JL, Saldeen TG, Rand K (1998) Interactive role of infection, inflammation and traditional risk factors in atherosclerosis and coronary artery disease. *J Am Coll Cardiol* 31: 1217–1225

# Role of infection in atherosclerosis and precipitation of acute cardiac events

*Francesco Romeo[1], Fabrizio Clementi[1], Tom Saldeen[2] and Jay L. Mehta[3]*

[1]Department of Cardiology, University of Rome "Tor Vergata", Rome, Italy; [2]Department of Surgical Sciences, University of Uppsala, Dag Hammarskjölds väg 17, 75237 Uppsala, Sweden; [3]VA Medical Center and Departments of Medicine and Physiology, University of Florida College of Medicine, and University of Arkansas for Medical Sciences, 4301 West Markham, Slot 532, Little Rock, AR 77205-7199, USA

## Introduction

Atherosclerotic vascular disease is now widely considered to be associated with inflammation. The earliest lesion in atherosclerosis, the so-called "fatty streak", is an inflammatory lesion consisting of monocyte-derived macrophages and T lymphocytes. As atherosclerosis proceeds, there is extensive infiltration of the blood vessels with T lymphocytes. The shoulder region of the rupture-prone plaque is characterized by extensive accumulation of inflammatory cells. These issues have been discussed in detail elsewhere in this book and in recent reviews [1–3].

Several investigators in the last two decades have directed their efforts toward the identification of the trigger/s that can initiate the inflammatory process. Many have suggested inflammation to be a key pathogenic trigger in atherosclerosis, since the traditional risk factors, such as hypercholesterolemia, hypertension, smoking and diabetes mellitus, are not present in a consistent fashion in all or even in a majority of patients with atherosclerosis. However, it has become clear that these risk factors can activate endothelium and leukocytes, and trigger the inflammatory process.

There has been a steady decline in atherosclerosis-related mortality and morbidity, particularly in the West [4], in parallel with the advent and widespread use of antibiotics. This observation has led many investigators to suggest that antibiotic-sensitive processes may be the basis of inflammation and atherosclerosis [5, 6]. Many experimental and clinical studies support the concept that infection may be a trigger that can initiate and sustain vascular inflammatory process. The infectious agents that could be involved in this process are viruses (Cytomegalovirus (CMV), Herpes simplex virus (HSV), Hepatitis A virus, etc.) and bacteria (*Chlamydia pneu-*

Inflammatory and Infectious Basis of Atherosclerosis, edited by Jay L. Mehta
© 2001 Birkhäuser Verlag Basel/Switzerland

*moniae, Helicobacter pylori*, etc.). This chapter deals with infection as a potential basis for atherosclerosis, at least in some selected patient populations.

## Cytomegalovirus (CMV), Herpes simplex virus (HSV) and Hepatitis A virus

An association of CMV and HSV, and more recently of Hepatitis A virus, with atherosclerosis has been described. High levels of antibody titers against these viruses have been found in patients with restenosis after coronary intervention and in patients with coronary artery disease (CAD) compared to controls [7, 8]. Patients with transplantation atherosclerosis have also been shown to have high antibody titers [9]. Many other studies have documented the presence of CMV or HSV nucleic acid and antigens in human atheromas [10–14].

Fabricant and colleagues [15] first described the pathogenic role of these viruses in atherosclerosis. Recently, the Atherosclerosis Risk in Communities (ARIC) study [16] documented a significant correlation between carotid intimal-medial thickness and the levels of anti-CMV antibodies, but found no correlation with antibodies against HSV Type I or Type II antigens. Zhu et al. [17] showed a correlation between titers of antibodies against Hepatitis A virus and CMV and the presence of CAD. Others have, however failed to show a consistent correlation of antibody levels against viruses with CAD. For example, Manegold et al. [18] found no correlation of prior CMV infection with chronic restenosis after conventional coronary balloon angioplasty. Morrow and Ridker [19], based on the analysis of blood from participants of the Physicians Health Study, failed to find a positive correlation between baseline titers of antibody directed against HSV or CMV and future risk of myocardial infarction or stroke in a 12-year follow-up. Adler et al. [20] failed to observe a correlation between prior infection with CMV and angiographically demonstrated CAD.

## *Helicobacter pylori*

There have been some reports relating *H. pylori* with the pathogenesis of atherosclerosis [21] as well as with serum lipid levels [22]. Others [23] have found a weak association between angiographically demonstrated CAD and co-nesting of serological evidence of infection with *H. pylori* and *C. pneumoniae*. However, most studies have failed to show any association of *H. pylori* serology with carotid or coronary atherosclerosis. A meta-analysis [24] of 18 studies failed to show any correlation of seropositivity against *H. pylori* with the presence or extent of CAD. Recent studies, however, suggest that the more virulent strain bearing the cytotoxin-associated gene-A (CagA) species may be relevant in atherosclerosis through low-grade, persistent inflammatory stimulation [25].

## Chlamydia pneumoniae

Many reports have linked *C. pneumoniae*, based on serum IgG and IgA antibody titers against *C. pneumoniae*, with the severity of CAD and with acute coronary syndromes. The first serological evidence of an association of *C. pneumoniae* with CAD was provided by Saikku et al. [26]. They examined serum samples from 40 male patients with acute myocardial infarction, 30 male patients with chronic CAD and 41 control subjects. 68% of patients with acute myocardial infarction and 50% of patients with chronic CAD had elevated IgG (> 1/128) and/or IgA (> 1/32) titers against *C. pneumoniae*. Only 17% of the control group had high titers. While many early studies correlated serum antibody levels with the presence and severity of coronary atherosclerosis [26–29], more recent studies [30–32] based on high quality measurements of IgG and IgA antibodies against *C. pneumoniae* have not confirmed the results of earlier studies. In a large group of patients with CAD from three different countries (Sweden, Italy and USA), we measured serum IgG and IgA titers against *C. pneumoniae* in patients with stable and unstable CAD as well as in subjects with minimal atherosclerosis. The IgG and IgA antibody titers were similar in patients with CAD, regardless of the activity of the disease, and control subjects. The antibody levels were higher in cases from Sweden as compared to those from Italy and USA, suggesting high infection rates in Nordic countries where people spend a significant portion of their time indoors which facilitates close inter-individual contact and spread of common organisms, such as *C. pneumoniae*.

The large Physicians Health Study also failed to provide a link between serum antibody titers against *C. pneumoniae* and the future risk of myocardial infarction [33]. Notably, measurement of markers of inflammation, such as C-reactive protein, did provide a statistically significant predictive value in this population.

Recent data from Argentina also failed to show a correlation between the presence of CAD and serum IgG levels, but other non-specific markers of inflammation, such as C-reactive protein and fibrinogen, correlated significantly with the presence of CAD and the risk of future cardiac events [31].

There has been much stronger evidence for the presence of *C. pneumoniae* in atheromatous coronary arteries. Several techniques, such as PCR, electron microscopy, immunostaining and culture of the organism have been used to examine the hypothesis of *Chlamydia*-mediated atherosclerosis. Many of these studies have indeed shown an association of the presence of *Chlamydia* within atherosclerotic regions. For example, Shor et al. [34] detected *C. pneumoniae* in fatty streaks and atheromatous lesions in seven autopsy cases. Kuo et al. [35] and Campbell et al. [36] demonstrated the presence of *Chlamydia* in coronary arteries of young adults. Muhlestein et al. [37] recently reported immunofluorescence positivity in 79% of 24 coronary artery specimens. Positivity for *C. pneumoniae* was found by immunochemistry in atherosclerotic tissues of patients in the ARIC study [38]. Others [39–41], however, could not find an association of *C. pneumoniae* with atherosclerosis. The quality and type of sections examined could explain discrepancy in data from different studies. We have recently examined coronary artery sections from 60 cases, of these 32 had severe atherosclerosis and 18 had mild atherosclerosis [30, 42]. Direct immunofluorescence was reactive in 86% of cases with severe atherosclerosis, but only in 6% of cases with mild atherosclerosis; whereas immunoperoxidase staining was reactive in 78% and 38% of cases with severe and mild atherosclerosis, respectively. Interestingly, there was no relationship between serum IgG and IgA antibody titers against *C. pneumoniae* and the severity of coronary artery atherosclerosis. We also measured serum lipoprotein (a) (Lp(a)) levels and HLA-DR genotypes. Lp(a) levels were $180 \pm 44$ mg/l in cases with severe atherosclerosis compared with $61 \pm 12$ mg/l in cases with mild atherosclerosis. Interestingly, 48% of cases with severe atherosclerosis were positive for HLA-Class II genotypes 13, 15 or 17 in the cardiac muscle compared with 19% of cases with mild atherosclerosis. This study suggested a correlation between severity of atherosclerosis, *Chlamydia* in coronary arteries, high Lp(a) levels and certain HLA-DR genotypes. Our hypothesis is that coronary atherosclerosis has a genetic and autoimmune component that may be triggered by an intracellular infection. Similar results were reported by Dahlén et al. [43, 44].

Overall analysis of data on the association of *C. pneumoniae* with atherosclerosis using immunochemistry and direct staining techniques shows a positivity rate of 70 and 100%. In contrast, there is a relatively low association of PCR positivity with the severity or presence of atherosclerosis. No consistent correlation has been observed between the presence of *C. pneumoniae* and antibody titers. The failure to observe such a relationship may be due to different levels of antibody titers used to correlate with the risk of CAD, relative lack of specificity of IgG (vs. IgA), and different methods to assay the antibodies. It is also quite likely that the variability in antibody titers caused by repeated infections is a cause of inconsistent relationship with a common disease such as CAD.

## Which pathogen is associated with atherosclerosis?

The association between CMV, HSV or *H. pylori* and atherosclerosis does not fulfill the Koch's criteria that should be met to link an infectious agent with the production of the disease [45, 46]. Evidence for *C. pneumoniae*, thus far, presents the strongest association with human atherosclerosis. On the basis of sero-epidemiological, pathological and laboratory data, this agent fulfills many of the Koch's criteria to be considered a pathogen in the genesis of atherosclerosis. In essence, *C. pneumoniae* has been isolated from human atherosclerotic plaques [35–37]; this agent can be identified in the atheromas by culture or directly by microscopy [47, 48]; this agent causes the disease on transfer to a susceptible host [49], and lastly, antibiotic therapy in some studies reduced the number of cardiovascular events.

The enthusiasm for implicating these pathogens in CAD has been dampened by the results of analysis of several studies. Danesh et al. [50] in a recent population-based, case-control study showed that after adjustment for age, sex, smoking, indicators of socioeconomic status and standard risk factors, the odds ratio (95% confidence intervals) for CAD seropositivity to *H. pylori* was 1.28 (confidence limits 0.93–1.75), to CMV 1.40 (0.96–2.05) and to *C. pneumoniae* 0.95 (0.66–1.36). They also found a strong correlation between *H. pylori* and *C. pneumoniae* IgG concentrations suggesting co-nesting of these infections [51]. These observations on seropositivity do not, however, rule out a role for *Chlamydia* or other organisms in initiating or perpetuating the atherosclerotic lesion in some genetically prone individuals, especially in those with other traditional risk factors [2].

## Mechanisms by which infection can cause atherosclerosis?

The precise mechanism/s by which infectious agents can play a role in atherogenesis is unclear. The pathogenic role of infectious agents could result from direct local infection of the vessel wall or from indirect action on initiation of a number of immunological responses.

There is a strong theoretical basis for the role of viruses in the pathogenesis of atherosclerosis. Human endothelial cells infected with HSV demonstrate increased thrombomodulin formation and enhanced adherence of platelets and granulocytes [52, 53]. CMV induces major histocompatibility class I antigen expression in human aortic smooth muscle cells [54]. Transfection with this virus and *Chlamydia* also causes expression of genes for several cytokines [55]. The failure to culture infectious virus particles from the atherosclerotic lesion is probably due to the "hit and run" mechanism of HSV-mediated disease [56]. These viruses may in theory provoke the disease, but not persist in the lesion. It has also been suggested that viruses, such as CMV, can infect a few endothelial cells, and thereafter a blast of cytokines from these infected cells can cause an explosive reaction in the neighboring cells [57]. This may relate to the inability to consistently demonstrate the presence of infectious pathogen in all or most cells.

Chronic bacterial infections can aggravate the preexisting plaque by enhancing T-cell activation and other inflammatory responses that may cause destabilization of the intimal fibrous cap with subsequent rupture and overlying thrombosis [1]. Recently Kol et al. [58] demonstrated that *C. pneumoniae* produces large amount of heat shock protein 60 (HSP60) during chronic, persistent infection. Endogenous HSP60 may play a role in atherogenesis. *C. pneumoniae* localizes predominantly within plaque macrophages. These authors and Mayr et al. [59] provided evidence that HSP60 colocalizes in plaque macrophages in human atherosclerotic lesions. This bacterial product stimulates macrophage function with the release of pro-inflammatory cytokines such as tumor necrosis factor α (TNFα) and matrix degrading metalloproteinases [60].

*Chlamydia* as well as CMV, induce production of cytokines (TNFα, IL-1, IL-2) [55]. These cytokines have a variety of tissue injurious effects. Cytokines are potent inducers of generators of free radicals, which facilitate oxidation of low-density lipoprotein (LDL), a key event in atherosclerosis, and attract monocytes and other inflammatory cells to the area of endothelial injury. Free radicals also stimulate platelet activation and leukocyte chemotaxis and may participate in the formation of a thrombus in atherosclerotically narrowed arteries. Cytokines also influence the coagulation cascade by disturbing the delicate balance between endogenous tissue plasminogen activator and its fast acting inhibitor-1, resulting in thrombus formation [61].

Cytokines decrease the synthesis of constitutive nitric oxide synthase [62], a hallmark of atherosclerosis, and may predispose to vasospasm, platelet aggregation and thrombosis. Conversely, *Chlamydia*l bacterial lipopolysaccharide is a potent stimulus for inducible nitric oxide synthase activity [62] leading to the formation of large amounts of nitric oxide which could cause endothelial dysfunction and disruption followed by deposition of monocyte and platelets on the vessel wall, release of growth factors and migration of smooth muscle cells.

As indicated earlier, presence of dyslipidemia markedly exacerbates the tissue damaging effect of *C. pneumoniae* [30]. While the role of *C. pneumoniae* in affecting lipid metabolism is unknown, many infectious agents, including *Chlamydia* and HSV, decrease the activity of cytoplasmic cholesteryl ester hydrolase, and promote accumulation of intracellular cholesteryl esters [63]. A recent study shows that the atherogenic effects of *Chlamydia* are dependent on the presence of cholesterol [63]. Others have also shown correlation of *Chlamydia* seropositivity with atherogenic lipid profile [64, 65].

Another mechanism by which infection can cause or aggravate atherosclerosis is inhibition of apoptosis [66], probably by the inhibition of the P53-modulated apoptotic progress. Fan et al. [67] showed that *Chlamydia*-infected cells are resistant to apoptosis. This effect could lead to excess accumulation of smooth muscle cells, thereby contributing to restenosis and atherosclerotic lesions. The stimulation of smooth muscle cell migration and proliferation is also achieved by the inhibition of the tumor-suppressor gene P53, and by the increase of growth factors or of the expression of growth factors receptors. The facilitation of migration of smooth muscle cells from the media and adventitia to the developing neointima is another mechanism that contributes to neointima formation in atherosclerosis. This mechanism has been demonstrated by Zhou et al. [68] in rats infected with human CMV and has been related to the enhanced smooth muscle cell-derived platelet-derived growth factor (PDGF) receptor expression [1]. All these animal and cell-based studies helped generate the hypothesis that infection can cause atherosclerosis. Many of these concepts are summarized in Figures 1–3. Nonetheless, it will be very difficult to demonstrate the relevance of these observations in humans.

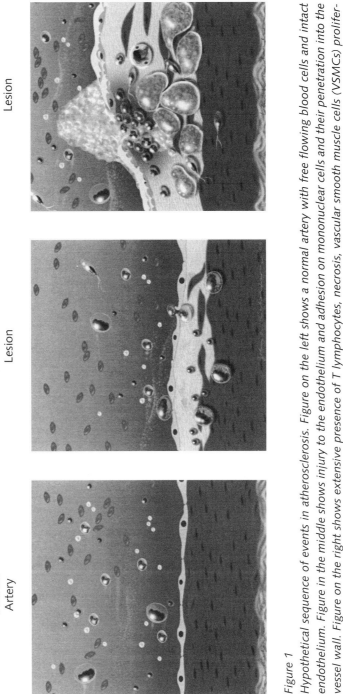

Normal Artery     Intermediate Lesion     Advanced Lesion

*Figure 1*

*Hypothetical sequence of events in atherosclerosis. Figure on the left shows a normal artery with free flowing blood cells and intact endothelium. Figure in the middle shows injury to the endothelium and adhesion on mononuclear cells and their penetration into the vessel wall. Figure on the right shows extensive presence of T lymphocytes, necrosis, vascular smooth muscle cells (VSMCs) proliferation, neovascularization, plaque rupture and formation of platelet-rich thrombosis.*

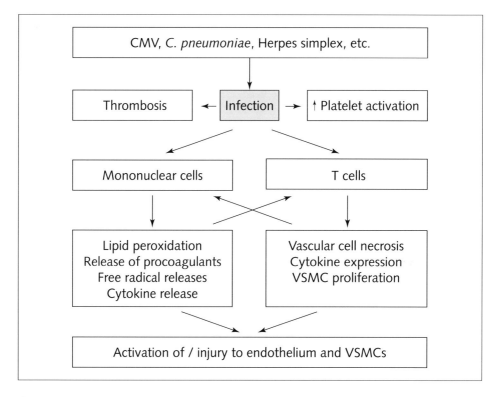

*Figure 2*
*Role of infection in inducing thrombosis, platelet activation, and mononuclear cell and T-cell activation with a number of events that lead to activation and injury to endothelium and VSMCs.*

## Clinical trials of antibiotics in atherosclerosis

If infection is the cause of atherosclerosis and its clinical manifestations, treatment with antibiotics should modify the frequency of clinical events.

Azithromycin is a potent azalide antibiotic, which has been shown to be very active against *Chlamydia*. The first small trial with azithromycin was carried out in survivors of an acute myocardial infarction in the UK. Gupta et al. [69], in a small number of patients, demonstrated a significant reduction in some markers of inflammation, such as monocyte-macrophage tissue factor and the surface adhesion molecule CD 11b, in patients treated with azithromycin. Azithromycin-treated patients also showed a significant reduction in cardiovascular events (p < 0.03), but the number of patients included and the number of cardiac events in the study were too

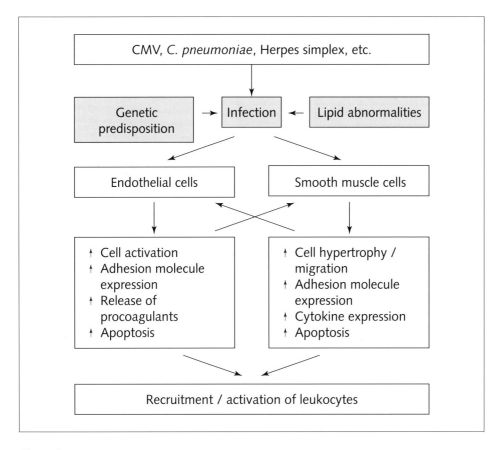

*Figure 3*
*Role of infection in activating endothelial and smooth muscle cells. A cascade of events leads to recruitment and activation of leukocytes.*

small to exclude the possibility that the observed benefits were mere chance observations.

Subsequently, Gurfinkel et al. [70] reported similar result in a pilot antibiotic trial from Argentina (ROXIS trial). They randomized 202 patients with unstable angina or none Q-wave myocardial infarction to roxithromycin, 150mg twice daily, or placebo for 30 days. All clinical events, such as angina, evolution of acute myocardial infarction and death, were reduced at one month in treated patients. The difference between treated and untreated patients tended to be of borderline significance. Follow up studies showed that the favorable effect of roxythromycin waned at 3–6 months. Importantly, levels of IgG antibody against *C. pneumoniae* remained unchanged, but the markers of inflammation, such as C-reactive protein, fell in both placebo- and roxythromycin-treated patients [71].

The results of these two small studies created much interest. However, these early observations were not confirmed by a somewhat larger clinical trial. In a double blind, randomized, secondary prevention study (ACADEMIC trial), 333 patients with serological evidence of prior *C. pneumoniae* exposure were included [72]. The dosage of azithromycin was 500 mg daily for three days, then 500 mg per week for three months. Antibody titers (IgG and IgA) and inflammatory markers, such as C-reactive protein, IL-1, IL-6 and TNFα, were analyzed at three and six months. Clinical end-points were cardiovascular death, resuscitated cardiac arrest, non-fatal myocardial infarction or stroke, unstable angina requiring hospitalization and need for coronary interventions. This study showed that in CAD patients with serological evidence of prior exposure to *C. pneumoniae*, markers of inflammation improved at six months with azithromycin, but no differences were observed in antibody titers and clinical events. These results stress the need for further investigation into large clinical trials, taking into consideration the multifactorial nature of the disease.

These recent negative clinical studies also suffer from many major methodological limitations. The patient population was heterogeneous and the main end-point was not the degree of atherosclerosis, but the clinical manifestations of atherosclerosis, which are widely variable and dependent on a variety of cofactors.

There are several other major clinical trials of antibiotics underway in CAD patients. For example, the WIZARD (weekly intervention with zithromax against atherosclerosis-related disorders) trial is enrolling 3500 subjects with prior myocardial infarction and *C. pneumoniae* antibody for three months. In this study, a 2.5-year observation period is planned. The ACES (Azithromycin Coronary Events Study), sponsored by the NHLBI, will include 4000 subjects with evidence of CAD, irrespective of antibody status, for one year, with a planned four-year observation period.

## Limitations of antibiotic therapy

The interest in antibiotic therapy stemmed from early reports suggesting a causative role for *C. pneumoniae* in atherosclerosis. Therein may lie the major limitation of this strategy. As discussed above, the seropositivity is not a true index of persistent infection.

Further, the infection rate with *C. pneumoniae* in the general population is about 2–3% per year. While it can be rationalized that infection could promote and maintain atherosclerosis in combination with other risk factors, and may be an important mechanism of atherogenesis in certain genetically predisposed individuals, studies based on serological markers are unlikely to yield evidence of benefit. This may also be the basis of contradictory results of preliminary studies. Treatment based on antibody titers may also be a limitation of the ACADEMIC study. Lack of correlation between serological markers of inflammation and activity of disease suggests that routine antibiotic therapy in all CAD patients or all patients with acute coronary syndromes is unlikely to yield beneficial effect. We believe that a cause-effect relationship between one single infectious agent and atherosclerosis remains unproven. We need to define the subset of patients in whom infection is the primary cause of atherogenesis, or instability of the disease, before a strong foundation for the use of antibiotics can be laid.

It is to be noted that some of the beneficial effect of macrolide antibiotics in CAD may be a result of independent anti-inflammatory properties [73]. This may explain the fall in C-reactive protein and other markers of inflammation in patients treated with antibiotics. Furthermore, prolonged use of antibiotics, particularly those that have a broad range of pathogen sensitivity, has significant epidemiological significance. Routine use of large doses in a large population may result in antibiotic resistance, which is of major public health concern, particularly when the relationship between infection and CAD is far from proven.

## Mosaic of inflammation, infection and atherosclerosis

A large body of evidence has in the past, supported the role of certain risk factors in the pathogenesis of atherosclerosis. Recently evidence has been presented for an infection and autoimmune nature of the disease. However, one major unanswered question remains: what causes or initiates the atherosclerotic process? Traditional risk factors do not explain the atherosclerotic process in a relatively large number of patients. Furthermore, infection is not present in all patients. Lastly, it is unlikely that a group of five or ten risk factors can explain the genesis of a malady that affects a third to half of the world population. What is clear is that inflammation occurs in response to some kind of injury and it perpetuates the atherosclerotic process, yet it is probably not the cause of atherosclerosis. Perhaps infectious agents, in the presence of traditional risk factors, such as dyslipidemia, can initiate the atherosclerotic process and lead to an inflammatory response. This may result in clinical CAD in genetically-prone or otherwise susceptible individuals. It is futile to think that infection with an ubiquitous organism, such as *C. pneumoniae*, is the cause of atherosclerosis in all individuals, and therefore, antibiotic therapy will be useful in all CAD patients.

## Conclusion

In conclusion, atherosclerosis is a multifactorial disease. Traditional risk factors are associated with this disease in a significant number of patients. We believe that there is only a weak association between infection and the precipitation of atherosclerosis or the acute manifestations of this complex disease entity. Further prospective large studies need to be conducted to study the association of infection with atherogenesis. If the infectious agent/s associated with atherosclerosis is/are clearly demonstrated, large studies on the treatment of the offending organism can be designed to assess the efficacy of antibiotics in a select group of patients in whom infection is the major underlying cause.

## Acknowledgment

This review was supported by funds from the VA Central Office and a contract with the Department of Defense, Washington, DC, the Anne C. Reeves Cardiology Research Endowment and A. Howard Stebbins III Cardiology Chair Endowment.

## References

1    Libby P (1995) Molecular bases of the acute coronary syndromes. *Circulation* 91: 2844–2850

2    Mehta JL, Saldeen TGP, Rand K (1998) Interactive role of infection, inflammation, and traditional risk factors in atherosclerosis and coronary artery disease. *J Am Coll Cardiol* 31: 1217–1225

3    Ross R (1999) Atherosclerosis – an inflammatory disease. *N Engl J Med* 340: 115–126

4    McGovern PG, Pankow JS, Shahar E, Doliszny KM, Folsom AR, Blackburn H, Luepker RV for the Minnesota Heart Survey Investigators (1996) Recent trends in acute coronary heart disease mortality, morbidity, medical care, and risk factors. *N Engl J Med* 334: 884–890

5    Buja LM (1996) Does atherosclerosis have an infectious etiology? *Circulation* 94: 872–873

6    Libby P, Egan D, Skarlatos S (1997) Roles of infectious agents in atherosclerosis and restenosis: an assessment of the evidence and need for future research. *Circulation* 96: 4095–4103

7    Zhou YF, Leon MB, Waclawiw MA, Popma JJ, Yu ZX, Finkel T, Epstein SE (1996) Association between prior cytomegalovirus infection and the risk of restenosis after coronary atherectomy. *N Engl J Med* 335: 624–630

8    Adam E, Melnick JL, Probtsfield JL, Petrie BL, Burek J, Bailey KR, McCollum CH, DeBakey ME (1987) High level of cytomegalovirus antibody in patients requiring vascular surgery for atherosclerosis. *Lancet* 2: 291–293

9    Loebe M, Schuler S, Zais O, Warnecke H, Fleck E, Hetzer R (1990) Role of cytomegalovirus infection in the development of coronary artery disease in the transplanted heart. *J Heart Transplant* 9: 707–711

10   Hendrix MG, Salimans MM, van Boven CP, Bruggeman CA (1990) High prevalence of

latently present cytomegalovirus in arterial walls of patients suffering from grade III atherosclerosis. *Am J Pathol* 136: 23–28

11    Wu TC, Hruban RH, Ambinder RF, Pizzorno M, Cameron DE, Baumgartner WA, Reitz BA, Hayward GS, Hutchins GM (1992) Demonstration of cytomegalovirus nucleic acids in the coronary arteries of transplanted hearts. *Am J Pathol* 140: 739–747

12    Hendrix MG, Dormans PH, Kitslaar P, Bosman F, Bruggeman CA (1998) The presence of cytomegalovirus nucleic acids in arterial walls of atherosclerotic and non-atherosclerotic patients. *Am J Pathol* 134: 1151–1157

13    Hendrix MG, Daemen M, Bruggeman CA (1991) Cytomegalovirus nucleic acid distribution within the human vascular tree. *Am J Pathol* 138: 563–567

14    Hosenpud JD, Chou SW, Wagner CR (1991) Cytomegalovirus-induced regulation of major histocompatibility complex class I antigen expression in human aortic smooth muscle cells. *Transplantation* 52: 896–903

15    Fabricant CG, Fabricant J, Litrenta MM, Minick CR (1978) Virus-induced atherosclerosis. *J Exp Med* 148: 335–340

16    Nieto FJ, Adam E. Sorlie P, Farzadegan H, Melnick JL, Comstock GW, Szklo M (1996) Cohort study of cytomegalovirus infection as a risk factor for carotid intimal-medial thickening, a measure of subclinical atherosclerosis. *Circulation* 94: 922–927

17    Zhu J, Quyyumi AA, Norman JE, Csako G, Epstein SE (199) Cytomegalovirus in the pathogenesis of atherosclerosis: the role of inflammation as reflected by elevated C-reactive protein levels. *J Am Coll Cardiol* 34: 1738–1743

18    Manegold C, Alwazzeh M, Jablonowski H, Adams O, Medve M, Seidlitz B, Heidland U, Haussinger D, Strauer BE, Heintzen MP (1999) Prior cytomegalovirus infection and the risk of restenosis after percutaneous transluminal coronary balloon angioplasty. *Circulation* 99: 1290–1294

19    Morrow DA, Ridker PM (2001) C-reactive protein – a prognostic marker of inflammation in atherothrombosis. In: JL Mehta: *Inflammatory and infectious basis of atherosclerosis*. Birkhäuser, Basel, 203–220

20    Adler SP, Hur JK, Wang JB, Vetrovec GW (1998) Prior infection with cytomegalovirus is not a major risk factor for angiographically demonstrated coronary artery atherosclerosis. *J Infect Dis* 177: 209–212

21    Birnie DH, Holme ER, McKay IC, Hood S, McColl KE, Hillis WS (1998) Association between antibodies to heat shock protein 65 and coronary atherosclerosis. Possible mechanism of action of *Helicobacter pylori* and other bacterial infections in increasing cardiovascular risk. *Eur Heart J* 19: 387–394

22    Laurila A, Bloigu A, Nayha S, Hassi J, Leinonen M, Saikku P (1999) Association of *Helicobacter pylori* infection with elevated serum lipids. *Atherosclerosis* 142: 207–210

23    Anderson JL, Carlquist JF, Muhlestein JB, Horne BD, Elmer SP (1998) Evaluation of C-reactive protein, an inflammatory marker, and infectious serology as risk factors for coronary artery disease and myocardial infarction. *J Am Coll Cardiol* 32: 35–41

24    Danesh J, Peto R (1998) Risk factors for coronary heart disease and infection with *Heliobacter pylori*: meta-analysis of 18 studies. *BMJ* 316: 1130–1132

25  Pasceri V, Cammarota G, Patti G, Cuoco L, Gasbarrini A, Grillo RL, Fedeli G, Gasbarrini G, Maseri A. (1998) Association of virulent Helicobacter pylori strains with ischemic heart disease. *Circulation* 97: 1675–1679

26  Saikku P, Leinonen M, Mattila K, Ekman MR, Nieminen MS, Makela PH, Huttunen JK, Valtonen V (1988) Serological evidence of an association of a novel *Chlamydia*, TWAR, with chronic coronary heart disease and acute myocardial infarction. *Lancet* 2: 983–986

27  Mendall MA, Carrington D, Strachan D, Patel P, Molineaux N, Levi J, Toosey T, Camm AJ, Northfield TC (1995) *Chlamydia pneumoniae*: risk factors for seropositivity and association with coronary heart disease. *J Infect* 30: 121–128

28  Thom DH, Wang SP, Grayston JT, Siscovick DS, Stewart DK, Kronmal RA, Weiss NS (1991) Chlamydia pneumoniae strain TWAR antibody and angiographically demonstrated coronary artery disease. *Arterioscler Thromb* 11: 547–551

29  Puolakkainen M, Kuo CC, Shor A, Wang SP, Grayston JT, Campbell LA (1993) Serological response to *Chlamydia pneumoniae* in adults with coronary arterial fatty streaks and fibrolipid plaques. *J Clin Microbiol* 31: 2212–2214

30  Saldeen TGP, Ericsson K, Lindquist O, Pahlson C, Lindblom B, Liu AJ, Mehta JL (1998) Chlamydia and HLA-DR genotypes in coronary atherosclerosis (abstract). *J Am Coll Cardiol* 31: 272A

31  Altman R, Rouvier J, Scazziota A, Absi RS, Gonzalez C (1999) Lack of association between prior infection with Chlamydia pneumoniae and acute or chronic coronary artery disease. *Clin Cardiol* 22: 85–90

32  Romeo F, Martuscelli E, Ericsson K, Saldeen TGP, Mehta JL (2000) Seropositivity against Chlamydia pneumoniae in patients with coronary atherosclerosis disease. *Clin Cardiol* 23: 327–330

33  Ridker PM, Kundin RB, Stampfer MJ, Poulin S, Hennekens CM (1998) A prospective study of *Chlamydia pneumoniae* IgG serpositivity and risk of future myocardial infarction (abstract). *Circulation* I–602

34  Shor A, Kuo CC, Patton DL (1992) Detection of *Chlamydia pneumoniae* in coronary arterial fatty streaks and atheromatous plaques. *S Afr Med J* 82: 158–161

35  Kuo CC, Coulson AS, Campbell LA, Cappuccio AL, Lawrence RD, Wang SP, Grayston JT (1997) Detection of *Chlamydia pneumoniae* in atherosclerotic plaques in the walls of arteries of lower extremities from patients undergoing bypass operation for arterial obstruction. *J Vasc Surg* 26: 29–31

36  Campbell LA, O'Brien ER, Cappuccio AL, Kuo CC, Wang SP, Stewart D, Patton DL, Cummings PK, Grayston JT (1995) Detection of *Chlamydia pneumoniae* TWAR in human coronary atherectomy tissues. *J Infect Dis* 172: 585–588

37  Muhlestein JB, Hammond EH, Carlquist JF, Radicke E, Thomson MJ, Karagounis LA, Woods ML, Anderson JL (1996) Increased incidence of *Chlamydia* species within the coronary arteries of patients with symptomatic atherosclerotic versus other forms of cardiovascular disease. *J Am Coll Cardiol* 27: 1555–1561

38  Melnick SL, Shahar E, Folsom AR, Grayston JT, Sorlie PD, Wang SP, Szklo M (1993) Past infection by *Chlamydia pneumoniae* strain TWAR and asymptomatic carotid ath-

erosclerosis. Atherosclerosis Risk in Communities (ARIC) Study Investigators. *Am J Med* 95(5): 499–504

39  Andreasen JJ, Farholt S, Jensen JS (1998) Failure to detect *Chlamydia pneumoniae* in calcific and degenerative arteriosclerotic aortic valves excised during open heart surgery. *APMIS* 106: 717–720

40  Paterson DL, Hall J, Rasmussen SJ, Timras P (1998) Failure to detect *Chlamydia pneumoniae* in atherosclerotic plaques of Australian patients. *Pathology* 30: 169–172

41  Weiss SM, Roblin PM, Gaydos CA, Cummings P, Patton DL, Schulhoff N, Shani J, Frankel R, Penney K, Quinn TC et al (1996) Failure to detect *Chlamydia pneumoniae* in coronary atheromas of patients undergoing atherectomy. *J Infect Dis* 173: 957–962

42  Ericson,K, Saldeen TGP, Lindquis O, Påhlson C, Mehta JL (2000) Relationship of *Chlamydia pneumoniae* infection with severity of human coronary atherosclerosis. *Circulation* 101: 2568–2571

43  Dahlén GH, Boman J, Birgander LS, Lindblom B (1995) Lp(a) lipoprotein, IgG, IgA and IgM antibodies to Chlamydia pneumoniae and HLA class II genotype in early coronary artery disease. *Atherosclerosis* 114: 165–174

44  Dahlén GH, Slunga L, Lindblom B (1994) Importance of Lp(a) lipoprotein and HLA genotypes in atherosclerosis and diabetes. *Clin Genet* 46: 46–56

45  Ossewaarde JM, Ferkens EJ, Devries A, Vallinga CE, Kromhout D (1998) *Chlamydia pneumoniae* is a risk factor for coronary heart disease in symptom-free elderly men, but *Helicobacter pylori* and cytomegalovirus are not. *Epidemiol Infect* 120: 93–99

46  Blasi F, Denti F, Erba M, Cosentini R, Raccanelli R, Rinaldi A, Fagetti L, Esposito G, Ruberti U, Allegra L (1996) Detection of *Chlamydia pneumoniae*, but not *Helicobacter pylori*, in atherosclerotic plaques of aortic aneurysms. *J Clin Microbiol* 34: 2766–2769

47  Ramirez JA (1996) Isolation of *Chlamydia pneumoniae* from the coronary artery of a patients with coronary atherosclerosis. The *Chlamydia pneumoniae*/atherosclerosis study group. *Ann Intern Med* 125: 979–982

48  Jackson LA, Campbell LA, Schmidt RA, Kuo C-C, Cappuccio AL, Lee MJ, Grayston JT (1997) Specificity of detection of *Chlamydia pneumoniae* in cardiovascular atheroma: evaluation of the innocent bystander hypothesis. *Am J Pathol* 150: 1785–1790

49  Muhlestein JB, Anderson JL, Hammond EH, Zhao L, Trehan S, Schwobe EP, Carlquist JF (1998) Infection with *Chlamydia pneumoniae* accelerates the development of atherosclerosis and treatment with azithromycin prevents it in a rabbit model. *Circulation* 97: 633–636

50  Danesh J, Wong Y, Ward M, Muir J (1999) Chronic infection with *Helicobacter pylori*, *Chlamydia pneumoniae*, or cytomegalovirus: population based study of coronary heart disease. *Heart* 81: 245–247

51  Danesh J, Wong YK, Ward M, Hawtin P, Murphy M, Muir J (1998) Strong correlation between *Helicobacter pylori* seropositivity and *Chlamydia pneumoniae* IgG concentrations. *J Epidemiol Community Health* 52: 821–822

52  Key NS, Vercellotti GM, Winkelmann JC, Moldow CF, Goodman JL, Esmon NL, Esmon CT, Jacob HS (1990) Infection of vascular endothelial cells with herpes simplex

virus enhances tissue factor activity and reduces thrombomodulin expression. *Proc Natl Acad Sci USA* 87: 7095–7099

53    Vercellotti GM (1998) Effects of viral activation of the vessel wall on inflammation and thrombosis. *Blood Coagul Fibrinolysis* 9 (Suppl 2): S3–6

54    Hosenpud JD, Chou SW, Wagner CR (1991) Cytomegalovirus-induced regulation of major histocompatibility complex class I antigen expression in human aortic smooth muscle cells. *Transplantation* 52: 896–903

55    Rasmussen SJ, Eckmann L, Quayle AJ, Shen L, Zhang YX, Anderson DJ, Fierer J, Stephens RS, Kagnoff MF (1997) Secretion of proinflammatory cytokines by epithelial cells in response to *Chlamydia* infection suggests a central role for epithelial cells in *Chlamydial* pathogenesis. *J Clin Invest* 99: 77–87

56    Galloway DA, McDougall JK (1983) The oncogenic potential of herpes simplex viruses: evidence for a 'hit-and-run' mechanism. *Nature* 302: 21–24

57    Waldman WJ (1998) Cytomegalovirus as a perturbing factor in graft/host equilibrium: Havoc at the endothelial interface. In: M Scoltz, HF Rabenau, HW Doerr, J Cinati Jr (eds): CMV-related immunopathology, Monogram Virology. Karger, Basel, 21: 54–66

58    Kol A, Sukhova GK, Lichtman AH, Libby P (1998) Chlamydial heat shock protein 60 localizes in human atheroma and regulates macrophage tumor necrosis factor-alpha and matrix metalloproteinase expression. *Circulation* 98: 300–307

59    Mayr M, Metzler B, Kiechl S, Willeit J, Schett G, Xu Q, Wick G (1999) Endothelial cytotoxicity mediated by serum antibodies to heat shock proteins of Escherichia coli and Chlamydia pneumoniae. *Circulation* 99: 1560–1566

60    Galis ZS, Sukhova GK, Lark MW, Libby P (1994) Increased expression of matrix metalloproteinases and matrix degrading activity in vulnerable regions of human atherosclerotic plaques. *J Clin Invest* 94: 2493–2503

61    Pober JS, Cotran RS (1990) Cytokines and endothelial cell biology. *Physiol Rev* 70: 427–451

62    Moncada S, Palmer RM, Higgs EA (1991) Nitric oxide: physiology, pathophysiology, and pharmacology. *Pharmacol Rev* 43: 109–142

63    Hu H, Pierce GN, Zhong G (1999) The atherogenic effects of Chlamydia are dependent on serum cholesterol and specific to *Chlamydia pneumoniae*. *J Clin Invest* 103: 747–753

64    Laurila A, Bloigu A, Nayha S, Hassi J, Leinonen M, Saikku P (1997) Chronic *Chlamydia pneumoniae* infection is associated with a serum lipid profile known to be a risk factor for atherosclerosis. *Arterioscler Thromb Vasc Biol* 17: 2910–2913

65    Murray LJ, O'Reilly DP, Ong GM, O'Neill C, Evans AE, Bamford KB (1999) *Chlamydia pneumoniae* antibodies are associated with an atherogenic lipid profile. *Heart* 81: 239–244

66    Ojcius DM, Souque P, Perfettini JL, Dautry-Varsat A (1998) Apoptosis of epithelial cells and macrophages due to infection with the obligate intracellular pathogen *Chlamydia psittaci*. *J Immunol* 161: 4220–4226

67    Fan T, Lu H, Hu H, Shi L, McClarty GA, Nance DM, Greenberg AH, Zhong G (1998) Inhibition of apoptosis in *Chlamydia*-infected cells: blockade of mitochondrial

cytochrome c- release and caspase activation. *J Exp Med* 187 (4): 487–496

68   Zhou YF, Yu ZX, Wanishsawad C, Shou M, Epstein SE (1999) The immediate early gene products of human cytomegalovirus increase vascular smooth muscle cell migration, proliferation, and expression of PDGF beta-receptor. *Biochem Biophys Res Commun* 256 (3): 608–613

69   Gupta S, Leatham EW, Carrington D, Mendall MA, Kaski JC, Camm AJ (1997) Elevated *Chlamydia pneumoniae* antibodies, cardiovascular events, and azithromycin in male survivors of acute myocardial infarction. *Circulation* 96: 404–407

70   Gurfunkel E, Bozovich G, Daroco A, Beck E, Mautner B (1997) Randomised trial of roxithromycin in non-q-wave coronary syndromes. *Lancet* 350: 404–407

71   Gurfinkel E, Bozovich G, Beck E, Testa E, Livellara B, Mautner B (1999) Treatment with the antibiotic roxithromycin in patients with acute non-Q-wave coronary syndromes. The final report of the ROXIS Study. *Eur Heart J* 20: 121–127

72   Anderson JL, Muhlestein JB, Carlquist J, Allen A, Trehan S, Nielson C, Hall S, Brady J, Egger M, Horne B et al (1999) Randomized secondary prevention trial of azithromycin in patients with coronary artery disease and serological evidence for *Chlamydia pneumoniae* infection: The azithromycin in coronary artery disease: Elimination of myocardial infection with *Chlamydia* (ACADEMIC) study. *Circulation* 99: 1540–1547

73   Martin D, Bursill J, Qui MR, Breit SN, Campbell T (1998) Alternative hypothesis for efficacy of macrolides in acute coronary syndromes. *Lancet* 351: 1858–1859

# C-reactive protein – a prognostic marker of inflammation in atherothrombosis

*David A. Morrow and Paul M. Ridker*

Cardiovascular Division, Department of Medicine, Brigham and Women's Hospital, 75 Francis Street, Boston, MA 02115, USA

## Introduction

Though significant advancements continue in the management of unstable ischemic heart disease, preventive interventions with a similar magnitude of benefit have the potential to reduce the number of cardiovascular deaths each year by more than 100,000 in the United States alone [1]. Epidemiological data have established important risk factors for atherosclerotic vascular disease, including advanced age, tobacco use, obesity, diabetes, hypertension and dyslipidemia. However, up to one third of first coronary events occur among individuals without these traditional risk factors [2]. Thus, efforts to identify additional indicators of cardiovascular prognosis that add to the predictive information from traditional risk factors, and that might aid in targeting therapy are central to improving the preventive strategies.

Research documenting the key processes driving the initiation, progression and destabilization of atherosclerotic vascular disease have guided these efforts [3]. In particular, pathological and experimental data have provided evidence for a fundamental role of inflammation in atherothrombosis [4], and directed attention to inflammatory markers as potential novel indicators of underlying atherosclerosis and increased cardiovascular risk [5]. Candidate markers have included proposed key participants in atherogenesis [4] such as cytokines [6–8] that promote the initial recruitment of inflammatory monocytes in response to endothelial cell dysfunction, intercellular adhesion molecules [9–11] which mediate the migration of activated monocytes into the subendothelial space, as well as enzymes [12] which might contribute to the compromise of the protective barrier between circulating blood and the highly pro-thrombotic core of the maturing atherosclerotic plaque. However, to date, the acute-phase inflammatory proteins have been the focus of the majority of clinical investigation, with particular attention to the prototypical acute-phase reactant, C-reactive protein (CRP).

Inflammatory and Infectious Basis of Atherosclerosis, edited by Jay L. Mehta
© 2001 Birkhäuser Verlag Basel/Switzerland

## C-reactive protein

CRP is a pentameric polypeptide initially described as a reactant to the somatic C-polysaccharide of *Streptococcus pneumonia* [13]. This acute-phase protein is produced exclusively by hepatocytes in response to stimulation by inflammatory cytokines, primarily interleukin-6 (IL-6) [13]. CRP levels are dependent on the rate of *de novo* hepatic production and remain stable over long periods of time in the absence of new stimuli [13, 14]. However, CRP rises several hundred-fold in response to acute injury, infection or other inflammatory stimuli, and when measured with traditional assays has been useful in following disease activity in chronic inflammatory conditions such as systemic lupus, inflammatory bowel disease and rheumatoid arthritis [13, 15]. Marked elevation of CRP in these disease processes may be adequately detected using semi-quantitative latex agglutination or standard turbidometric methods. However, the development of high-sensitivity assays for CRP (hs-CRP) has now enabled evaluation of CRP within the normal range for apparently healthy individuals [15, 16]. Further, the introduction of automated methods (particle-enhanced nephelometry) with high analytical sensitivity and reproducibility has provided a simple clinical tool for the detection of low levels of systemic inflammation [15, 17].

## Association of hs-CRP, atherosclerosis and cardiovascular risk

### hs-CRP and prevalent coronary heart disease

Informed by pathological data supporting the role of inflammation in the initiation, progression and complications of atherosclerosis, clinical investigators have explored the association between inflammatory markers and the presence of atherosclerotic vascular disease [3]. Cross-sectional data have documented a positive correlation between elevated levels of hs-CRP and prevalent coronary heart disease (CHD). For example, among middle-aged men in Great Britain, Mendall and colleagues demonstrated a 1.5-fold increase in the prevalence of CHD for each doubling in the levels of hs-CRP [18]. Elevated levels of CRP have also been found among patients with acute myocardial ischemia [19] and infarction [20]. However, concentrations of hs-CRP may also increase with age, body-mass index and tobacco use [18, 21], and retrospective or cross-sectional data such as these can not exclude the possibility of important confounding by these as well as other variables [22]. Further, in the absence of prospective data it is not possible to establish whether elevation of the inflammatory marker is a result or related to the cause of atherothrombosis [22].

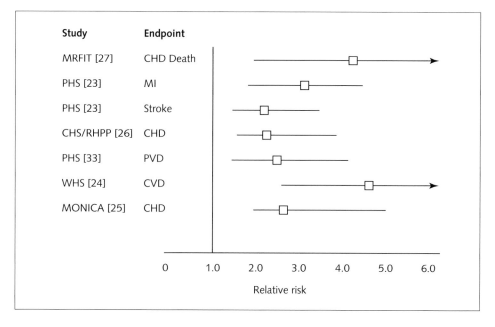

| Study | Endpoint |
|-------|----------|
| MRFIT [27] | CHD Death |
| PHS [23] | MI |
| PHS [23] | Stroke |
| CHS/RHPP [26] | CHD |
| PHS [33] | PVD |
| WHS [24] | CVD |
| MONICA [25] | CHD |

*Figure 1*
*Prospective studies of C-reactive protein as a risk factor for cardiovascular disease among apparently healthy individuals. CHD, coronary heart disease; MI, myocardial infarction; PVD, peripheral vascular disease; CVD, cardiovascular disease. Adapted from [2].*

## hs-CRP in cardiovascular risk assessment

In contrast, a series of prospective studies that can control for such confounders have been able to establish that baseline elevation of hs-CRP is a strong and consistent predictor of future cardiovascular morbidity among apparently healthy individuals free of clinical vascular disease [23-26], as well as those with multiple vascular risk factors [27] or recognized coronary artery disease [28–31] (Fig. 1).

Several studies have shown a prognostic capacity for hs-CRP among individuals either recognizable as high risk for or already symptomatic with cardiovascular disease. Among men with multiple vascular risk factors followed in the Multiple Risk Factor Intervention Trial (MRFIT) study, those with the highest baseline levels of hs-CRP were at nearly three-fold higher risk of CHD mortality (RR 2.8; 95% CI 1.4–5.4) over 17 years of follow-up [27]. Investigators from the Cardiovascular Health Study and Rural Health Promotion Project demonstrated a two to three-fold higher risk of coronary events among elderly men and women with evidence of preclinical atherosclerotic vascular disease and baseline levels of hs-CRP in the highest quartile [26]. Further, the European Concerted Action on Thrombosis and Disabilities Study (ECAT) Group showed a 45% increase in the relative risk of non-fatal myocardial infarction (MI) or sudden cardiac death (95% CI for RR 1.15–1.83) with each standard deviation increase in baseline hs-CRP among patients with angina followed for an average of two years [28]. Finally, in a nested case-control analysis of individuals with stable CHD post-myocardial infarction in the Cholesterol and Recurrent Events (CARE) trial, hs-CRP was predictive of higher risk for recurrent non-fatal MI or fatal coronary events (75% higher relative risk in the highest vs. lowest quintile of hs-CRP) [31].

While these studies provide consistent evidence of a prognostic relationship between hs-CRP and future events among persons already recognizable as high risk, three studies have extended these observations to individuals at seemingly low risk who may present a particular challenge to clinicians planning strategies for primary CHD prevention [23–25]. The Physicians Health Study (PHS) followed 22,071 apparently healthy men with no clinical vascular disease and low rates of cigarette consumption [32]. In a nested case-control analysis, investigators from the PHS found significantly elevated levels of baseline hs-CRP among participants who developed arterial vascular events compared with matched controls [23]. Moreover, individuals in the highest quartile of hs-CRP had a two-fold increased risk of future stroke (RR 1.9, 95% CI 1.1–3.3), a three-fold higher risk of future MI (RR 2.9, 95% CI 1.8–4.6) (Fig. 2, left) [23], and a four-fold higher risk of developing severe peripheral arterial disease (RR 4.1, 95% CI 1.2–6.0) [33]. In contrast with data from the MRFIT study [27], these risk estimates were not modified by smoking status [23]. Further, adjustment for other cardiovascular risk factors including total and high-density lipoprotein (HDL) cholesterol, triglycerides, diabetes, fibrinogen, and lipoprotein(a) did not significantly alter the predictive capacity of hs-CRP.

The MONICA (Monitoring Trends and Determinants in Cardiovascular Disease) Augsberg Cohort Study offers corroborating evidence for the prognostic association of hs-CRP and vascular events from a large prospective study of individuals initially free of cardiovascular disease [25]. In a random sample of 936 middle-aged healthy men, a one standard deviation increase in log-normalized baseline hs-CRP was associated with a 1.7-fold higher risk of a first major coronary event (95% CI 1.29–2.17) [25]. Similar to findings in the PHS, this hazard rate ratio was not significantly altered after adjustment for multiple potential confounders, including age and smoking status.

Findings from the Women's Health Study (WHS) show that the association between hs-CRP and cardiovascular risk among initially healthy individuals is not limited to men. In a nested case control analysis, post-menopausal women who subsequently developed a first cardiovascular event had significantly higher baseline levels of hs-CRP compared with age- and smoking-matched control subjects who remained free of vascular disease during three years of follow-up [24]. Those with the highest levels of hs-CRP (4th quartile) were at nearly five times the risk of any

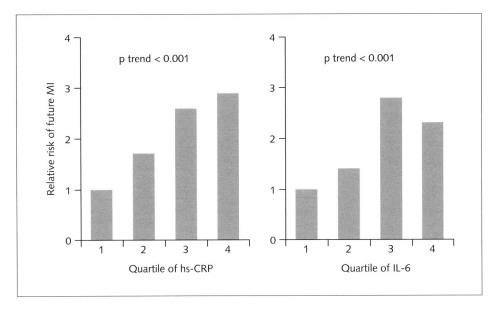

*Figure 2*

*Relative risk of first myocardial infarction (MI) in apparently healthy men stratified by quartile of baseline high-sensitivity c-reactive protein (hs-CRP) (left) and interleukin-6 (IL-6) (right). Adapted from [23, 47].*

vascular event (RR 4.8, 95% CI 2.3–10.1), and seven times the risk of myocardial infarction or stroke (RR 7.3, 95% CI 2.7–19.9) [24]. Consistent with findings in men, these risk estimates were independent of other recognized cardiovascular risk factors and persisted among the multiple low risk subgroups examined (Fig. 3).

Additional subgroup analyses did, however, demonstrate an association between elevated hs-CRP and the use of hormonal replacement therapy (HRT) [34]. Median levels of hs-CRP were two times higher among women using HRT compared with women on no HRT (0.27 vs. 0.14 mg/dl, p = 0.001). Though median hs-CRP levels in the WHS [24] were greater than those observed in prior studies consisting only of men, stratification by use of hormonal replacement revealed that women on no HRT had a distribution of baseline CRP similar to men (Fig. 4) [34]. The association between elevated hs-CRP and HRT was present among all subgroups evaluated, regardless of the form of HRT used, and is consistent with findings from a prospective analysis of a similar group of women in the Postmenopausal Estrogen/Progestin Interventions Study [35] and the population of elderly women in the Cardiovascular Health Study [36]. It has been hypothesized [35, 36] that these data point to a possible mechanism for a transient increase in thrombotic risk associated with initiation of HRT suggested by results from the

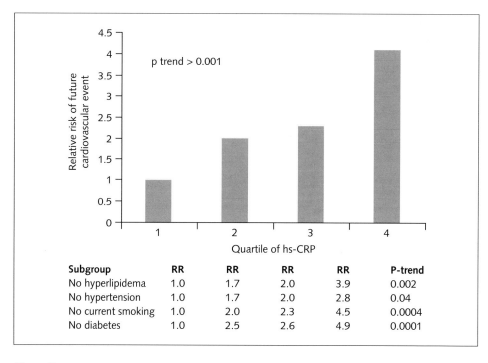

*Figure 3*

*Adjusted relative risk (RR) of future cardiovascular events among apparently healthy women stratified by quartile of baseline hs-CRP concentration both among all subjects (chart) and among specific low-risk subgroups (below). Adapted from [24].*

Heart and Estrogen/progestin Replacement Study (HERS) [37]. However, further investigation in carefully conducted clinical studies will be important for evaluating whether these observations supporting the possibility of pro-inflammatory effects of HRT are clinically relevant [34].

## hs-CRP and established risk markers

If inflammatory markers such as hs-CRP are to become useful in clinical practice, it is important that they contribute prognostic information beyond that offered by established markers of cardiovascular risk [22]. In each of the large prospective studies among healthy individuals, the association of baseline hs-CRP with increased risk for future cardiovascular morbidity has been shown to persist after adjustment for traditional risk factors including age, hypertension, diabetes, body mass index and smoking status [23–25]. Further, both in the PHS and WHS, hs-CRP

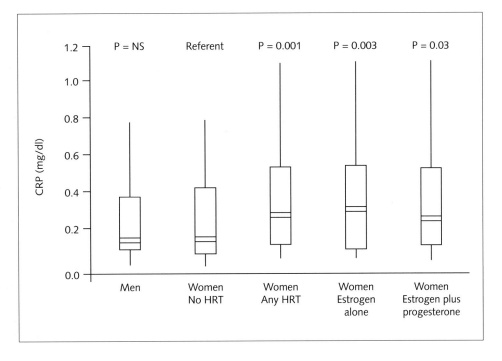

*Figure 4*
*Distributions of hs-CRP among study participants according to gender and hormone replacement therapy (HRT) status. Box plots show $10^{th}$, $25^{th}$, $50^{th}$, $75^{th}$ and $90^{th}$ percentiles of the hs-CRP distribution for each group. mg/dl = milligram per deciliter. From [34].*

was a strong predictor of future MI among those at low as well as high risk on the basis of lipid parameters alone, and added to the predictive information offered by the total to high density cholesterol ratio (TC:HDL) [24, 38]. Moreover, the PHS comparison with other traditional (TC and TC:HDL) and "novel" (lipoprotein(a), homocysteine, fibrinogen and tissue plasminogen activator (t-PA) antigen) markers of cardiovascular risk, showed the combination of hs-CRP and the TC:HDL ratio to be the strongest predictor of first myocardial infarction (Fig. 5) [22].

## Other inflammatory markers

The pathobiological mechanisms through which elevation of the acute phase reactants relate to vascular risk are as yet undefined. Though CRP may exert direct effects on the expression of tissue factor [39], activation of complement [40], and adhesion of leukocytes [41], it remains plausible that the marker is primarily a pas-

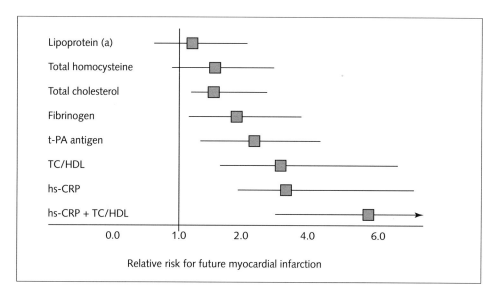

**Figure 5**
*Relative risk for future myocardial infarction among apparently healthy individuals. t-PA, tissue plasminogen activator; TC/HDL, total cholesterol to high density lipoprotein ratio. From [22].*

sive indicator of inflammatory processes central to atherogenesis. Consistent with this notion, elevation of several inflammatory mediators/participants have also been associated with incident CHD.

As the primary stimulant for CRP production, interleukin-6 (IL-6) levels correlate closely with hs-CRP in non-cardiovascular conditions [42]. In addition, IL-6 has a broad range of humoral and cellular immune effects [43], and may stimulate coagulation [44, 45]. Elevated levels of IL-6 have been demonstrated in stable [8] as well as unstable ischemic heart disease [6] and may be associated with increased risk for early adverse outcomes [46]. In addition, baseline elevation of IL-6 has been associated with increased risk of all cause mortality during seven years of follow-up in a subgroup of high-functioning elderly men and women from the Iowa 65+ Rural Health Study [7]. Data from the PHS, have further shown that among healthy men with low rates of cigarette consumption, the relative risk of a first MI increased with increasing quartiles of IL-6, with a 2.3-fold higher risk of MI (95% CI 1.3–4.3, p = 0.005) among those with the highest levels of IL-6 (Fig. 2, right) [47]. This risk relationship was present after adjustment for baseline differences in total cholesterol, HDL cholesterol, body mass index, blood pressure, and diabetes and was stable among all low risk groups evaluated, including non-smokers. Further, the relationship between IL-6 and MI remained statistically significant even after controlling for

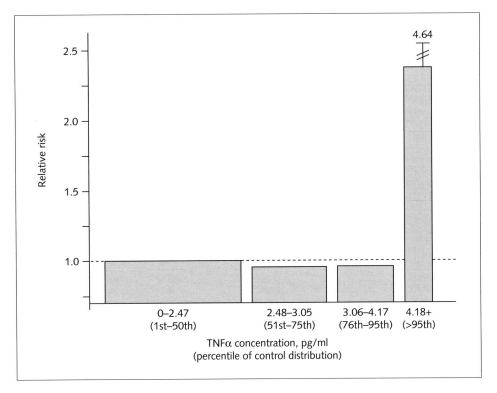

*Figure 6*
*Relative risk of death and recurrent non-fatal myocardial infarction (MI) among patients sta-
bilized post-myocardial infarction according to baseline levels of TNFα. pg/ml, picograms
per milliliter. From [49].*

baseline concentrations of hs-CRP [47]. In light of these data, it is not surprising
that several acute phase proteins (CRP, serum amyloid A, albumin and fibrinogen)
produced in response to hepatic stimulation by IL-6 have all been associated with
increased cardiovascular risk [48].

In addition, other inflammatory cytokines have been found to correlate with
myocardial ischemia [8] and increased risk of recurrent events among those with
unstable [46] and stable coronary artery disease [49]. For example, investigators
from the CARE study measured tumor necrosis factor α (TNFα) at least three
months post-MI among 272 individuals who subsequently suffered a recurrent
event and among the same number of age and gender-matched study participants
and found that TNFα was significantly elevated among cases compared with controls (p = 0.02) [49]. Further, the relative risk of experiencing a recurrent cardiac
event was 2.7-fold higher (P = 0.004) among individuals with TNFα levels greater

than the 95<sup>th</sup> percentile of the control distribution (Fig. 6) [49]. As such, these data add to the accumulating evidence that sensitive markers of systemic inflammation may be useful in detecting individuals at higher risk for future first or recurrent cardiac events.

Finally, prospective analyses have shown an association between elevated levels of vascular adhesion molecules, such as soluble intercellular adhesion molecule-1 (ICAM-1), and future cardiovascular events [9, 10]. In contrast to non-specific markers of systemic inflammation such as the acute phase proteins, vascular adhesion molecules are integral participants in vascular endothelial activation and inflammation and point more directly to a fundamental contribution of inflammation in atherothrombosis [10]. Further investigation directed at elucidating the precise relationships between elevation of inflammatory markers and adverse prognosis will advance our understanding of the pathobiology of atherogenesis as well as potentially introduce new targets for therapeutic intervention.

## hs-CRP and preventive interventions

Though elevated hs-CRP identifies individuals at increased cardiovascular risk, the inflammatory marker is likely to have little impact on clinical strategies for primary or secondary prevention if the associated risk can not be modified by available therapies. Thus, data suggesting important interactions between hs-CRP and specific pharmacological therapies are of particular clinical as well as experimental interest.

## hs-CRP and clinical risk reduction

In the PHS, participants were randomly assigned to low-dose aspirin (325 mg, orally, every other day (POQOD)) or placebo with a 44% reduction in the risk of first MI associated with aspirin use (p < 0.001) [32]. In subgroup analyses, stratification by quartiles of baseline hs-CRP revealed an increasing gradient of benefit with aspirin therapy from the lowest to highest quartile of hs-CRP (Fig. 7, top) [23]. Those with the highest levels of hs-CRP realized a 55.7% reduction in the risk of future myocardial infarction (p = 0.02), whereas those in the lowest quartile showed only a 13.9% risk reduction (p = 0.77) [23]. Analogously, in the CARE trial where therapy with 40 mg of daily pravastatin was associated with a 24% reduction in the risk of recurrent coronary events compared with placebo [50], a nested case-control analysis revealed significant variation in the magnitude of risk reduction in association with baseline hs-CRP (Fig. 7, bottom) [31]. Although pravastatin therapy was found to benefit both those with and without evidence of inflammation, the risk reduction attributable to pravastatin therapy was greatest among those with elevation of inflammatory markers (54 vs. 25%) despite nearly identical lipid parameters

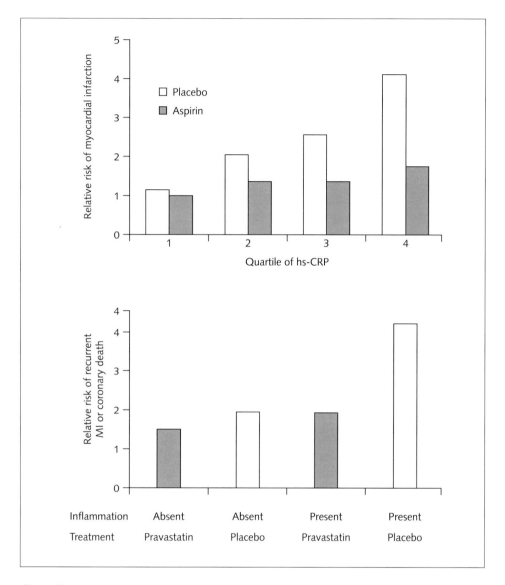

*Figure 7*
*Efficacy of aspirin (top) and pravastatin (bottom) therapy and interaction with evidence of inflammation. MI = myocardial infarction. Adapted from [23, 31].*

in each group [31]. In addition, the association between inflammation and risk of recurrent events was attenuated among those treated with pravastatin (RR 1.29, p = 0.5) as compared with those taking placebo (RR 2.1, p = 0.048) [31].

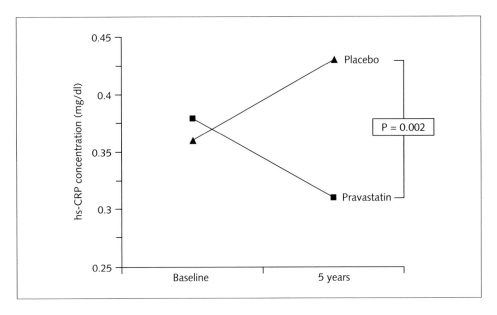

Figure 8

Mean levels of hs-CRP at baseline and 60 months according to placebo or pravastatin assignment. mg/dl = milligrams per deciliter. Adapted from [59].

Together, findings from these two clinical studies support several observations relevant to the evaluation of hs-CRP for use in routine cardiovascular risk assessment. First, the increase in cardiovascular risk associated with elevation of inflammatory markers appears to be modified by specific therapies. Second, baseline measurement of inflammatory markers such as hs-CRP may prove useful in targeting certain preventive and therapeutic interventions . Further, though the pathophysiological basis for these interactions are not established, findings from the PHS and CARE lend support to speculation that the anti-inflammatory properties of aspirin may be contributing in part to its efficacy in the prevention of coronary events, [8] and to the possible clinical relevance of laboratory observations demonstrating non-lipid effects of the 3-hydroxy-3-methylglutaryl coenzyme A (HMG-CoA) reductase inhibitors [51, 52].

## Inflammation as a target for therapy

The convergence of pathological and clinical data indicating the importance of inflammation in atherogenesis has motivated researchers to evaluate possible anti-inflammatory or immunoregulatory actions of several established therapies as well as to explore potential novel interventions targeted at interrupting the inflammatory pathways which may contribute to atherothrombosis [5].

Experimental data have demonstrated several non-lipid actions of the HMG-CoA reductase inhibitors, such as modulation of immune function [51, 53], antiproliferative effects on vascular smooth muscle [54, 55], and antithrombotic properties [52, 56], as well as morphological effects on the atherosclerotic plaque [57, 58]. Data from human studies using these agents provide evidence for the possible clinical importance of these actions. Samples collected at baseline and five years after randomization in 476 participants from CARE who remained free of vascular events demonstrate a significant fall in median hs-CRP concentration (–17.4%, P = 0.004) among those treated with pravastatin compared with a trend toward rising median hs-CRP (+ 4.2%, P = 0.2) among those allocated to placebo (Fig. 8) [59]. These trends in the levels of hs-CRP were independent of the magnitude of change in lipid parameters with only slight attenuation of the effect of pravastatin on the change in hs-CRP in analyses controlled for LDL cholesterol, and no reduction in hs-CRP among patients allocated to placebo who had a fall in LDL levels during the follow-up period [59]. Together with data from animal studies demonstrating that both dietary and statin-induced lipid lowering results in a reduction in the activity of metalloproteinases proposed to contribute to plaque compromise [60, 61], these data from CARE suggest that statin therapy may achieve a reduction in cardiovascular events through both lipid-dependent and lipid-independent effects on inflammatory-cell function and related plaque vulnerability.

## Conclusions

Pathological and experimental data suggest that atherosclerosis is a fundamentally inflammatory disease. A series of prospective epidemiological studies support this notion providing consistent evidence of an association between sensitive markers of systemic inflammation and the risk of future cardiovascular events. In particular, high-sensitivity testing for CRP appears to identify apparently healthy individuals who are at higher risk for vascular events at five or more years after blood sampling, as well as patients with stable and unstable coronary disease who are more likely to suffer recurrent adverse events. In each of these settings, measurement of hs-CRP adds to the prognostic information offered by traditional vascular risk factors. Further, clinical studies suggest that increased risk associated with elevation of hs-CRP may be modified by aspirin or HMG-CoA reductase inhibitors. Experimental data demonstrate that such agents modulate inflammatory processes or mediators which may be central to atherothrombosis [8, 61]. Taken together, these data support the possibilty that anti-inflammatory therapies might come to play a role in the prevention and treatment of cardiovascular disease and that inflammatory markers such as hs-CRP may prove clinically useful in targeting therapy to those patients who will derive the greatest benefit.

# References

1   Manson JE, Ridker PM, Gaziano JM, Hennekens CH (1997) *Primary prevention of myocardial infarction*. Oxford University Press, New York

2   Ridker PM, Haughie P (1998) Prospective studies of C-reactive protein as a risk factor for cardiovascular disease. *J Investig Med* 46: 391–395

3   Ridker P (1997) Fibrinolytic and inflammatory markers for arterial occlusion: the evolving epidemiology of thrombosis and hemostasis. *Thromb Haemost* 78: 53–59

4   Ross R (1999) Atherosclerosis – An inflammatory disease. *N Engl J Med* 340: 115–126

5   Morrow DA, Ridker PM (1999) Inflammation in cardiovascular disease. In: E Topol (ed): *Textbook of cardiovascular medicine updates*. Lippincott Williams & Wilkins, Cedar Knolls, 1–12

6   Biasucci LM, Vitelli A, Liuzzo G, Altamura S, Caligiuri G, Monaco C, Rebuzzi AG, Ciliberto G, Maseri A (1996) Elevated levels of interleukin-6 in unstable angina. *Circulation* 94: 874–877

7   Harris TB, Ferrucci L, Tracy RP, Corti MC, Wacholder S, Ettinger WH Jr, Heimovitz H, Cohen HJ, Wallace R (1999) Associations of elevated interleukin-6 and C-reactive protein levels with mortality in the elderly. *Am J Med* 106: 506–512

8   Ikonomidis I, Andreotti F, Economou E, Stefanadis C, Toutouzas P, Nihoyannopoulos P (1999) Increased proinflammatory cytokines in patients with chronic stable angina and their reduction by aspirin. *Circulation* 100: 793–798

9   Hwang SJ, Ballantyne CM, Sharrett AR, Smith LC, Davis CE, Gotto AM Jr, Boerwinkle E (1997) Circulating adhesion molecules VCAM-1, ICAM-1, and E-selectin in carotid atherosclerosis and incident coronary heart disease cases: the Atherosclerosis Risk In Communities (ARIC) study. *Circulation* 96: 4219–4225

10  Ridker PM, Hennekens CH, Roitman-Johnson B, Stampfer MJ, Allen J (1998) Plasma concentration of soluble intercellular adhesion molecule 1 and risk of future myocardial infarction in apparently healthy men. *Lancet* 351: 88–92

11  Aukrust P, Mu F, Ueland T, Berget T, Aaser E, Brunsvig A, Solum NO, Forfang K, Froland SS, Gullestad L (1999) Enhanced levels of soluble and membrane-bound CD40 ligand in patients with unstable angina. Possible reflection of T lymphocyte and platelet involvement in the pathogenesis of acute coronary syndromes. *Circulation* 100: 614–620

12  Kai H, Ikeda H, Yasukawa H, Kai M, Seki Y, Kuwahara F, Ueno T, Sugi K, Imaizumi T (1998) Peripheral blood levels of matrix metalloproteases-2 and -9 are elevated in patients with acute coronary syndromes. *J Am Coll Cardiol* 32: 368–372

13  Pepys MB, Baltz ML (1983) Acute phase proteins with special reference to C-reactive protein and related proteins (pentaxins) and serum amyloid A protein. *Adv Immunol* 34: 141–212

14  Macy E, Hayes T, Tracy R (1997) Variability in the measurement of C-reactive protein in healthy subjects: implications for reference interval and epidemiologic applications. *Clin Chem* 43: 52–58

15    Ledue TB, Weiner DL, Sipe JD, Poulin SE, Collins MF, Rifai N (1998) Analytical eval-
      uation of particle-enhanced immunonephelometric assays for C-reactive protein, serum
      amyloid A and mannose-binding protein in human serum. *Ann Clin Biochem* 35: 745–
      753

16    Wilkins J, Gallimore R, Moore E, Pepys M (1998) Rapid automated high sensitivity
      enzyme immunoassay of C-reactive protein. *Clin Chem* 44: 1358–1361

17    Rifai N, Tracy RP, Ridker PM (1999) Clinical efficacy of an automated high-sensitivity
      C-reactive protein assay. *Clin Chem* 45: 2136–2141

18    Mendall MA, Patel P, Ballam L, Strachan D, Northfield TC (1996) C reactive protein
      and its relation to cardiovascular risk factors: a population based cross sectional study.
      *BMJ* 312: 1061–1065

19    Berk BC, Weintraub WS, Alexander RW (1990) Elevation of C-reactive protein in
      "active" coronary artery disease. *Am J Cardiol* 65: 168–172

20    Pietila K, Harmoinen A, Poyhonen L, Ruosteenoja R (1986) C-reactive protein in suben-
      docardial and transmural myocardial infarcts. *Clin Chem* 32: 1596–1597

21    Tracy RP, Psaty BM, Macy E, Bovill EG, Cushman M, Cornell ES, Kuller LH (1997)
      Lifetime smoking exposure affects the association of C-reactive protein with cardiovas-
      cular disease risk factors and subclinical disease in healthy elderly subjects. *Arterioscler
      Thromb Vasc Biol* 17: 2167–2176

22    Ridker PM (1999) Evaluating novel cardiovascular risk factors: can we better predict
      heart attacks? *Ann Intern Med* 130: 933–937

23    Ridker PM, Cushman M, Stampfer MJ, Tracy RP, Hennekens CH (1997) Inflammation,
      aspirin, and the risk of cardiovascular disease in apparently healthy men. *N Engl J Med*
      336: 973–979

24    Ridker PM, Buring JE, Shih J, Matias M, Hennekens CH (1998) Prospective study of C-
      reactive protien and the risk of future cardiovascular events among apparently healthy
      women. *Circulation* 98: 731–733

25    Koenig W, Sund M, Froehlich M, Fischer H, Lowel H, Doering A, Hutchinson W, Pepys
      M (1999) C-reactive protein, a sensitive marker of inflammation, predicts future risk of
      coronary heart disease in initially healthy middle-aged men: Results from the MONICA
      (Monitoring trends and determinants in cardiovascular disease) Augsberg Cohort Study,
      1984 to 1992. *Circulation* 99: 237–242

26    Tracy RP, Lemaitre RN, Psaty BM, Ives DG, Evans RW, Cushman M, Meilahn EN,
      Kuller LH (1997) Relationship of C-reactive protein to risk of cardiovascular disease in
      the elderly. Results from the Cardiovascular Health Study and the Rural Health Promo-
      tion Project. *Arterioscler Thromb Vasc Biol* 17: 1121–1127

27    Kuller LH, Tracy RP, Shaten J, Meilahn EN (1996) Relation of C-reactive protein and
      coronary heart disease in the MRFIT nested case-control study. Multiple Risk Factor
      Intervention Trial. *Am J Epidemiol* 144: 537–547

28    Haverkate F, Thompson SG, Pyke SD, Gallimore JR, Pepys MB (1997) Production of C-
      reactive protein and risk of coronary events in stable and unstable angina. European

Concerted Action on Thrombosis and Disabilities Angina Pectoris Study Group. *Lancet* 349: 462–466

29  Liuzzo G, Biasucci LM, Gallimore JR, Grillo RL, Rebuzzi AG, Pepys MB, Maseri A (1994) The prognostic value of C-reactive protein and serum amyloid a protein in severe unstable angina. *N Engl J Med* 331: 417–424

30  Morrow DA, Rifai N, Antman EM, Weiner D, McCabe CM, Cannon CP, Braunwald E (1998) C-Reactive protein is a potent predictor of mortality independently and in combination with troponin T in acute coronary syndromes. *J Am Coll Cardiol* 31: 1460–1465

31  Ridker PM, Rifai N, Pfeffer MA, Sacks FM, Moye LA, Goldman S, Flaker GC, Braunwald E (1998) Inflammation, pravastatin, and the risk of coronary events after myocardial infarction in patients with average cholesterol levels. Cholesterol and Recurrent Events (CARE) Investigators. *Circulation* 98: 839–844

32  Steering Committee of the Physicians' Health Study Research G (1989) Final report on the aspirin component of the ongoing Physicians' Health Study. *N Engl J Med* 321: 129–135

33  Ridker PM, Cushman M, Stampfer MJ, Tracy RP, Hennekens CH (1998) Plasma concentration of C-reactive prtoein and risk of developing peripheral vascular disease. *Circulation* 97: 425–428

34  Ridker PM, Hennekens CH, Rifai N, Buring JE, Manson JE (1999) Hormone replacement therapy and increased plasma concentration of C-reactive protein. *Circulation* 100: 713–716

35  Cushman M, Legault C, Barrett-Connor E, Stefanick ML, Kessler C, Judd HL, Sakkinen PA, Tracy RP (1999) Effect of postmenopausal hormones on inflammation-sensitive proteins: the Postmenopausal Estrogen/Progestin Interventions (PEPI) Study. *Circulation* 100: 717–722

36  Cushman M, Meilahn EN, Psaty BM, Kuller LH, Dobs AS, Tracy RP (1999) Hormone replacement therapy, inflammation, and hemostasis in elderly women. *Arterioscler Thromb Vasc Biol* 19: 893–899

37  Hulley S, Grady D, Bush T, Furberg C, Herrington D, Riggs B, Vittinghoff E (1998) Randomized trial of estrogen plus progestin for secondary prevention of coronary heart disease in postmenopausal women. Heart and Estrogen/progestin Replacement Study (HERS) Research Group. *JAMA* 280: 605–613

38  Ridker PM, Glynn RJ, Hennekens CH (1998) C-reactive protein adds to the predictive value of total and HDL cholesterol in determining risk of first myocardial infarction. *Circulation* 97: 2007–2011

39  Cermak J, Key NS, Bach RR, Balla J, Jacob HS, Vercellotti GM (1993) C-reactive protein induces human peripheral blood monocytes to synthesize tissue factor. *Blood* 82: 513–520

40  Wolbink GJ, Brouwer MC, Buysmann S, ten Berge IJ, Hack CE (1996) CRP-mediated activation of complement *in vivo*: assessment by measuring circulating complement-C-reactive protein complexes. *J Immunol* 157: 473–479

41    Zouki C, Beauchamp M, Baron C, Filep J (1997) Prevention of *in vitro* neutrophil adhesion to endothelial cells through shedding of L-selectin by C-reactive protein and peptides derived from C-reactive protein. *J Clin Invest* 100: 522–529

42    Bataille R, Klein B (1992) C-reactive protein levels as a direct indicator of interleukin-6 levels in humans *in vivo*. *Arthritis & Rheumatism* 35: 982–984

43    Van Snick J (1990) Interleukin-6: an overview. *Ann Rev Immunol* 8: 253–278

44    Mestries JC, Kruithof EK, Gascon MP, Herodin F, Agay D, Ythier A (1994) In vivo modulation of coagulation and fibrinolysis by recombinant glycosylated human interleukin-6 in baboons. *European Cytokine Network* 5: 275–281

45    Stouthard JM, Levi M, Hack CE, Veenhof CH, Romijn HA, Sauerwein HP, van der Poll T (1996) Interleukin-6 stimulates coagulation, not fibrinolysis, in humans. *Thromb Haemost* 76: 738–742

46    Biasucci LM, Liuzzo G, Fantuzzi G, Caligiuri G, Rebuzzi AG, Ginnetti F, Dinarello CA, Maseri A (1999) Increasing levels of interleukin (IL)-1Ra and IL-6 during the first 2 days of hospitalization in unstable angina are associated with increased risk of in-hospital coronary events. *Circulation* 99: 2079–2084

47    Ridker PM, Rifai N, Stampfer MJ, Hennekens CH (2000) Plasma concentration of interleukin-6 and the risk of future myocardial infarction among apparently healthy men. *Circulation* 101: 1767–1772

48    Danesh J, Collins R, Appleby P, Peto R (1998) Association of fibrinogen, C-reactive protein, albumin, or leukocyte count with coronary heart disease: meta-analyses of prospective studies. *JAMA* 279: 1477–1482

49    Ridker PM, Rifai N, Pfeffer M, Sacks F, Lepage S, Braunwald E (2000) Elevation of tumor necrosis factor-alpha and increased risk of recurrent coronary events following myocardial infarction. *Circulation* 101: 2149–2153

50    Sacks FM, Pfeffer MA, Moye LA, Rouleau JL, Rutherford JD, Cole TG, Brown L, Warnica JW, Arnold JM, Wun CC et al (1996) The effect of pravastatin on coronary events after myocardial infarction in patients with average cholesterol levels. Cholesterol and Recurrent Events Trial investigators. *N Engl J Med* 335: 1001–1009

51    Vaughan CJ, Murphy MB, Buckley BM (1996) Statins do more than just lower cholesterol. *Lancet* 348: 1079–1082

52    Corsini A, Bernini F, Quarato P, Donetti E, Bellosta S, Fumagalli R, Paoletti R, Soma VM (1996) Non-lipid-related effects of 3-hydroxy-3-methylglutaryl coenzyme A reductase inhibitors. *Cardiology* 87: 458–468

53    Kurakata S, Kada M, Shimada Y, Komai T, Nomoto K (1996) Effects of different inhibitors of 3-hydroxy-3-methylglutaryl coenzyme A (HMG-CoA) reductase, pravastatin sodium and simvastatin, on sterol synthesis and immunological functions in human lymphocytes *in vitro*. *Immunopharmacology* 34: 51–61

54    Munro E, Patel M, Chan P, Betteridge L, Clunn G, Gallagher K, Hughes A, Schachter M, Wolfe J, Sever P (1994) Inhibition of human vascular smooth muscle cell proliferation by lovastatin: the role of isoprenoid intermediates of cholesterol synthesis. *Eur J Clin Invest* 24: 766–772

55    Rogler G, Lackner KJ, Schmitz G (1995) Effects of fluvastatin on growth of porcine and human vascular smooth muscle cells *in vitro*. *Am J Cardiol* 76: 114A–116A

56    Rosenson RS, Tangney CC (1998) Antiatherothrombotic properties of statins: implications for cardiovascular event reduction. *JAMA* 279: 1643–1650

57    Shiomi M, Ito T, Tsukada T, Yata T, Watanabe Y, Tsujita Y, Fukami M, Fukushige J, Hosokawa T, Tamura A (1995) Reduction of serum cholesterol levels alters lesional composition of atherosclerotic plaques. Effect of pravastatin sodium on atherosclerosis in mature WHHL rabbits. *Arterioscler Thromb Vasc Biol* 15: 1938–1944

58    Williams JK, Sukhova GK, Herrington DM, Libby P (1998) Pravastatin has cholesterol-lowering independent effects on the artery wall of atherosclerotic monkeys. *J Am Coll Cardiol* 31: 684–691

59    Ridker PM, Rifai N, Pfeffer MA, Sacks FM, Braunwald E (1999) Long-term effects of pravastatin on plasma concentration of C-reactive protein. *Circulation* 100: 230–235

60    Aikawa M, Rabkin E, Okada Y, Voglic SJ, Clinton SK, Brinckerhoff CE, Sukhova GK, Libby P (1998) Lipid lowering by diet reduces matrix metalloproteinase activity and increases collagen content of rabbit atheroma: a potential mechanism of lesion stabilization. *Circulation* 97: 2433–2444

61    Aikawa M, Voglic S, Rabkin E, Shiomi M, Libby P (1998) An HMG-CoA reductase inhibitor (cervistatin) supresses accumulation of macrophages expressing matrix metalloproteinases and tissue factor in atheroma of WHHL rabbits. *Circulation* 98: I–47

# Inflammation as a marker of outcome in myocardial ischemia

*Luigi M. Biasucci, Dominick J. Angiolillo and Giovanna Liuzzo*

Institute of Cardiology, Catholic University, Largo Vito, 00168 Roma, Italy

## Introduction

Ischemic heart disease (IHD) is a major health problem, and accounts for almost 50% of all deaths and for a large part of hospitalization and health system costs [1, 2]. IHD is also a devastating problem for the individuals affected by this disease. One of the problems related to IHD is the relative lack of reliable and affordable methods for risk stratification. IHD represents a clinical spectrum ranging from sudden death to mild stable angina. Clinical data are sufficient to judge that the outcome of patients with a large anterior myocardial infarction (MI), a very low ejection fraction (EF) and in New York Heart Association (NYHA) class III or IV is very different from that of patients with angina in NYHA class 1 and no coronary risk factors. However, it is often difficult to predict the prognosis of patients with IHD. The clinical data, and the non-invasive and invasive diagnostic tests are of little help in many patients. Traditional risk factors can explain only one half of all causes of MI. Further, the majority of MIs develop in the presence of non-significant coronary stenoses. Recently, growing evidence indicates that markers of inflammation may provide a more accurate prognostic stratification of IHD patients [3–5].

## Inflammatory markers: the rationale

Atherosclerosis is nowadays considered to be an inflammatory disease [6]. Activated macrophages presenting human major histocompatibility (HLA)-DR antigens are common in coronary atherosclerotic plaques of IHD patients [7], and are more frequent in patients with acute coronary syndromes [8]. Macrophages are not the only inflammatory cells present within the plaque, as lymphocytes and mast cells are also present in the atherosclerotic regions [9, 10]. These cells were found to be particularly abundant in the shoulder region of the plaques, an area with predilection for disruption [11–13]. The presence of inflammatory cells is likely to be of crucial importance in the mechanisms leading to plaque activation and rupture, since macrophages are capable of degrading extracellular matrix by secreting proteolytic enzymes such as plasminogen activators and matrix metalloproteinases, that may weaken the fibrous cap [11, 14].

The abundance of inflammatory cells in plaques of patients with IHD clearly suggests that an inflammatory component may be part of the pathophysiological process leading to unstable conditions. This process may also be reflected in the systemic circulation, as pro-inflammatory cytokines produced by inflammatory cells can be measured directly in the peripheral blood or, indirectly, by the measurement of acute phase proteins, such as C-reactive protein (CRP), fibrinogen and serum amyloid A (SAA) protein, whose production is induced by pro-inflammatory cytokines in the liver [15–18].

In this chapter, we discuss various circulating markers of inflammation in relation to IHD.

## Circulating markers of inflammation

Several circulating markers of inflammation can be measured in the peripheral venous blood, and these markers may be used as prognostic markers [3–5].

### Leukocyte counts and activation products

It has been known since the 1970s that an increased leukocyte count carries an increased risk of IHD [19]. More recently, leukocyte activation has been assessed with specific methods, such as release of specific enzymes or presentation of activation molecules on their surfaces. Mehta et al. showed that these markers of leukocyte activation are expressed more often in unstable than in stable coronary syndromes. However, these markers do not seem to have a prognostic power [20].

Dinerman et al. have assessed protease elastase as a marker of granulocyte activation and found that it was higher in the plasma of unstable angina (UA) patients and MI patients vs. controls [21]. Our group has shown elevated levels of granulocyte protease myeloperoxidase release in UA and MI patients [20]. Activation of monocytes and lymphocytes has also been shown in patients with IHD, with a gradient from stable to unstable syndromes [22, 23]. Intriguingly, Caligiuri et al. [26] have shown that lymphocyte activation is inversely related to the amount of inflammatory reaction in acute unstable angina. They showed increased expression of IL-2SR, a marker of lymphocyte activation, in patients with stable angina or those without restenosis after percutaneous transluminal coronary angioplasty (PTCA) than in patients with unstable angina or those with a high rate of restenosis. These observations suggest that lymphocyte activation may, at least in part, be protective, possibly by secretion of anti-inflammatory cytokines such as IL-4 and IL-10 [24].

## Fibrinogen

Fibrinogen is a well established risk factor for IHD and a good prognostic marker in patients affected by IHD. A number of studies have shown that fibrinogen is associated with a greater risk of death and MI in stable and unstable patients, however, it has always been considered as a marker of haemostatic activation, rather than of inflammation. For this reason fibrinogen will not be discussed in detail in this chapter. However, although fibrinogen is a pivotal haemostatic protein, it is produced by the liver under IL-6 and IL-1 stimulation following infections and/or an inflammatory status and therefore it must also be considered a part of the inflammatory acute phase reaction [25–27].

## C-reactive protein and serum amyloid A

There is growing evidence that CRP is a reliable prognostic marker in IHD. CRP is a pentameric protein involved with complement activation and opsonization and represents the prototypic acute phase response protein, as its levels increase rapidly after an inflammatory stimulus (6 h) and may rise several-fold depending on the intensity of the stimulus [28, 29]. Moreover, CRP is not consumed in any process, as happens for example with fibrinogen in the coagulation process, therefore its concentration is dependent simply on the rate of production and excretion, with a half-life of 19 h, which makes CRP levels quite stable over time. CRP is also a protein that is not released or degraded *ex vivo*, making this protein stable in blood samples even at room temperature [25]. Finally, CRP can be measured precisely by commercially available methods offering high volume, low cost and high sensitivity measurements. CRP is a well known and widely used marker of disease activity and of prognosis in infectious and in inflammatory diseases, and it came to the cardiologists' attention for the first time almost twenty years ago when van de Beer et al. [30] reported that CRP was elevated in patients with IHD, particularly in unstable angina pectoris (UAP) and MI. These observations were confirmed in 1990 by Berk et al who found CRP to be elevated in the majority of patients with UAP [17]. At the same time the ECAT (European Concerted Action on Thrombosis) group was actively enrolling patients for a study on the prognostic value of CRP as well as of others biochemical markers [31].

In 1994 our group presented the first paper demonstrating a significant association between CRP levels and prognosis in unstable angina. Our study included patients without an elevation in troponin T to rule out any effect of myocardial cell necrosis on inflammation [3]. We observed that a level of CRP > 3 mg/l (90° percentiles) was associated with an increased risk of the combined end-points, i.e. recurrent angina, death, and MI (Fig. 1). Although the hard endpoint of death and MI was also frequent in the group with elevated CRP (6 vs. 0), the small sample size

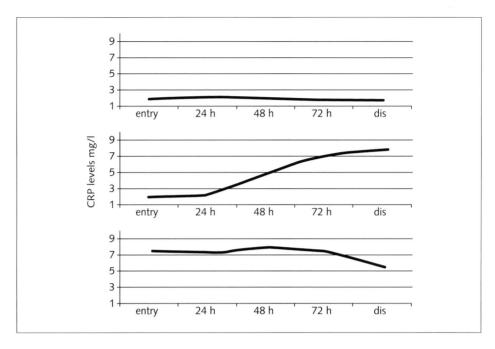

*Figure 1*
*C-reactive protein (CRP) levels and short-term outcome in unstable angina. CRP levels in mg/l, data are reported at entry, 24, 48, 72 h and at discharge. Upper panel: patients with low (<3 mg/l) in this group no events were observed. Middle panel: 2 patients with low entry levels of CRP and subsequent elevation in CRP starting at 48 h, in these 2 patients refractory angina developed at 72 h. Lower panel: patients with CRP >3 mg/l, 21/19 of this group had coronary events [3].*

did not allow for a statistical significance. Interestingly, no patient in the low CRP level group, except for two who presented with CRP elevation after admission, had in-hospital complications. A CRP level > 10 mg/l had a 100% sensitivity for in-hospital cardiovascular events. Also SAA protein, another acute phase protein, was found to correlate with prognosis in this study, but to a less significant extent than CRP. This study for the first time demonstrated that CRP is a prognostic marker able to differentiate UAP patients into two groups, one with low CRP levels and low in-hospital risk and the other with high CRP levels and high in-hospital risk. These results provided strong evidence in favor of a pathogenetic role of inflammation in IHD and in acute coronary syndromes.

The ECAT study confirmed these observations in a much larger population [31]. In this study, 2300 patients with either stable or unstable angina were enrolled and followed for two years. Major cardiovascular events were significantly associated with levels of fibrinogen, but the significance with CRP, which was measured with a less sensitive method, was borderline (p = 0.05). This same group re-analysed the data with CRP measurements using an ultra-sensitive method [4]. In this case patients in top quintiles of CRP showed a 3.5-fold increased risk of major cardiovascular events during follow-up. Also in this study, SAA was associated in a less significant way than CRP to events. Toss and colleagues [32] in an analysis of the fragmin during instability in coronary artery disease (FRISC) study found that elevated CRP levels (> 10 mg/L) were associated with an 8% rate of death and non-fatal MI in UAP and non-q wave MI patients at 150 days (vs. 2% in patients with CRP < 2 mg/l). This group [33] has recently confirmed these observations in an extended follow-up at two years.

The importance of CRP in the assessment of mid- to long-term follow-up of patients with unstable coronary artery disease has been confirmed by two other studies. We have followed patients discharged from the hospital with a diagnosis of UA for one year. In these patients blood samples were taken at entry, discharge and at three and 12 months during follow-up [5]. This study gave two important pieces of information: (1) CRP remained elevated for 12 months in 39% of patients, demonstrating the persistence of the inflammatory stimulus in two-thirds of UAP patients, (2) patients with elevated CRP at discharge (> 3 mg/l at discharge) had an odds ratio for recurrent unstable events, including death, MI and new hospitalization, of 8.7 in a multivariate analysis independent of fibrinogen levels, age, family history, diabetes, and hypertension. Intriguingly the difference in the one year outcome between patients with low and high CRP levels persisted also when the patients were subgrouped according to medical or surgical therapy, suggesting that the inflammatory response might be more important than the choice of an invasive or medical therapy. This observation, if confirmed in larger studies, suggests that a more aggressive medical therapy in patients with high CRP. This is also suggested by the recent observation that elevated CRP levels (> 3 mg/l) are associated with an increased risk of restenosis and of acute complications after balloon angioplasty either in stable and unstable angina (Fig. 2) and that CRP (> 3 mg/l) is associated with an increased risk of new ischemic events up to eight years after coronary artery bypass graft (CABG) [34, 35].

Other recent studies have confirmed our observations. Ferreiros and colleagues [36] have reported a follow-up study of patients with UAP and non-q wave MI and confirmed that elevated levels of CRP are associated with an elevated risk (CRP at discharge odds ratio 20.89) at 90 days. In this study a cut-off value of 15 mg/l was chosen on the basis of a receiver/operator characteristic curve. These authors reported that 48.5% of patients had elevated levels of CRP during hospitalization, a figure very similar to our 49%. However, Ferreiros and colleagues did not find a correlation between CRP levels at entry and in-hospital outcome, in agreement with Toss [32], Montelascot and Oltrona [37, 38], but at variance from Liuzzo [3] and Morrow [39]. It is possible that different patient selection and methods used for

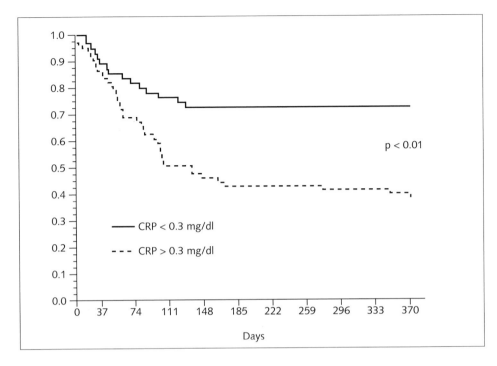

*Figure 2*
*CRP levels and one-year risk of restenosis after PTCA. Patients (stable and unstable angina)*
*with low CRP levels (<3 mg/l) (filled line) had less than 20% restenosis rate at one year*
*(p<0.001 vs. patients with CRP >3 mg/l [34].*

CRP level determination might have played a role in the inconsistent results. It must be considered that risk, in particular of death and MI is not only related to disease activity, but also to the comorbid conditions (such as previous MI, low EF, diabetes, renal insufficiency, and age) which all represent additional risk factors also in the short term.

In conclusion, the value of CRP as a marker of short term (in-hospital) prognosis is still debatable, however, multiple studies confirm the utility of CRP for the mid to long-term prognostic stratification of patients who survived an acute coronary syndrome.

## Other markers of inflammation: cytokines and adhesion molecules

Although pro-inflammatory cytokines are the major cause for the rise in acute phase protein levels and have direct procoagulant and vasoactive properties and may induce plaque destabilization, their use as prognostic markers in UAP is less appealing than that of the acute phase protein for a number of reasons: cytokines are more expensive and time consuming to measure, the measurement itself is less reliable, and many cytokines, such as IL-1β and IFNγ, circulate at very low concentrations in the peripheral blood, so that stimulation of isolated monocytes or of whole blood may be necessary to assess their levels, unless more complex methods, such as fluorocytometry, are used. The half-life of many cytokines is also so short that the role of chance may be very important in determining the likelihood of finding them. We have determined levels of two cytokines with a relatively long half-life (~ 6 h) in the peripheral circulation. These include IL-6 and the receptor antagonist of IL-1 (IL-1Ra), the latter being also a good marker of TNFα levels. In two different studies, these two cytokines were found to be elevated in UAP and were significantly associated with prognosis [18, 40]. Of note, both IL-6 and IL-1Ra were elevated at entry in patients with a poor in-hospital prognosis and further increased in this group of patients, but remained stable, or slightly decreased, in those with a good outcome: this finding is similar to what has been observed in sepsis, burn, severe inflammatory disease and in SIRS (systemic inflammatory reaction syndrome) [41]. Other studies have also shown elevated IL-6 levels in acute MI and the association of elevated IL-6 levels with platelet activation [42]. Overall, for the above mentioned reasons, measurement of interleukins seems to be more of a research interest rather than playing a real practical role in the clinical arena.

A similar comment may be attributed to the measurement of adhesion molecules, which, under inflammatory stimulation, are expressed on leukocyte, platelet or endothelial cell surface. The adhesion molecules, such as intercellular adhesion molecules (ICAM), vascular cells adhesion molecules (VCAM), and the E-selectin expressed by endothelial cells, L-selectin by leukocytes and P-selectins by platelets, mediates adhesion and activation of circulating cells to the endothelium and may be part of the process that initiates or amplifies the inflammatory events in acute coronary syndromes [43]. Although a number of studies have shown that these molecules are associated with unstable disease, and may be involved with the mechanism of disease since P-selectin levels in the coronary sinus increase with ischemic episodes [44,45], their clinical role is not yet well defined, and these measurements suffer from the same methodological limitations as cytokines.

## Role of inflammatory markers in a troponin era

Troponins (T and I) are specific myocardial proteins released following myocardial damage. Both troponins have been demonstrated to be very specific and a good sensitive marker of myocardial ischemic damage, and are released and become detectable in the blood after a minor myocardial injury, such as that which may be present in the case of UAP. Several studies confirm the utility of both troponins in

227

the short and mid-term risk stratification in UA and non-q wave MI [46–48]. The proven value of troponins, with their much higher specificity for acute coronary syndromes than inflammatory markers, raises the question of whether the latter, and specifically CRP, are of additional value for the prognostic stratification of these syndromes. In the study by Liuzzo et al. [3] and in the subsequent study by Biasucci et al. [5] we excluded all patients with positive troponin-T levels (> 0.2 ng/ml), in order to avoid any pro-inflammatory role of myocardial damage. The early studies to address the issue of the additional value of CRP over troponins were published in 1998. Morrow and colleagues [39] in a TIMI 11A substudy showed that CRP and troponins had additive value in the prognosis of patients with UAP and non-q wave MI, in particular low levels of CRP and negative levels of toponin-T were associated with a less than 1% risk of death at 14 days, when high CRP (15 mg/L) and early positivity of bed-side troponin-T were present. Rebuzzi and colleagues [49] studied 102 patients with UAP and assessed the additive role of CRP in relation to troponin-T, electrocardiographic change and symptoms. In this study CRP was of little value in patients with positive troponin-T, but significantly increased the possibility of detecting patients at risk of MI at 3 T negative patients, 15% of those with CRP positive (> 3 mg/l) had MI vs. less than 2% of those with CRP < 3 mg/l) (Fig. 3). These observations have been confirmed recently in a number of studies [50, 51], except in one [52], and show the additive role of CRP to the predictive value of troponins. Troponins are more specific, and may be more useful than CRP in determining short term prognosis, as they indicate the presence of complicated and thrombi-rich coronary lesions from which micro-emboli may arise. Conversely, CRP is more sensitive and may represent the underlying ongoing disease. Thus CRP is probably a better marker of long term prognosis. Overall the combination of the two markers, one more sensitive, the other more specific, may be of clinical importance.

## Inflammatory markers and acute coronary syndromes: culprits or markers?

With the accumulating data on the importance of inflammatory markers, and in particular CRP, in acute coronary syndromes, there is a growing interest in the real meaning of these markers. Are these markers a sign of the disease activity, or do they play an active pathophysiological role? This question is important, since new strategies may be developed to modulate the inflammatory reaction if it were the pathogenic villain. We have studied the relation between inflammatory markers and possible pro-inflammatory events and found that levels of inflammatory markers were not associated with myocardial damage (as troponin-T was negative in our patients), ischemic events (as CRP was < 3 mg/l in various angina patients with a greater ischemic burden than UAP patients) and thrombus formation (as CRP levels did not change after an ischemic episode characterized by a rise in markers of

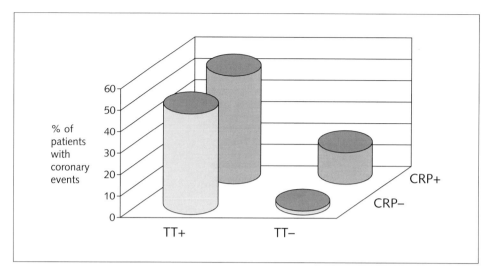

*Figure 3*
*Incremental prognostic value of CRP on top of troponin-T (TT). On the left: in patients with positive (>0.2 mg/dl) TT (TT+), positive CRP (>3 mg/l) was associated with a little increase in risk. On the right: patients with TT <0.2 mg/dl (TT–) and CRP <3 mg/l (CRP–) had a very low risk of events, in TT–- group, CRP+ patients had a significantly higher risk of events [49].*

thrombin formation, such as thrombin-anti-thrombin complex and prothombin fragment 1 + 2) [53]. Inflammatory markers, including IL-6, also do not seem to be related to plaque rupture, as we have found that CRP and IL-6 were detectable only in UAP with elevated CRP undergoing intracoronary procedure, suggesting that plaque rupture is not, *per se*, a cause of systemic inflammatory response [54]. More intriguingly, similar results were observed in patients undergoing coronary angiography, where no plaque rupture is caused, suggesting that an inflammatory hyper-responsiveness may represent a cause of destabilization in acute coronary syndromes [55].

There is consistent evidence that inflammatory markers are elevated years before the index event in apparently healthy individuals [56], suggesting that the elevation of these markers is not secondary to any acute ischemic, thrombotic or necrotic event, but one cannot rule out the possibility that inflammation reflects the total atherosclerotic burden. However, no data support this possibility, as markers of inflammation do not correlate with the extension of coronary artery disease, or with the severity of the peripheral arterial disease. Preliminary data from our group suggest that a similar amount of inflammation is present in an UA patient with a single coronary vessel disease and in patients with diffuse and severe peripheral vascular disease [57]. CRP levels are also associated with a number of risk factors, including smoking, obesity, diabetes, age, and thus could reflect the total "risk burden" of individuals. However, others have found the CRP level to be an independent cardiovascular risk. Pro-inflammatory cytokines, and CRP itself, also have an important role in regulating the immune reaction and take part in the coagulation process. The ability of CRP to bind to complement or to induce tissue factor [58] or pro-inflammatory cytokines [59, 60] has been thought to play a causative role of the genesis of in acute coronary syndromes.

## Conclusions

Inflammatory markers are associated with acute coronary syndromes and are likely to play a major pathophysiological role in these syndromes. CRP, in particular, because of its stability, relatively long half life, linearity of production and elimination, low-cost and high efficiency of high-sensitivity methods for its measurement, seems to represent a clinically useful tool for risk stratification. CRP may be of additive value to troponins in the short term risk stratification in UAP and Q and non-q wave MI, and may serve as a reliable marker of mid- to long-term prognostication in patients with coronary disease. CRP measurements may be useful to discriminate patients at risk from restenosis or recurrent ischemic events after PTCA or CABG. Other inflammatory markers such as adhesion molecules or cytokines are of great interest for the understanding of the disease, and growing data support their role as causative agents in plaque destabilization, thrombus formation and disease progression, but at present they have a limited clinical role due to expensive and time consuming measurements. Further studies are required to better define the role of inflammatory markers in the pathophysiology of atherosclerosis. This information may lead to novel therapeutic approaches.

*Acknowledgments*
This study was supported by a grant from Centro Ricerche Coronariche, per il cuore, onlus. Roma, Italy. The authors are indebted to Professor Attilio Maseri for his discussion and advice and for having always supported this line of research, and to all the people working with us in the wards and in the laboratories.

## References

1    National Center for Health Statistics (1987) *Vital and health statistics. Detailed diagnostic and procedures for patients discharged from short stay hospital.* US Department of Health and Human Services, Public Health Service, series 13, n°90, Hyattsville, Md,

2    Johnson CL, Rigkind BM, Sempos CT, Canal MD, Bacharik PS, Briefel RC, Gordon DJ, Burt VL, Brown CD, Lippel K et al (1993) The national health and nutrition examination surveys. *JAMA* 269 (23): 3002–3008

3    Liuzzo G, Biasucci LM, Gallimore RJ, Grillo RL, Rebuzzi AG, Pepys MB, Maseri A (1994) The prognostic value of C-reactive protein and serum amyloid A protein in severe unstable angina. *N Engl J Med* 331: 417–425

4    Haverkate F, Thompson SG, Pike SDM, Gallimore JR, Pepys MB (1997) for the European Concerted Action on Thrombosis and Disabilities Angina Pectoris Study Group: Production of C-reactive protein and risk of coronary events in stable and unstable angina. *Lancet* 349: 462–466

5    Biasucci LM, Liuzzo G, Grillo RL, Caligiuri G, Rebuzzi AG, Buffon A, Summaria F, Ginnetti F, Fadda G, Maseri A (1999) Elevated levels of C-reactive protein at discharge in patients with unstable angina predict recurrent instability. *Circulation* 99 (7): 855–860

6    Ross R (1993) The pathogenesis of atherosclerosis: A perspective for 1990s. *Nature* 362: 801–808

7    Jonasson L, Holm J, Skalli O, Gabbiani G, Hansson GK (1985) Expression of class II transplantation antigen on vascular smooth muscle cells in human atherosclerosis. *J Clin Invest* 76: 125–31

8    van der Wal AC, Becker AE van der Loos CM, Das PK (1994) Site of intimal rupture or erosion of thrombosed coronary atherosclerotic plaque is characterized by an inflammatory process irrespective of the dominant plaque morphology. *Circulation* 89: 36–44

9    Hansson GK, Jonasson L, Holm J (1989) Detection of activated T Lymphocytes in the human atherosclerotic plaque. *Am J Pathol* 135: 169–175

10   Jonasson L, Holm J, Skalli O, Bondjers G, Hansson GK (1986) Regional acccumulations of T cells, macrophages and smooth cells in the human atherosclerotic plaque. *Atherosclerosis* 6: 131–138

11   Moreno PR, Falk E, Palacios IF, Newell JB, Fuster V, Fallon JT (1994) Macrophage infiltration in acute coronary syndromes: implication for plaque rupture. *Circulation* 90: 775–778

12   Sato T, Takebayaschi S, Kohchi K (1987) Increased subendothelial infiltration of the coronary arteries with monocytes/macrophages in patients with unstable angina. *Atherosclerosis* 68: 191–197

13   Kaartinen M, Penttila A, Kovanene PT (1994) Accumulation of activated mast cells in the shoulder region of human coronary atheroma, the predilection site of atheromatous rupture. *Circulation* 90: 1669–1678

14   Henney AM, Wakeley PR, Davis MJ, Foster K, Hembry T, Murphy G, Humphries S (1992) Location of stromelysin gene in atherosclerotic plaques using in situ hybridization. *Proc Natl Acad Sci USA* 88: 8154–8158

15   Pepys MB (ed) (1989) *Acute phase proteins in the acute response.* Springer-Verlag, London

16   De Beer FC, Hind CRK, Fox KM, Allan RM, Maseri A, Pepys MB (1982) Measurement

of serum C-reactive protein concentration in myocardial ischemia and infarction. *Br Heart J* 47: 239–243

17    Berk BC, Weintraub WS, Alexander RW (1990) Elevation of C-reactive protein in "active" coronary artery disease. *Am J Cardiol* 65: 168–172

18    Biasucci LM, Vitelli A, Liuzzo G, Altamura S, Caligiuri G, Monaco C, Rebuzzi AG, Ciliberto G, Maseri A (1996) Elevated Levels of Interleukin-6 in Unstable Angina. *Circulation* 94: 874–877

19    Metha J, Dinerman, Metha P, Salden TGP, Lawson D, Donnellty WH, Wallin R (1989) Neutrophil function in ischemic heart disease. *Circulation* 79: 549–556

20    Biasucci LM, D'Onofrio G, Liuzzo G, Zini G, Monaco C, Caligiuri G, Tommasi M, Rebuzzi AG, Bizzi B, Maseri A (1996) Intracellular neutrophil myeloperoxidase is reduced in unstable angina and acute myocardial infarction, but its reduction is not related to ischemia. *J Am Coll Cardiol* 27: 611–616

21    Dinerman JL, Metha JL, Salden TGP, Emerson S, Wallin R, Davda R, Davidson A (1990) Increased neutrophil elastase release in unstable angina pectoris and acute myocardial infarction. *J Am Coll Cardiol* 15: 1559–1563

22    Neri Serneri GG, Prisco D, Martini F, Gori AM, Brunelli T, Poggesi L, Rostagno C, Gensini GF, Abbate R (1997) Acute T-cell activation is detectable in unstable angina. *Circulation* 95: 1806–1812

23    Mazzone A, De Servi S, Ricevuti G, Mazzucchelli I, Fossati G, Pasotti D, Bramucci E, Angoli L, Marisco F, Specchia G et al (1993) Increased expression of neutrophil and monocytes adhesion molecules in unstable coronary artery disease. *Circulation* 88: 358–363

24    Caligiuri G, Liuzzo G, Biasucci LM, Maseri A (1998) Immune system activation follows inflammation in unstable angina pathogenetic implications. *J Am Coll Cardiol* 32 (5): 1295–1304

25    Pepys MB, Baltz ML (1983) Acute phase proteins with special reference to C-reactive Protein and related proteins (pentaxins) and plasma amyloid A protein. *Adv Immunol* 34: 141–212

26    Baumann H, Gauldie J (1994) The acute phase response. *Immunol Today* 15: 74–80

27    Geisterfer M, Richards C, Baumann M, Fey G, Gywnne D, Gauldie J (1993) Regulation of Il-6 and the hepatic Il-6 receptor in acute inflammation *in vivo*. *Cytokine* 5: 1–7

28    Schultz DR, Arnold PI (1990) Properties of four acute phase proteins: C-reactive protein, serum amyloid A protein, α1-acid glycoprotein, and fibrinogen. *Seminar in Arthritis and Rheumatism* 20 (3): 129–147

29    Kushner I (1982) The phenomenon of the acute phase response. *Ann NY Acad Sci* 389: 39–48

30    De Beer FC, Hind CRK, Fox KM, Allan RM, Maseri A, Pepys MB (1992) Measurement of serum C-reactive protein concentration in myocardial ischemia and infarction. *Br Heart J* 47: 239–243

31    Thompson SG, Kienast J, Pyke SDM, Haverkate F, van de LOO JC (1995) for the European Concerted Action on Thrombosis and Disabilities Angina Pectoris Study Group:

Haemostatic factor and the risk of myocardial infarction or sudden death in patients with angina pectoris. *N Engl J Med* 332: 635–641

32   Toss H, Lindahl B, Siegbahm A, Wallentin L (1997) Prognostic influence of increased fibrinogen and C-reactive Protein levels in unstable coronary artery disease FRISC Study Group-Fragmin during instability in coronary artery disease. *Circulation* 96 (12): 4204–4210

33   Lindahl B, Toss H, Siegbahn L, Wallentin L (1999) C-reactive protein and fibrinogen in unstable coronary artery disease are related to long-term cardiac mortality. *Eur Heart J* 20: 593; 3189 (Abstract)

34   Buffon A., Liuzzo G, Biasucci LM, Pasqualetti P, Ramazzotti V, Rebuzzi AG, Crea F, Maseri A (1999) Pre-procedural serum levels of C-reactive protein predict early complications and late restenosis following coronary angioplasty. *J Am Coll Cardiol* 34 (5): 1512–1521

35   Milazzo D, Biasucci LM, Luciani N, Martinelli L, Canosa C, Schiavello R, Maseri A, Possati G (1999) Elevated levels of C-reactive protein before coronary artery bypass grafting predict recurrence of ischemic events. *Am J Cardiol* 84 (4): 459–461, A9

36   Ferreiros ER, Boissonet CP, Pizzaro R, Merletti PF, Corrado G, Cagide A, Bazzino OO (1999) Independent prognostic value of elevated C-reactive protein in unstable angina. *Circulation* 100 (19): 1958–1963

37   Montelascot G, Philippe F, Ankri A, Vincent E, Bearez E, Paulard JE, Cavie D, Flammeng D, Dutart A, Careyon A et al (1998) Early increase of von Willebrand factor predicts adverse outcome in unstable coronary artery disease: beneficial effects of enoxofarm. French Investigators of the ESSENCE Trial. *Circulation* 98 (4): 294–299

38   Oltrona L, Ardissino D, Merlini PA, Spinola A, Chiodo F, Pezzano A (1997) C-reactive Protein elevation and early outcome in patients with unstable angina pectoris. *Am J Cardiol* 80 (8): 1002–1006

39   Morrow DA, Rifai N, Antmann E, Weiiner DL, McCabe CH, Cannon CP, Braunwald E (1998) C-reactive protein is a potent predictor of mortality independently of and in combination with troponin-T in acute coronary syndromes. A TIMI 11A substudy. Thrombolysis in myocardial infarction. *J Am Coll Cardiol* 31: 1460–1465

40   Biasucci LM, Liuzzo G, Fantuzzi G, Caligiuri G, Rebuzzi AG, Ginnetti F, Dinarello CA, Maseri A (1999) Increasing levels of IL1Ra and of Il-6 during the first two days of Hospitalization in unstable angina are associated with increased risk of in-hospital coronary events. *Circulation* 99 (16): 2079–2084

41   Cannon JG, Tompkins RG, Gelfand JA, Michie HR, Stanford GG, van der Meer JWM, Endres S, Lonnemann G, Corsetti J, Chernow B et al (1990) Circulating interleukin-1 and tumor necrosis factor in septic shock and experimental endotoxin fever. *J Infect Dis* 161: 79–84

42   Marx H, Neumann FJ, Ott I, Gawaz M, Koch W, Pinkauti T, Schnig A (1997) Induction of cytokine expression in leucocytes in acute myocardial infarction. *J Am Coll Cardiol* 30 (1): 165–170

43   Crockett-Torabi E, Fontane JC (1995) The selectins: insights into selectin-induced intra-cellular signaling in leukocytes. *Immunol Res* 14: 237–251

44   Inoue T, Hoshi K, Yaguchi I, Imasaki Y, Takayanagi K, Morooka S (1999) Serum levels of circulating adhesion molecules after coronary angioplasty. *Cardiology* 91 (4): 236–242

45   Tenaglia AN, Buda AJ, Wilkins RG, Barron MK, Jefford pR, Vo K, Jordan MO, Kusnick BA, Lefer DJ (1997) Levels of expression of P-selectin, E-selectin, and intercellular adhesion molecule-1 in coronary atherectromy specimens from patients with stable and unstable angina pectoris. *Am J Cardiol* 79 (6): 742–747

46   Hamm CW, Goldmann BU, Heeschen C, Kraymann G, Berger J, Meinertz T (1997) Emergency room triage of patients with acute chest pain by means of rapid testing for cardiac troponin-T or troponin-I. *N Engl J Med* 337 (23): 1648–1653

47   Hamm CW, Ravkide J, Gerhardt W, Jorgensen P, Peheim E, Ljungdahl L, Goldmann B, Katus HA (1992) The prognostic value of serum troponin-T in unstable angina. *N Engl J Med* 327 (3): 146–150

48   Olatidoye AG, Wu AH, Feug YJ, Waters D (1998) Prognostic role of Tn-T versus Tn-I in UAP pectoris for cardiac events with meta-analysis comparing published studies. *Am J Cardiol* 81 (12): 1405–1410

49   Rebuzzi AG, Quaranta G, Liuzzo G, Caligiuri G, Lanza GA, Gallimore R, Grillo RL, Cianflone D, Biasucci LM, Maseri A (1998) Incremental prognostic value of serum levels of troponin-T and C-reactive protein on admission in patients with unstable angina pectoris. *Am J Cardiol* 82: 715–719

50   de Winter RJ, Bholasingh R, Lijmer JG, Koster RW, Gorgels JP, Schouter Y, Hoek FJ, Sanders GT (1999) Independent prognostic value of C-reactive protein and troponin-I in patients with unstable angina or non-Q-wave myocardial infarction. *Cardiovascular Res* 42 (1): 240–245

51   Heeschen C, Hamm CW, Bruemer J, Goldmann BU, Simoons ML, Deu A (1999) C-reactive protein and troponin-T independently predict mortality in patients with unstable refractory angina. *Eur Heart J* 20: 594; 3190 (Abstract)

52   Benamer H, Steg PG, Benessiano J, Vicaut E, Gaultier CJ, Boccara A, Aubry P, Nicaise P, Brochet E, Juliard JM et al (1998) Comparison of the prognostic value of C-reactive protein and troponin-I in patients with unstable angina pectoris. *Am J Cardiol* 82 (7): 845–850

53   Biasucci LM, Liuzzo G, Caligiuri G, quaranta G, Andreotti F, Sperti G, Van de Greef W, Rebuzzi AG, Kluft C, Maseri A (1996) Temporal relation between ischemic episodes and activation of the coagulation system in unstable angina. *Circulation* 93 (121): 2121–2127

54   Liuzzo G, Buffon A, Biasucci LM, Gallimore JR, Caligiuri G, Vitelli A, Altamura S., Ciliberto C, Rebuzzi AG, Crea F et al (1998) Enhanced inflammatory response to coronary angioplasty in patients with severe unstable angina. *Circulation* 98 (22): 2370–2376

55   Liuzzo G, Angiolillo DJ, Ginnetti F, Rizzello V, Caligiuri G, Petrone E, Kol A, Sperti G,

Biasucci LM, Maseri A (1998) Monocytes of patients with recurrent unstable angina are hyper-responsive to lypopolysaccharide challenge. *J Am Coll Cardiol* 31: 272A (Abstract)

56  Ridker PM, Cushman M, Stampfer MJ, Tracy RP, Hennekens CH (1997) Inflammation, aspirin, and the risk of developing peripheral vascular disease. *Circulation* 97: 425–428

57  Monaco C, Rossi E, Milazzo D, Liuzzo G, Caligiuri G, Angiolillo DJ, Rizzello V, Summaria F, Petrone E, Ginnetti F et al (1997) The inflammatory acute phase response in unstable angina is unrelated to extension and severity of atherosclerosis. *Thrombosis and Haemostasis* (Suppl): 185 (Abstract)

58  Cermak J, Key NS, Bach RR, Balla J, Jacob HS, Vercellotti GM (1993) C-reactive protein induces human peripheral blood monocytes to synthesize tissue factor. The American Society of Hematology. *Blood* 82 (2): 513–520

59  Ballou SP, Lozanski G (1992) Induction of inflammatory cytokine release from cultured human monocytes by C-reactive protein. *Cytokine* 4: 361–368

60  Pue CA, Mortensen RF, Marsh CB, Pope HA, Wewers MD (1996) Acute phase levels of C-reactive protein enhance IL-1β and IL-1ra production by human blood monocytes but inhibit IL-1β and IL-1ra production by alveolar macrophages. *J Immunol* 156: 1594–1600

# Antibiotics in the prevention of coronary heart disease: review of the randomised trials

*John Danesh and Rory Collins*

Clinical Trial Service Unit and Epidemiological Studies Unit, Nuffield Department of Clinical Medicine, University of Oxford, Radcliffe Infirmary, Oxford OX2 6HE, UK

## Introduction

Over the past few decades, several different persistent infectious agents (including *Chlamydia pneumoniae*, *Helicobacter pylori*, and cytomegalovirus) have been investigated as possible causes of vascular disease [1], but so far randomized trials have reported only on anti-chlamydial treatments in relation to clinical events. *Chlamydia pneumoniae* is an intracellular bacterium of the lung that was identified in 1986, and recognized as a treatable cause of acute respiratory diseases (such as pneumonia) [2]. The organism is probably spread by respiratory droplets, and about one-third to one-half of middle-aged Westerners have serological evidence of previous exposure [3]. The first reported association between seropositivity to *C. pneumoniae* and coronary heart disease (CHD) appeared in 1988 [4]; and, a few years later, *C. pneumoniae* elementary bodies were directly observed by electron micrography in coronary plaques [5]. Since then, dozens of seroepidemiological and pathology-based studies have reported on possible associations between *C. pneumoniae* infection and vascular disease [1, 6, 7]. These observational studies have encouraged trials of antibiotics to determine whether *C. pneumoniae* may be a treatable cause of CHD. This chapter provides a brief review of the major randomized studies that have reported or are known to be in progress.

## Intervention trials of antibiotics and CHD

By the year 2000, three randomized, placebo-controlled trials of antibiotics had reported on the prevention of CHD events (Tab. 1). These trials were conducted in the United Kingdom [8], Argentina [9, 10], and the United States [11], and each involved only a few hundred patients. Two of the trials involved patients with stable CHD and high serum concentrations of *C. pneumoniae* IgG antibodies [8, 11], whereas the other involved patients with recent unstable angina or non-Q-wave myocardial infarction irrespective of *C. pneumoniae* serum antibody titres [9, 10].

Inflammatory and Infectious Basis of Atherosclerosis, edited by Jay L. Mehta

Each trial put patients on brief courses of oral macrolides (such as roxithromycin) or of macrolide-derivatives (such as azithromycin). These antibiotics have anti-chlamydial and, possibly, anti-inflammatory effects. All of the trials involved measurement of some potential vascular intermediates in blood samples collected at baseline and after at least six months of follow-up, as well as recording vascular events (such as fatal CHD, non-fatal myocardial infarction, coronary re-vascularization procedures, and/or prolonged episodes of angina).

Each study reported a reduction in the level of at least one blood factor possibly related to inflammation following antibiotic treatment (Tab. 1). These apparent effects were not, however, generally highly statistically significant (with most less than 2.5 standard deviations away from zero), and are of uncertain relevance, since they were based on small sample sizes, lacked adjustment for multiple comparisons, and may have been reported only after an exploration of the data had suggested extreme findings. The plausibility of any such effects is also weakened by the absence in larger observational studies of strong correlations between *C. pneumoniae* IgG titres and these putative vascular intermediates (such as C-reactive protein) [12, 13].

The first reported trial recorded a total of only eight CHD events, and yielded a non-significant result (although the investigators reported a four-fold reduction in CHD on the basis of an inappropriate non-randomized comparison) [8]. The second trial recorded 22 CHD events, and it too yielded non-significant results after six months of follow-up [10] (hence, in retrospect, its earlier claim of a four-fold reduction in CHD at one month was probably due to chance and/or selective reporting of an interim analysis [9]). The third trial recorded 16 events and yielded non-significant results (again, reported in an interim analysis) [11]. However, even though these "pilot" trials were too small, and the duration of follow-up too brief, to provide good evidence for, or against, a role for *C. pneumoniae* in CHD, they have prompted interest in conducting further randomized trials of anti-infective strategies.

## Observational studies of *C. pneumoniae* and CHD

Several trials are now in progress that involve larger sample sizes, lengthier antibiotic treatment periods, and longer follow-up (Tab. 2). Even these trials, however, may only be able to provide somewhat limited information about any effects of anti-chlamydial treatment in CHD. The reason for this is that there is considerable uncertainty as to the strength of any independent association between persistent *C. pneumoniae* infection and CHD that might exist, with different types of observational studies yielding substantially different estimates. Whereas pathology-based studies that have assessed human arterial specimens for endovascular markers of *C. pneumoniae* (i.e., DNA, antigens, elementary bodies or viable organisms) give a

Table 1 - Reported randomised trials of anti-infective treatment strategies in the prevention of CHD events

| Ref. | Drug/ Duration (days) | Nos. allocated Active/Placebo | Follow-up (months) | Biochemical intermediates reported to be altered | Nos. of CHD events Active vs Placebo |
|---|---|---|---|---|---|
| [8] | Azithromycin/4-7 | 112/111 | 18 | Fibrinogen; monocyte markers; tissue factor | 3 vs. 5 |
| [9, 10] | Roxithromycin/30 | 102/100 | 6 | C-reactive protein | 8 vs. 14 |
| [11] | Azithromycin/90 | 151/151 | 6 | C-reactive protein; Interleukin-6 | 9 vs. 7 |

Table 2 - Some larger randomised trials of anti-infective strategies currently in progress in the prevention of CHD events

| Study | Location | Planned size | Entry criteria | Drugs/ Duration (months) | Planned follow-up (years) |
|---|---|---|---|---|---|
| ACES* | USA | 4000 | Previous MI or coronary revascularization | Azithromycin/12 | 4 |
| PROVE IT* | USA | 4000 | Acute coronary syndrome | Gatifloxacin/18 | 1.5 |
| WIZARD** | USA | 3800 | Previous MI or coronary revascularization | Azithromycin/3 | 3 |
| MARBLE* | UK | 1300 | Waiting for coronary artery by-pass graft surgery | Azithromycin/3 | 1 |
| STAMINA* | UK | 600 | Previous MI | Azithromycin + anti-Helicobacter pylori drugs/0.5 | 1.5 |

*Patients randomised irrespective of C. pneumoniae serostatus.
**Only patients with C. pneumoniae IgG titres ≥ 1:16 are to be randomised.
MI, myocardial infarction

combined weighted odds ratio for atherosclerosis of about 20 (95% confidence interval (CI) 15–32) [5–7], prospective studies involving more than 3000 cases of CHD death or non-fatal myocardial infarction give a combined odds ratio of only 1.15 (95% CI 0.97–1.36) in *C. pneumoniae* IgG seropositive individuals [14].

What might account for this 20-fold discrepancy between observational studies involving different methods? The pathology-based studies have been retrospective thereby creating uncertainty as to whether local *C. pneumoniae* infection is a cause or consequence of atheroma, whereas the prospective serological studies assessed evidence of infection several years before the onset of CHD. Most of the pathology-based studies have been prone to selection biases and lacked any adjustment for possible confounders, such as age, sex and smoking [5–7], but this could not plausibly explain much of the 20-fold difference. It is also unclear to what extent the discrepancy can be accounted for by the different definitions of vascular disease (atheroma vs CHD events) and the different markers of infection (endovascular markers such as DNA and antigens vs circulating antibody titres) used in these different sets of studies.

## Implications for future intervention trials

Such epidemiological uncertainties have implications for the numbers needed in clinical trials to assess any effects of *C. pneumoniae* eradication strategies on CHD appropriately reliably. For example, if the 20-fold odds ratio reported in the pathology-based studies mainly reflected a causal effect that was largely reversible (rather than some artefact of confounding or reverse association), then anti-chlamydial treatments might be expected to reduce CHD event rates very substantially. To confirm or refute such large effects, trials of similar size to the previous "pilot" trials (Tab. 1) may be needed, although follow-up might need to be much longer. If, however, the prospective serological studies provide a more reliable guide to the likely strength of any association between *C. pneumoniae* and CHD, then trials would need to involve much larger numbers than those previously conducted or currently in progress. Even if there is a 10% excess risk of CHD due to *C. pneumoniae* that is fully reversible by antibiotics, none of the existing trials would be large enough to confirm or refute its existence: for example, the two largest current trials, ACES and WIZARD, can only detect reductions in CHD events of at least 25% [15]. Some future meta-analysis of these trials would be more powerful than any of them individually, but much larger new trials may eventually be needed.

Given the tentative nature of the current evidence for associations of *C. pneumoniae* with CHD, an appropriate research strategy for future trials might be to "factor" anti-infective strategies into much larger trials of unrelated interventions that are already being conducted among people at high risk of CHD with long-term follow-up, and to test interventions that might be effective against more than one infection. For example, regimens involving a macrolide plus a second broad spectrum antibiotic and a gastric acid-suppressing agent should eliminate not just *C. pneumoniae* but also *Helicobacter pylori* [1] (as in STAMINA: Tab. 2). If such trials randomized individuals irrespective of antibody status, with baseline blood samples stored for future testing either in all patients or in a "retrospective case-control" subset of them, this would allow the use of any improved assay methods available only at the end of the trial. Measurement of various circulating "inflammatory" markers in these blood samples might also suggest whether any benefits of anti-infective treatments increase with increasing evidence of baseline inflammation [16].

Thus, as yet, there is no good epidemiological evidence for a causative association between *C. pneumoniae* infection and CHD, and the initial randomised trials of anti-infective strategies have been inconclusive. Even if a causal link exists, the effects of persistent infection on CHD risk may not be strong and may not be rapidly and fully reversible by antibiotic treatments. In such circumstances, anti-infective interventions studies should probably aim to randomize larger numbers of individuals than in current studies, and to observe them for longer periods, in order to assess reliably any realistically moderate effects on CHD.

## Acknowledgements

Dr. Danesh is supported by a Merton College fellowship and the Frohlich Trust. Professor Collins holds a British Heart Foundation personal chair.

## References

1   Danesh J, Collins R, Peto R (1997) Chronic infections and coronary heart disease: is there a link? *Lancet* 350: 430–436

2   Grayston JT, Kuo CC, Wang SP, Altman J (1986) A new *Chlamydia psittaci* strain, TWAR, isolated in acute respiratory tract infections. *N Engl J Med* 315: 161–168

3   Saikku P (1992) The epidemiology and significance of *Chlamydia pneumoniae. J Infection* 25 (Suppl. 1): 27–34

4   Saikku P, Leinonen M, Mattila K, Ekman MR, Nieminen MS, Makela PH, Huttunen JK, Vattonen V (1988) Serological evidence of an association of a novel *Chlamydia*, TWAR, with chronic coronary heart disease and acute myocardial infarction. *Lancet* 2: 983–986

5   Shor A, Kuo CC, Patton DL (1992) Detection of *Chlamydia pneumoniae* in coronary arterial fatty streaks and atheromatous plaques. *S Afr Med J* 82: 158–161

6   Danesh J, Appleby P (1998) Persistent infection and vascular disease: a systematic review. *Expert Opin Invest Drugs* 7: 691–713

7   Wong YK, Gallagher PJ, Ward ME (1999) *Chlamydia pneumoniae* and atherosclerosis. *Heart* 81: 232–238

8   Gupta S, Leatham EW, Carrington D, Mendall MA, Kaski JC, Camm AJ (1997) Ele-

vated *Chlamydia pneumoniae* antibodies, cardiovascular events, and azithromycin in male survivors of myocardial infarction. *Circulation* 96: 404–407

9  Gurfinkel E, Bozovich G, Daroca A, Beck A, Mautner B (1997) Randomised trial of roxithromycin in non-Q-wave coronary syndromes: ROXIS pilot study. *Lancet* 350: 404–407

10  Gurfinkel E, Bozovich G, Beck E, Testa E, Livellara B, Mautner B (1999) Treatment with the antibiotic roxithromycin in patients with acute non-Q-wave coronary syndromes: the final report of the ROXIS study. *Eur Heart J* 20: 121–127

11  Anderson JL, Muhlestein JB, Carlquist J, Allen A, Trehon S, Nielson C, Hall S, Brady J, Egger M, Horne B, Lim T (1999) Randomized secondary prevention trial of azithromycin in patients with coronary artery disease and serological evidence for *Chlamydia pneumoniae* infection: the azithromycin in coronary artery disease: elimination of myocardial infection with chlamydia (ACADEMIC) study. *Circulation* 99: 1540–1547

12  Ridker PM, Kundsin RB, Stampfer MJ, Poulin S, Hennekens CH (1999) Prospective study of *Chlamydia pneumoniae* IgG seropositivity and risks of future myocardial infarction. *Circulation* 99: 1161–1164

13  Danesh J, Whincup PH, Walker M, Lennon L, Thomson A, Appleby P, Gallimore JR, Pepys MB (2000) Low-grade inflammation and coronary heart disease: prospective study and updated meta-analysis. *BMJ* 321: 199–204

14  Danesh J, Whincup PH, Walker M, Lennon L, Thomson A, Appleby P, Wong Y-K, Bernardes-Silva M, Ward M (2000) *Chlamydia pneumoniae* IgG titres and coronary heart disease: prospective study and meta-analysis. *BMJ* 321: 208–213

15  Grayston JT (1999) Antibiotic treatment trials for secondary prevention of coronary artery disease events. *Circulation* 99: 1538–1539

16  Danesh J (1999) Smoldering arteries? Low-grade inflammation and coronary heart disease. *JAMA* 282: 2169–2171

# Fish oil – a potential therapy for inflammatory atherosclerosis

*Tom Saldeen[1] and Jay L. Mehta[2]*

[1]Department of Surgical Sciences, University of Uppsala, Dag Hammarskjölds väg 17, 752 37 Uppsala, Sweden; [2]VA Medical Center and Departments of Medicine and Physiology, University of Florida College of Medicine, and University of Arkansas for Medical Sciences, 4301 West Markham, Slot 532, Little Rock, AR 77205-7199, USA

## Introduction

Inflammation plays an important role in both the initiation of atherosclerosis and the development of atherothrombotic events [1]. An anti-inflammatory effect of n-3 fatty acids in fish oil was suggested by epidemiological studies which show that Greenland Eskimos, who consume large quantities of fish oils rich in long-chain n-3 fatty acids, have a very low incidence not only of atherosclerosis and coronary artery disease but also of inflammatory and autoimmune disorders such as rheumatoid arthritis, psoriasis, asthma, inflammatory bowel disease, type I diabetes mellitus, thyrotoxicosis and multiple sclerosis [2].

## Effect of fish oil in coronary artery disease (CAD)

Fifteen large studies enrolling more than 60,000 subjects have shown a decreased mortality in CAD as well as in total mortality of about 20–30% after intake of fish oil, fatty fish or n-3 fatty acids [3–18]. In a randomized controlled trial on the effect of intake of fatty fish or natural fish oil, 2033 men who had recovered from myocardial infarction were studied for two years [8]. The fish/fish oil group showed a 29% reduction in two year all-cause mortality. In another study enrolling 11,324 patients surviving a recent myocardial infarction [18], intake of 1 g daily of n-3 fatty acids in 2,836 patients for 3.5 years resulted in a 20% decrease in total deaths, a 30% decrease in cardiovascular deaths and a 45% decrease in sudden deaths. Interestingly, these patients already had conventional treatment with aspirin, beta-blockers and angiotensin converting enzyme inhibitors and were already exposed to a healthy Mediterranean diet. Thus, there seems to be no doubt that fish oil has a beneficial effect on CAD. Part of the effect seems to be due to reduced incidence and severity of cardiac arrhythmia [19–22]. The anti-arrythmic effect may relate to a direct effect of the fish oil on the heart. Arrhythmias can be induced by thromboxane and prevented by prostacyclin. The increased prostacyclin/thromboxane ratio after intake of fish oil [23] may thus be of importance for this effect.

Fish oil also has an effect on blood lipids. Hypertriglyceridaemia has been identified as an independent risk factor for CAD, and probably is an important factor in the development of atherosclerosis. Intake of fish oil usually results in a marked decrease in triglycerides. Different preparations have different effects. Whereas a daily intake of 15 ml natural stable fish oil containing about 5 g n-3 fatty acids for 6 months resulted in a decrease in triglycerides by 64% [24], daily intake of six capsules highly concentrated, unstable fish oil, also containing about 5 g n-3 fatty acids, for six months resulted in a decrease in triglycerides by only 27% [25], and no change in total or high-density lipoprotein (HDL) cholesterol. Similar results were obtained when two natural fish oils, one stable and one unstable, were compared. Intake of the stable fish oil resulted in a much stronger decrease in triglycerides [26]. Stable fish oil was also more potent than unstable fish oil in decreasing low-density lipoprotein (LDL) cholesterol [27], total cholesterol and lipoprotein (a), and in increasing HDL cholesterol [28]. In addition to its effect on the plasma concentration of the various cholesterols, fish oil was also shown to make the LDL cholesterol particle larger and less dense and thus less prone to induce atherosclerosis. Lipoprotein (a) (Lp(a)) is believed to be one of the most important risk factors for CAD. It is a lipoprotein with structural similarities to both LDL cholesterol and plasminogen, an important protein in the fibrinolytic system. When Lp(a) replaces plasminogen in the thrombus the risk of developing myocardial infarction is increased. Few compounds other than fish oil have been shown to lower plasma Lp(a). Nicotinic acid (vitamin B3) is such a substance but has certain side effects in contrast to fish oil, which has been found to have no serious side effects.

A major mechanism behind the effect of fish oil on CAD may also be an influence on the inflammatory atherosclerosis process.

## Fish oil and atherosclerosis

We have found an altered fatty acid pattern in human coronary arteries in sudden cardiac death [29]. The concentration of n-3 fatty acids is decreased and the concentration of saturated fatty acids increased. It is therefore logical to investigate the effect of supplementation with fish oil containing n-3 fatty acids on atherosclerosis. Human studies have shown a decrease in coronary atherosclerosis due to intake of fish oil [30]. Thus, patients with CAD who ingested 1.5 g of n-3 fatty acids daily for two years had less progression and more regression of CAD on coronary angiography than did patients who ingested placebo.

Intake of fish oil has been shown to decrease atherosclerosis in several experimental studies [31–36]. In some studies fish oil was shown to have no effect [37, 38] and in a few studies was even found to increase atherosclerosis [39, 40], probably due to increased lipid peroxidation [40]. Addition of exogenous antioxidants has been shown to block this potentially negative effect of fish oil in some studies [34]. If fish oil has a positive effect on this inflammatory process it could also influence other inflammatory diseases.

## Fish oil and other inflammatory diseases

A meta-analysis of 400 cases has shown that fish oil improves rheumatoid arthritis, a common inflammatory disease [41]. Thus, the number of tender joints and duration of morning stiffness decreased significantly after intake of fish oil. Several clinical studies have also shown beneficial effects of fish oil on other inflammatory conditions such as psoriasis, atopic dermatitis, ulcerative colitis, Crohn's disease, bronchitis and IgA-mediated nephropathy. There are probably several different mechanisms behind the effect of fish oil on inflammation.

## Fish oil and cell membrane fluidity

Fish oil intake increases the fluidity of the cell membranes due to the structure of the fatty acids. While saturated fatty acids have a straight structure, omega-3 fatty acids like EPA and DHA are markedly curved (Fig. 1) because of their double bonds. Saturated, straight fatty acids are closely packed together in the cell membrane, which becomes stiff, while curved fatty acids such as EPA and DHA can't be packed so closely (Fig. 2). They need more space and make the cell membrane more plastic and less stiff. This is of importance for enzyme function and function of receptors. Some membrane-bound enzymes have been shown to be particularly sensitive to their fatty acid environments such as adenylate cyclase, 5'-nucleotidase and $Na^+/K^+$ ATPase. Among the receptors, adrenergic and insulin receptors are particularly sensitive to the fatty acid environment.

## Fish oil and eicosanoids

Intake of fish oil results in replacement of arachidonic acid in the phospholipids of the cell membranes by the n-3 fatty acid provided, resulting in less production of arachidonic acid-derived eicosanoids, 2-series prostaglandins and 4-series leukotrienes and increased production of EPA-derived eicosanoids, 3-series prostaglandins and 5-series leukotrienes. These latter compounds are often less biologically potent than the arachidonic acid derived analogues. This results in significant effects on processes of importance for inflammation such as platelet aggregation, vasoconstriction, neutrophil function and immunity. Fish oil alters the function of

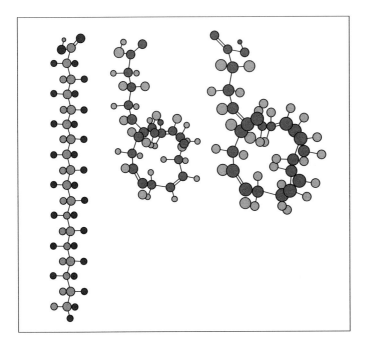

Figure 1
*Straight structure of saturated fatty acid (left) and markedly curved structure of n-3 fatty acids EPA and DHA.*

several mediators involved in the communication between cells (eicosanoids, cytokines, nitric oxide (NO)) and alters the expression of molecules involved in direct cell-to-cell contact such as adhesion molecules. The production of cytokines and of NO is partly regulated by eicosanoids. However, many of the effects of fish oil seem to be exerted in an eicosanoid-independent manner e.g. by expression of key genes.

## Fish oil and cytokines

Intake of fish oil has been shown to increase mRNA for cytokines IL-2, IL-4 and transforming growth factor β (TGFβ) and decrease mRNA for oncogenes c-myc and c-ras and of IL-1β and IL-6 [37]. The decrease in IL-1b mRNA level is not due to increased degradation but to decreased synthesis. Fish oil also decreased tumor necrosis factor α (TNFα) mRNA levels. Nuclear factor-κB (NF-κB) regulates the synthesis of cytokines such as IL-1, IL-2 , IL-6, TNFα and INFβ and is activated by the phosphorylation and subsequent dissociation of one of its three subunits,

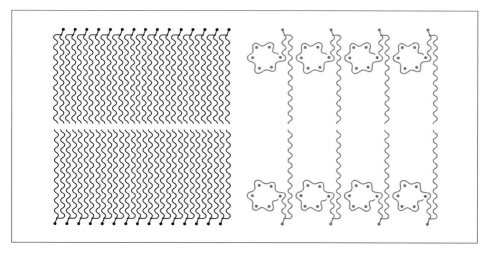

*Figure 2*
*Saturated fatty acids are closely packed into a stiff cell membrane (left), while curved n-3*
*fatty acids such as EPA and DHA make the cell membrane more plastic.*

inhibitory κB, leaving the remaining dimer free to translocate to the nucleus and bind to appropriate response elements on target genes [42]. Prostaglandin $E_2$ ($PGE_2$) acts on T lymphocytes to reduce the formation of interferon γ (IFNγ) without affecting the formation of IL-4. Fish oil decreases $PGE_2$ and therefore increases IFNγ.

## Fish oil and expression of adhesion molecules

Induction in endothelial cells of adhesion molecules for circulating leukocytes and of inflammatory mediators by cytokines has been suggested to contribute to the early phases of atherogenesis. Atheroma formation requires the adhesion of circulating leukocytes to the endothelium and their subsequent transendothelial migration. This process depends on the endothelial expression of endothelial leukocyte adhesion molecules, such as vascular cell adhesion molecule 1 (VCAM-1), intracellular adhesion molecule 1 (ICAM-1) and E-selectin. DHA has been shown to decrease cytokine-induced expression of endothelial leukocyte adhesion molecules, secretion of inflammatory mediators, and leukocyte adhesion to endothelial cells. Thus, DHA decreased the expression of VCAM-1, ICAM-1 and E-selectin [43]. DHA also decreased the secretion of IL-6 and IL-8. Cyclogenase inhibition did not block the effect of DHA on VCAM-1. DHA also reduced VCAM-1 mRNA induction by the cytokines indicating that the effect is pretranslational, and reduced the adhesion of human monocytes to cytokine-stimulated endothelial cells. An effect of DHA on cytokine-induced nuclear translocation of specific transcription factors such as NF-κB was suggested to be a likely possibility behind the effect [43]. Fish oil intake decreases the expression of various adhesion-molecules such as CD11a and CD54 on peripheral-blood monocytes. It has also been shown that DHA decreases mRNA for CD106, an adhesion molecule.

## Fish oil and nitric oxide

Endothelium-dependent vasorelaxation has been found to be reduced in patients with atherosclerosis [44]. N-3 fatty acids have been shown to improve endothelium-dependent vasorelaxation [45, 46] partly due to an increased NO production, and a decrease in superoxide with a prolonged half-life of NO production. We found that increased vascular NO activity after intake of fish oil is mainly due to a decreased breakdown of NO [47]. DHA decreases mRNA for inducible NO synthase due to inhibition of transcription. Overall, it seems that n-3 fatty acids increase the activity of constitutive NO in the endothelial cells mainly by decreasing superoxide production but also by decreasing the inducible NO activity, mainly by inhibiting NO synthase. These dual effects of fish oil may be beneficial in atherosclerosis.

## Fish oil and gene expression

Fish oil fatty acids like EPA and DHA can reduce phospholipase C (PLC) activity resulting in reduced diacylglycerol (DAG) and inositol-1,4,5-triphosphate (IP3) generation (Fig. 3), decreased intracellular free Ca and a reduced activation of protein kinase C (PKC) isoforms [42]. These fatty acids can thus prevent activation of NF-κB and suppress expression of certain genes including those for cytokines, adhesion molecules, and inducible nitric oxide synthase (iNOS). N-3 fatty acids can also decrease gene expression for growth factors thought to play a role in the pathogenesis of atherosclerosis, such as platelet-derived growth factor and monocyte chemoattractant protein-1 [48, 49].

## Fish oil and neutrophils

Fish oil has been shown to decrease generation of superoxide in neutropils [50], without involvement of the cyclogenase pathway and without altering neutrophil lysosomal enzyme release [50]. Fish oil has also been found to decrease chemotaxis [51], which is probably of importance for the effect of fish oil on CAD and other

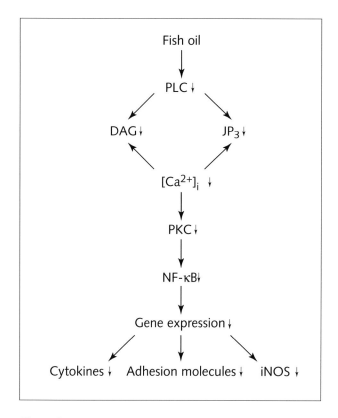

*Figure 3*
*Mechanisms by which fish oil fatty acids decrease gene expression of cytokines, adhesion molecules and inducible nitric oxide synthase. PLC, phospholipase C; DAG, diacylglycerol; PKC, protein kinase C; iNOS, inducible nitric oxide synthase.*

inflammatory conditions. Activated neutrophils seem to play an important role in the pathogenesis of CAD as well as in other inflammatory conditions. A decrease in superoxide generation by neutrophils and in neutrophil chemotaxis may thus partly explain the cardioprotective and anti-inflammatory effects of fish oil. However, the stability of the fish oil seems to be of great importance since an unstable fish oil can increase, instead of decrease, superoxide generation.

## Fish oil and macrophages

Macrophages play an important role in physiological and pathophysiological immune reactions, are key cells in the pathogenesis of atherosclerosis, and contribute to the vulnerability of the atherosclerotic plaque. We have found [52] that EPA decreased the production of inducible nitric oxide in macrophages stimulated with INFγ and lipopolysaccharide, and improved the viability of the stimulated cells. Cell death after stimulation could also be prevented by NO synthase inhibitors, indicating that NO can contribute to cell death. Peroxynitrite and hydroxyl radicals formed in the reaction between NO and superoxide may also contribute to the cell death as addition of superoxide dismutase (SOD) improved cell viability. The cell death observed seems to be apoptotic. The effects of fish oil on NO activity and on cell viability in macrophages and other cells may contribute to the anti-atherogenic and anti-inflammatory effects of fish oil. Rupture of an atherosclerotic plaque is believed to be the precipitating event in most heart attacks. Most ruptures occur in the plaque periphery, at sites heavily infiltrated with macrophages. It has been suggested that the release of proteolytic enzymes from the macrophages may contribute to the weakening of the collagen cap. N-3 fatty acids have been shown to suppress the release of proteolytic enzymes from the macrophages. A high content of n-3 fatty acids in the plaque macrophages could therefore make the plaque less vulnerable.

## Fish oil and intracellular calcium

EPA and DHA have been shown to inhibit receptor-mediated calcium influx in T cells [53] by acting directly on receptor-operated Ca channels. Reduced IP3 levels as a result of diminished phospholipase activity can also contribute to decreased intracellular free Ca concentrations, which in turn would reduce the activity of some isoforms of PKC [42].

## Other effects of fish oil

Recently the interaction of free fatty acids with steroid hormone receptors has received much attention [54, 55]. Long chain n-3 fatty acids have been shown to activate PPAR (peroxisome proliferator-activated receptors). It has been proposed that the interaction of n-3 as well as n-6 fatty acids with these receptors might strongly contribute to the hypolipidemic and anti-inflammatory actions of these fatty acids [56]. The interaction of free fatty acids with steroid receptors is considered to be a new frontier in nutritional research for this new century [57]. Of interest for the anti-atherosclerotic effect of fish oil is that n-3 fatty acids have been found to decrease mitogen-induced vascular endothelial cell proliferation [58]. Fish oil also has an anti-thrombotic effect [59, 60], which may be partly due to decreased platelet aggregation and increased levels of superoxide dismutase (SOD) after intake of fish oil [59, 61].

## Importance of stability for the effects of fish oils

Oxidizing free radicals provoke degradation of the double bonds of polyunsaturated fatty acids in cellular membranes resulting in the formation of short-chain fatty aldehydes such as malondialdehyde (MDA) which can be used as an index of oxidative damage. Red blood cell (RBC) MDA increases the rigidity and decreases deformability of RBC. Polyunsaturated fatty acids are highly suseptible to auto-oxidation because of their realtively weak C-H methylene bonds which readily undergo free-radical-mediated hydrogen abstraction. Fish oils containing highly unsaturated n-3 fatty acids in pure form are readily susceptible to auto-oxidation under aerobic conditions. Studies on human urine and plasma have shown that levels of lipid peroxidation products are increased after intake of certain fish oils. Studies have also shown a decrease in tissue vitamin E content and an increase in *in vitro* susceptibility to lipid peroxidation in tissues after intake of some fish oils. The *in vitro* stability of different commercially available fish oil preparations vary markedly (Tab. 1). Table 1 shows that the stability of 14 different fish oil preparations vary between one and 200 days. Chemically modified, highly concentrated fish oils are usually markedly more unstable than natural fish oils. As seen, most fish oil products available today are unstable, i.e., they become rancid when exposed to air, and after intake they can induce consumption of antioxidants such as vitamin E. This will lead to formation of free radicals, which can cause cellular injury. There is no direct association, however, between the content of vitamin E in the fish oils and their stability (Tab. 1). Even fish oil preparations containing large amounts of vitamin E can be very unstable. The problem with the instability of fish oils has not become widely known until recently. Oily fish, crude fish oil preparations and even some commercially available fish oils contain toxic contaminants such as pesticides and mercury. These have to be removed and during this process the antioxidants in the fish oils are lost and have to be restored in order to keep the stability of the fish oil. The effects observed after intake of an unstable fish oil are the net effects of the positive actions of the n-3 fatty acids and the negative results of the formation of free radicals.

Recently it has been shown [62] that intake of highly concentrated n-3 fatty acid preparations can have adverse effects. Thus, intake of such preparations for 6 months almost doubled the frequency of angina pectoris and significantly increased markers of inflammation and atherosclerotic activity, such as soluble E-selectin and soluble VCAM-1. Also, the use of nitrates was significantly higher in the group treated with highly concentrated n-3 fatty acid preparations compared to controls. The adverse effects were ascribed to the increased lipid peroxidation with increased thiobarbituric acid-reactive substances seen in these patients. It was also pointed out that highly concentrated n-3 fatty acid preparations induce oxidation far more easily than natural fish oil. NF-κB, which is an important transcription factor in chronic inflammatory diseases because it acts on different genes that encode for pro-inflammatory substances such as E-selectin and VCAM-1, is activated by oxidants.

*Table 1 - Stability of different fish oils* [*]

|  | Stability (days) | Vitamin E (IU/g) |  | Stability (days) | Vitamin E (IU/g) |
|---|---|---|---|---|---|
| Fish oil 1[**] | 1 | 6.8 | Fish oil 8 | 14 | 1.0 |
| Fish oil 2[**] | 3 | 20.0 | Fish oil 9 | 14 | 1.5 |
| Fish oil 3[**] | 4 | 4.4 | Fish oil 10 | 14 | 8.5 |
| Fish oil 4[**] | 4 | 5.0 | Fish oil 11 | 14 | 3.7 |
| Fish oil 5 | 6 | 4.4 | Fish oil 12 | 16 | 0.3 |
| Fish oil 6 | 10 | 1.4 | Fish oil 13 | 21 | 1.5 |
| Fish oil 7 | 13 | 1.0 | Natural stable fish oil | 200 | 4.5 |

[*]*Stability = time to rancidity (peroxide value 20) after exposure of the oil to air at room temperature*
[**]*Chemically modified fish oils. Other fish oils are natural.*

Intake of highly concentrated n-3 fatty acid preparations resulting in increased amounts of oxidants can thus induce increased levels of the inflammatory markers *via* the NF-κB pathway [25].

Hau et al. [63] showed that highly concentrated, unstable fish oil preparations increased the susceptibility of LDL to oxidation. Similar effects were found by Lussier-Cacan et al. [64]. Fish oil in the natural, stable form also had a marked effect not only on triglycerides, but also on cholesterol, fibrinogen and blood pressure [65]. Interestingly, stable fish oil also seems to have more beneficial effects on the inflammatory process than unstable fish oil. Thus, intake of stable fish oil had better effects than unstable fish oil on joint stiffness [27, 66, 67] and on the decrease in plasma fibrinogen [26].

The *in vitro* stability of fish oils has been shown to be inversely correlated to *in vivo* lipid peroxidation as measured by plasma levels of MDA and correlated to the ratio between the vasodilator prostacyclin and the vasoconstrictor thromboxane A2 [68]. Intake of several different fish oil products have been found to increase blood glucose probably due to increased lipid peroxidation in the pancreas, with decreased production of insulin. After intake of stable fish oil no such increase in blood glucose is seen [69, 70].

## Conclusion

In conclusion, stable fish oil has many interesting effects suggesting a major role for this oil as a potential therapy for inflammatory atherosclerosis.

## *Acknowledgement*

This review was supported by a grant from the Swedish Medical Research Council.

## References

1    Ross R (1999) Atherosclerosis an inflammatory disease. *N Engl J Med* 340: 115–126
2    Kromann N, Green A (1980) Epidemiological studies in the Upernavak District, Greenland: incidence of some chronic diseases 1959–1974. *Acta Med Scand* 208: 401–406
3    Curb JD, Reed DM (1985) Fish consumption and mortality from coronary heart disease. *N Engl J Med* 313: 821–822
4    Kromhout D, Bosschieter EB, de Lezenne CC (1985) The inverse relationship between fish consumption and 20-year mortality from coronary heart disease. *N Engl J Med* 312: 1205–1209
5    Shekelle RB, Missell L, Paul O, Shryock AM, Stamler J (1985) Fish consumption and mortality from coronary heart disease. *N Engl J Med* 313: 820
6    Vollset SE, Heuch I, Bjelke E (1985) Fish consumption and mortality from coronary heart disease. *N Engl J Med* 313: 820–821
7    Norell SE, Ahlbom A, Feychting M, Pedersen NL (1986) Fish consumption and mortality from coronary heart disease. *Br Med J* 293: 426
8    Burr ML, Fehily AM, Gilbert JF, Rogers S, Holliday RM, Sweetnam PM, Elwood PC, Deachman NM (1989) Effects of changes in fat, fish, and fibre intakes on death and myocardial reinfarction: diet and reinfarction trial (DART). *Lancet* 334: 757–761
9    Singh RB, Rastogi SS, Verma R, Laxmi B, Singh R, Ghosh S, Winz MA (1992) Randomised controlled trial of cardioprotective diet in patients with recent acute myocardial infarction: results of one year follow up. *Br Med J* 304: 1015–1019
10   Dolecek TA (1992) Epidemiological evidence of relationship between dietary polyunsaturated fatty acids and mortality in the Multiple Risk Factor Intervention Trial. *Proc Soc Exp Biol Med* 200: 177–182
11   Siscovick DS, Raghunathan TE, King I, Weinmann S, Wicklund KG, Albright J, Bovbjerg VE, Arbogast P, Smith H, Kushi LH (1995) Dietary intake and cell membrane levels of long-chain n-3 polyunsaturated fatty acids and the risk of primary cardiac arrest. *JAMA* 274: 1363–1367
12   Kromhout D, Feskens EJ, Bowles CH (1995) The protective effect of a small amount of fish on coronary heart mortality in an elderly population. *Int J Epidemiol* 24: 340–345
13   Ascherio A, Rimm EB, Stampfer MJ, Giovannucci EL, Willett WC (1995) Dietary intake of marine n-3 fatty acids, fish intake and the risk of coronary disease among men. *N Engl J Med* 332: 977–982
14   Rodriguez BL, Sharp DS, Abbott RD, Buvchfiel CM, Masaki K, Chyou PH, Huang B, Yano K, Curb JA (1996) Fish intake may limit the increase in risk of coronary heart disease morbidity and mortality among heavy smokers: The Honolulu Heart Program. *Circulation* 94: 952–956

15  Daviglus ML, Stamler J, Orencia AJ, Dyer AR, Liu K, Greenland P, Walsh MK, Morris D, Shekelle RB (1997) Fish consumption and the 30-year risk of fatal myocardial infarction. *N Engl J Med* 336: 1046–1053

16  Albert CM, Hennekens CH, O'Donnell CJ, Ajani UA, Carey VJ, Willett WC, Ruskin JN, Manson JE (1998) Fish consumption and risk of sudden cardiac death. *JAMA* 279: 23–28

17  De Logeril M, Salen P, Martin J-L, Moniaud I, Delaye J, Marmelle N (1999) Mediterranean diet, traditional risk factors, and the rate of cardiovascular complications after myocardial infarction: final report of the Lyon, Diet Heart Study. *Circulation* 99: 779–785

18  GISSI-Prevenzione Investigators (1999) Dietary supplementation with n-3 polyunsaturated fatty acids and vitamin E after myocardial infarction: results of the GISSI-Prevenzione trial. *Lancet* 354: 447–455

19  Charnock J (1994) Lipids and cardiac arrhytmia. *Prog Lipid Res* 33: 355–385

20  Yang BC, Saldeen TGP, Bryant JL, Nichols WW, Mehta JL (1993) Long-term dietary fish oil supplementation protects against ischemia-reperfusion-induced myocardial dysfunction in isolated rat hearts. *Am Heart J* 126: 1287–1292

21  Yang BC, Saldeen TGP, Nichols WW, Mehta JL (1993) Dietary fish oil supplementation attenuates myocardial dysfunction caused by global ischemia and reperfusion in isolated rat hearts. *J Nutrition* 123: 2067–2074

22  Yang B (1996) Protective effects of platelets and stable fish oil against ischemia/reperfusion injury: Role of nitric oxide and antioxidants. *Compr Sum Upps Diss Med Fac* 634, Doctoral thesis, Uppsala University

23  Engström K, Luostarinen R, Saldeen T (1996) Whole blood production of thromboxane prostacyclin and leukotriene B4 after dietary fish oil supplementation in men. Effect of vitamin E. *Prostaglandins, Leukot Essent Fatty Acids* 54: 419–425

24  Haglund O, Wallin R, Luostarinen R, Saldeen T (1990) Effects of a new fluid fish oil concentrate, Eskimo-3, on triglycerides, cholesterol, fibrinogen and blood pressure. *J Internal Med* 227:347–353

25  Johansen O, Brekke M, Seljeflot I, Adelnoor M, Arnesen H (1999) N-3 fatty acids do not prevent restenosis after coronary angioplasty: Results from the CART study. *J Am Coll Cardiol* 33: 1619–1626

26  Haglund O, Luostarinen R, Wallin R, Wibell L, Saldeen T (1991) The effects of fish oil on triglycerides, cholesterol, fibrinogen and malondialdehyde in humans supplemented with vitamin E. *J Nutr* 121: 165–169

27  Engström K, Alving B, Wallin R, Saldeen T (1996) Stable fish oil has better effect on cholesterol and joint stiffness than ordinary fish oil. *Hygiea* 105: 373

28  Haglund O, Luostarinen R, Wallin R, Saldeen T (1992) Effects of fish oil on triglycerides, cholesterol, lipoprotein(a), atherogenic index and fibrinogen. Influence of degree of purification of the oil. *Nutr Res* 12: 455–468

29  Luostarinen R, Boberg M, Saldeen T (1993) Fatty acid composition in total phosplipids of human coronary arteries in sudden cardiac death. *Atherosclerosis* 99: 187–193

30  Von Schacky C, Angerer P, Kothny W, Theisen K, Mudra H (1999) The effect of dietary w-3 fatty acids on coronary atherosclerosis. *Ann Intern Med* 130: 544–562

31  Zhu BQ, Smith DL, Sievers RE, Isenberg WM, Parmley WW (1988) Inhibition of atherosclerosis by fish oil in cholesterol-fed rabbits. *J Am Coll Cardiol* 12: 1073–1078

32  Zhu BQ, Sievers RE, Isenberg WM, Smith DL, Parmaly WW (1990) Regression of atherosclerosis in cholesterol-fed rabbits: effects of fish oil and verapamil. *J Am Coll Cardiol* 15: 231–237

33  Davis HR, Bridenstine RT, Vesselinovitch D, Wissler RW (1987) Fish oil inhibits development of atherosclerosis in rhesus monkeys. *Arteriosclerosis* 7: 441–449

34  Chen MF, Hsu HC, Liau CS, Lee YT (1999) The role of vitamin E on the anti-atherosclerotic effect of fish oil in diet-induced hypercholesterolemic rabbits. *Prostaglandins Other Lipid Mediat* 57: 99–111

35  Mortensen A, Hansen BF, Hansen JF, Frandsen H, Bartinikowska E, Andersen PS, Bertelsen LS (1998) Comparison of the effects of fish oil and olive oil on blood lipids and aortic atherosclerosis in Watanabe heritable hyperlipidaemic rabbits. *Br J Nutr* 80: 565–573

36  Reiner G, Skramene E, de Sancitis J, Radzioch D (1988) Dietary n-3 polyunsaturated fatty acids prevent the development of atherosclerosis. *Arteriosclerosis Thromb* 13: 1515–1524

37  Kristensen SD, Roberts KM, Lawry J, Martin JF (1988) The effect of fish oil on atherogenesis and thrombopoiesis in rabbits on high cholesterol diet. *Artery* 15: 250–258

38  Campos CT, Michalek VN, Matts JP, Buchwald H (1989) Dietary marine oil supplements fail to affect cholesterol metabolism or inhibit atherosclerosis in rabbits with diet-induced hypercholesterolemia. *Surgery* 106: 177–184

39  Rich S, Miller JF, Charous S, Davis HR, Shanks P, Glagov S, Lands WE (1989) Development of atherosclerosis in genetically hyperlipidemic rabbits during chronic fish-oil ingestion. *Arteriosclerosis* 9: 189–194

40  Thiery J, Seidel D (1987) Fish oil feedings results in an enhancement of cholesterol-induced atherosclerosis in rabbits. *Arteriosclerosis* 63: 53–56

41  Fortin PR, Lew RA, Liang MH, Wrighit EA, Beckett LA, Chalmers TC, Sperling RI (1995) Validation of a meta-analysis: the effects of fish oil in rheumatoid arthritis. *J Clin Epidemiol* 48: 1379–1390

42  Miles EA, Calder PC (1998) Modulation of immune function by dietary fatty acids. *Proc Nutr Soc* 57: 277–292

43  De Caterina R, Cybulsky MA, Clinton SK, Gimonbrone MA, Libby P (1990) Omega-3 fatty acids and endothelial leukocyte adhesion molecules. *Prostaglandins, Leukotrienes and Essential Fatty Acids* 52: 191–195

44  Chester AH, O'Neil GS, Moncada S, Tadjakarimi S, Yacoub MH (1990) Low basal and stimulated release of nitric oxide in atherosclerotic epicardial coronary arteries. *Lancet* 336: 897–900

45  Lawson DL, Mehta JL, Saldeen K, Mehta P, Saldeen TGP (1991) Omega-3 polyunsatu-

rated fatty acids augment endothelium-dependent vasorelaxation by enhanced release of EDRF and vasodilator prostaglandins. *Eicosanoids* 4: 217–223

46   Lawson D. Experimental studies on ischemic heart disease (1992) *Compr Sum Upps Diss Med Fac* 369, Doctoral thesis, Uppsala University

47   Bryant J, Yang B, Mehta P, Saldeen T, Mehta J (1993) Dietary fish oil decreases superoxide radical generation without affecting nitric oxide synthase activity: a mechanism of vasorelaxation. *J Am Coll Cardiol* 21: 430 A

48   Kaminski WE, Jendraschak E, Kiefl R, von Schacky C (1993) Dietary omega-3 fatty acids lower levels of platelet-derived growth factor mRNA in human mononuclear cells. *Blood* 81: 1871–1879

49   Baumann KH, Hessel F, Larass I, Müller T, Angerer P, Kiefl R, v Schacky C (1999) Dietary w-3, w-6, and w-9 unsaturated fatty acids and growth factor and cytokine gene expression in unstimulated and stimulated monocytes; a randomized volunteer study. *Arterioscler Thromb Vasc Biol* 19: 59–66

50   Luostarinen R, Saldeen T (1996) Dietary fish oil decreases superoxide generation by human neutrophils: relation to cyclooxygenase pathway and lysosomal enzyme release. *Prostaglandins, Leukotriens and Essential Fatty Acids* 55: 167–172

51   Luostarinen R, Siegbahn A, Saldeen T (1992) Effect of dietary fish oil supplemented with different doses of vitamin E on neutrophil chemotaxis in healthy volunteers. *Nutr Res* 12: 1419–1430

52   Haglund O, Dutertre Y, Saldeen T (1993) EPA decreases nitric oxide activity and increases cell viability in stimulated macrophages. Possible importance for the effect of w-3 fatty acids in prevention of cardiovascular disease and inflammatory conditions. *Hygiea* 102: 343

53   Chow SC Ansotegui IJ, Jondal M (1990) Inhibition of receptor mediated calcium influx in T cells by unsaturated non-esterified fatty acids. *Biochem J* 267: 727–732

54   O'Malley B (1990) The steroid receptor superfamily: more excitement predicted for the future. *Mol Endocrinol* 4: 363–369

55   Nunez EA (1993) Free fatty acids as modulators of the steroid hormone message. *Prostaglandins, Leukotriens and Essential Fatty Acids* 48: 63–70

56   Göttlicher M, Widmark E, Li Q, Gustafsson JÅ (1992) Fatty acids activate a chimera of the clofibric acid-activated receptor and the glucocorticoid receptor. *Proc Natl Acad Sci USA* 89: 4653–4657

57   Nair PP (1993) Nutrients and the human genome: New frontiers for the next century. *FASEB J* 7: 501–502

58   Pakala R, Pakala R, Sheng WL, Benedict CR (1999) Serotonin fails to induce proliferation of endothelial cells preloaded with eicosapentaenoic acid and docosahexaenoic acid. *Atherosclerosis* 145: 137–146

59   Chen LY, Jokela R, Li DY, Bowry A, Sandler H, Sjöqvist M, Saldeen T, Mehta JL (2000) Effect of stable fish oil on arterial thrombosis, platelet aggregation and superoxide dismutase activity. *J Cardiovasc Pharmacol* 35: 502–505

60   Chen L (1999) Experimental studies on thrombosis and thrombolysis. With special ref-

erence to importance of lys-plasminogen, active site thrombin inhibitors and stable fish oil. *Compr Sum Upps Diss Med Fac* 847, Doctoral thesis, Uppsala University.

61    Luostarinen R, Wallin R, Saldeen T (1997) Dietary (n-3) fatty acids increase superoxide dismutase activity and decrease thromboxane production in the heart. *Nutr Res* 17: 163–175

62    Johansen O (1999) Studies on coronary angioplasty, restenosis and very long chain n-3 fatty acids. Doctoral thesis. Department of Cardiology. Ullevål Hospital, University of Oslo

63    Hau MF, Smelt AH, Bindels AJ, Sijbrands EJ, Van der Laarse A, Onkenhout W, van Duyvenvoorde W, Princen HM (1996) Effects of fish oil on oxidation resistance of VLDL in hypertriglyceridemic patients. *Arterioscler Thromb Vasc Biol* 16: 1197–1202

64    Lussier-Cacan S, Dubreuil-Quidoz S, Roederer G, Leboeuf N, Boulet L, de Langavant GC, Davignon J, Naruszewicz M (1993) Influence of probucol on enhanced LDL oxidation after fish oil treatment of hypertriglyceridemic patients. *Arterioscler Thromb* 13: 1790–1797

65    Haglund O (1993) Effect of fish oil on risk factors for cardiovascular disease. *Compr Sum Upps Diss Med Fac* 428, Doctoral thesis, Uppsala University.

66    Saldeen T, Engström K, Jokela R, Wallin R (1999) Importance of *in vitro* stabilty for *in vivo* effects of fish oil. In: *Natural antioxidants and anticarcinogens in nutrition, health and disease*. The Royal Society of Chemistry, Cambridge UK. Special Publication 240: 326–330

67    Saldeen T (1997) *Fish oil and health with focus on natural stable fish oil*. Swede Health Press, Uppsala, Sweden, 1–63

68    Jokela R, Engström K, Wallin R, Saldeen T (1998) Effect of in vivo stability of dietary fish oil on lipid peroxidation and prostanoids *in vivo*. *Uppsala J Med Sci* 103: 213–222

69    Luostarinen R, Wallin R, Wibell L, Saldeen T (1995) Vitamin E supplementation counteracts the fish oil induced increase of blood glucose in humans. *Nutr Res* 15: 953–968

70    Luostarinen R (1995) Studies on (n-3) polyunsaturated fatty acids. With special reference to cardiovascular disease. *Compr Sum Upps Diss Fac Med* 558, Doctoral thesis, Uppsala University

# Index

# The PIR-Series
# Progress in Inflammation Research

Homepage:
http://www.birkhauser.ch

Up-to-date information on the latest developments in the pathology, mechanisms and therapy of inflammatory disease are provided in this monograph series. Areas covered include vascular responses, skin inflammation, pain, neuroinflammation, arthritis cartilage and bone, airways inflammation and asthma, allergy, cytokines and inflammatory mediators, cell signalling, and recent advances in drug therapy. Each volume is edited by acknowledged experts providing succinct overviews on specific topics intended to inform and explain. The series is of interest to academic and industrial biomedical researchers, drug development personnel and rheumatologists, allergists, pathologists, dermatologists and other clinicians requiring regular scientific updates.

**Available volumes:**
*T Cells in Arthritis*, P. Miossec, W. van den Berg, G. Firestein (Editors), 1998
*Chemokines and Skin*, E. Kownatzki, J. Norgauer (Editors), 1998
*Medicinal Fatty Acids*, J. Kremer (Editor), 1998
*Inducible Enzymes in the Inflammatory Response*, D.A. Willoughby, A. Tomlinson (Editors), 1999
*Cytokines in Severe Sepsis and Septic Shock*, H. Redl, G. Schlag (Editors), 1999
*Fatty Acids and Inflammatory Skin Diseases*, J.-M. Schröder (Editor), 1999
*Immunomodulatory Agents from Plants*, H. Wagner (Editor), 1999
*Cytokines and Pain*, L. Watkins, S. Maier (Editors), 1999
In Vivo *Models of Inflammation*, D. Morgan, L. Marshall (Editors), 1999
*Pain and Neurogenic Inflammation*, S.D. Brain, P. Moore (Editors), 1999
*Anti-Inflammatory Drugs in Asthma*, A.P. Sampson, M.K. Church (Editors), 1999
*Novel Inhibitors of Leukotrienes*, G. Folco, B. Samuelsson, R.C. Murphy (Editors), 1999
*Vascular Adhesion Molecules and Inflammation*, J.D. Pearson (Editor), 1999
*Metalloproteinases as Targets for Anti-Inflammatory Drugs*, K.M.K. Bottomley, D. Bradshaw, J.S. Nixon (Editors), 1999
*Free Radicals and Inflammation*, P.G. Winyard, D.R. Blake, C.H. Evans (Editors), 1999
*Gene Therapy in Inflammatory Diseases*, C.H. Evans, P. Robbins (Editors), 2000
*New Cytokines as Potential Drugs*, S. K. Narula, R. Coffmann (Editors), 2000
*High Throughput Screening for Novel Anti-inflammatories*, M. Kahn (Editor), 2000
*Immunology and Drug Therapy of Atopic Skin Diseases*, C.A.F. Bruijnzeel-Komen, E.F. Knol (Editors), 2000
*Novel Cytokine Inhibitors*, G.A. Higgs, B. Henderson (Editors), 2000
*Inflammatory Processes. Molecular Mechanisms and Therapeutic Opportunities*, L.G. Letts, D.W. Morgan (Editors), 2000
*Cellular Mechanisms in Airways Inflammation*, C. Page, K. Banner, D. Spina (Editors), 2000